A Clinical Guide to Stem Cell and Bone Marrow Transplantation

The Jones and Bartlett Series in Oncology

A Clinical Guide to Stem Cell and Bone Marrow Transplantation

Terry Wikle Shapiro RN-C, MSN, CFNP
University of Arizona Adult and Pediatric Bone Marrow
Transplantation Program, Tucson, AZ

Deborah Branney Davison RP-C, MSN, CRNP
Western Pennsylvania Cancer Institute, Pittsburgh, PA

Deborah M. Rust RN, MSN, CRNP, OCN
University of Pittsburgh School of Nursing, Oncology Subspecialty,
Nurse Practitioner Program, Pittsburgh, PA

Jones and Bartlett Publishers
Sudbury, Massachusetts
Boston   London   Singapore

Editorial, Sales, and Customer Service Offices

Jones and Bartlett Publishers
40 Tall Pine Drive
Sudbury, MA 01776
1-800-832-0034
508-443-5000

Jones and Bartlett Publishers International
Barb House, Barb Mews
London W6 7PA
UK

Acquisitions Editor: Robin Carter
Production Editor: Nindy LeRoy
Manufacturing Buyer: Jenna Sturgis
Design: Kenneth Hollman
Editorial Production Service: Ellipsis Inc.

Illustration: Horizon Design
Typesetting: Ellipsis Inc.
Cover Design: Hannus Design Associates
Printing and Binding: Courier
Cover Printing: John Pow Company

Library of Congress Cataloging-in-Publication Data

Shapiro, Terry Wikle.
  A clinical guide to stem cell and bone marrow transplantation /
Terry Wikle Shapiro, Deborah Branney Davison, Deborah M. Rust.
    p. cm.
  Includes bibliographical references and index.
  ISBN 0-7637-0217-X (alk. paper)
  1. Bone marrow--Transplantation--Handbooks, manuals, etc.
  2. Hematopoietic stem cells--Transplantation--Handbooks, manuals, etc.
  I. Davison, Deborah Branney. II. Rust, Deborah M. III. Title.
  [DNLM: 1. Stem Cells--transplantation--handbooks. 2. Bone Marrow
Transplantation--handbooks. 3. Tissue Transplantation--nursing--handbooks.
QH 581.2 S529c 1997]
RD123.5.S535 1997
617.4'4--dc21
DNLM/DLC
for Library of Congress   97-9563

Printed in the United States of America
01 00 99 98 97   10 9 8 7 6 5 4 3 2 1

Disclaimer

The nature of clinical bone marrow transplantation information is that it is constantly evolving because of ongoing research and clinical experience and is often subject to interpretation. While great care has been taken to ensure the accuracy of the information presented, the reader is advised that the authors, editors, reviewers, contributors, and publishers cannot be responsible for the continued currency of the information, for any errors or omissions in this handbook, or for any consequences arising therefrom. Because of the dynamic nature of clinical bone marrow transplantation, readers are advised that decisions regarding therapy must be based on the independent judgment of the clinician, changing information about a drug (e.g., as reflected in the literature and manufacturer's most current product information), and changing medical practices.

Contributors

Deborah Branney Davison, MSN, RP-C, CRNP
    Coordinator, Western Pennsylvania Cancer Institute
Cynthia Monheim, BA
    Graduate Student, Department of Clinical Psychology,
    University of Arizona
Deborah M. Rust, RN, MSN, CRNP, OCN
    Program Manager, Oncology Nurse Practitioner Program, University
    of Pittsburgh School of Nursing
    Nurse Practitioner, Adult Bone Marrow Transplant Program,
    University of Pittsburgh Cancer Institute
Daniel E. Shapiro, PhD, Assistant Professor, Department of Psychiatry,
    College of Medicine, University of Arizona
Terry Wikle Shapiro, RN-C, MSN, CFNP
    Pediatric and Adult Nurse Practitioner, Bone Marrow Transplant
    Program, University Medical Center, University of Arizona

Dedication

To Patricia Schaefer, RN, MD, who gave us the push we needed to see this project become a reality. We also cannot thank our families enough–our husbands Daniel, Dan, and Keith, and our children Alexandra, Derek, and Leah, who lent support and sanity in our times of need…we love you!

Preface

As the science and technology of clinical stem cell and bone marrow transplantation has grown, so has the need for a comprehensive guide to caring for these complex patients. As the number of advanced practice nurses, specialty nurses, physician's assistants, fellows, residents, and medical students who care for such patients grows, so does the need for relevant and practical information. We decided to put our combined 30-plus years of stem cell and bone marrow transplant experience to good use, and thus, this handbook was developed. The concept of this handbook also arose as a result of multiple pleas for a comprehensive "nuts and bolts" guide from colleagues intimately involved in the day-to-day management of patients undergoing stem cell and bone marrow transplantation.

In summary, we have attempted to provide the clinician with a pocket guide to assist in quick-referencing clinical issues and problems common to stem cell and bone marrow transplantation. In our experience, no single clinical handbook currently provides the bone marrow transplantation clinician with comprehensive information relevant to stem cell and bone marrow transplantation. Although we doubt this will be "the only handbook you'll ever need," we do think it will save the bone marrow transplantation clinician time and frustration when looking up clinical information specific to bone marrow transplantation.

The user should keep in mind that the content included in this text is general information extrapolated from the literature, and that program and institutional differences are bound to occur. In addition, stem cell and bone marrow transplantation technology changes at a rapid pace. Clearly, discoveries will be made before this text is published that will alter the accuracy of the information in this handbook. Nevertheless, it is our hope that this handbook will assist clinicians who provide day-to-day management to these challenging patients, providing an easier way to obtain the critical information they need to care for their patients.

Terry Wikle Shapiro, RN-C, MSN, CFNP

Contents

Chapter 7 Formulary 291
Terry Wikle Shapiro, Deborah Branney Davison

Chapter 8 Therapeutic Data 381
Deborah M. Rust, Terry Wikle Shapiro

Chapter 9 Long-Term Follow-Up 411
Deborah Branney Davison

Chapter 10 Psychosocial Issues 419
Daniel Shapiro, Cynthia Monheim

Index 440

Introduction to Stem Cell and Bone Marrow Transplantation

The pluripotent stem cells from which all committed blood cells arise (Figure I.1) are located in the bone marrow space, the peripheral blood, and the blood in the umbilical cord of newborns. All of these sites can be used as a source of bone marrow stem cells, whether for autologous or allogeneic marrow transplantation.

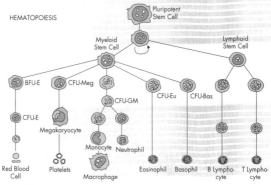

Figure I.1 Depicts hematopoiesis.

I. Allografting

A. Allografting involves transplanting marrow, peripheral blood stem cells (PBSCs), or umbilical cord blood (UCB) to a recipient who is genetically different.

B. Allografting using a monozygotic twin as a donor is termed a *syngeneic transplant.*

C. The most common and preferred situation is for marrow to be donated by a six out of six-antigen, human leukocyte antigen (HLA)-matched, (HLA-identical) sibling.

D. Partially matched family members or matched unrelated donors from a volunteer panel may also be used as donors.

E. UCB may be used as a source of allogeneic stem cells in the matched sibling donor as well as in the unrelated donor.

F. Allograft sources of marrow/blood cells
    1. Matched sibling donor
        a) Marrow
        b) PBSCs
        c) UCB
    2. Identical twin donor
        a) Marrow
        b) PBSCs
        c) UCB
    3. Partially-matched related donor
        a) Marrow
        b) PBSCs
        c) UCB
    4. Matched unrelated donor
        a) Marrow
        b) UCB
    5. Partially-matched unrelated donor
        a) Marrow
        b) UCB

G. Allografts are indicated for some congenital abnormalities of bone marrow function or where there is disease involving the marrow not amenable to cure with standard treatment.

1. Leukemias
   a) Acute myelogenous leukemia (AML)
   b) Acute lymphoblastic leukemia (ALL)
   c) Chronic myelogenous leukemia (CML)
   d) Myelodysplastic syndromes (MDS)
   e) Acute myelofibrosis
2. Lymphoproliferative disorders
   a) Hodgkin's disease
   b) Non-Hodgkin's lymphoma
   c) Multiple myeloma
   d) Chronic lymphocytic leukemia
3. Hematologic disorders
   a) ß-Thalassemia
   b) Sickle cell anemia (SCA)
   c) Congenital neutropenias
   d) Osteopetrosis
4. Bone marrow failure syndromes
   a) Severe aplastic anemia (SAA)
   b) Fanconi's anemia (FA)
   c) Reticular dysgenesis
5. Immunodeficiencies
   a) Severe combined immunodeficiencies
   b) Wiskott-Aldrich syndrome
   c) Miscellaneous immunodeficiencies
6. Nonhematologic genetic disorders
   a) Mucopolysaccharidosis
   b) Leukodystrophies
   c) Miscellaneous metabolic disorders

II. Autografting

A. Autografting involves transplanting marrow or PBSCs back into the person from whom the blood cells originated.

B. Since a marrow or stem cell source for allografting cannot always be found or may be too risky, autologous bone marrow or PBSC transplantation is also used as a method for treating a number of malignant disorders.
    1. Leukemias
        a) AML
        b) ALL
        c) CML
    2. Lymphoproliferative disorders
        a) Hodgkin's disease
        b) Non-Hodgkin's lymphoma
        c) Multiple myeloma
        d) Chronic lymphocytic leukemia
    3. Solid tumors
        a) Neuroblastoma
        b) Ewing's sarcoma
        c) Breast cancer
        d) Testicular cancer
        e) Melanoma
        f) Osteosarcoma
        g) Cerebral tumors
        h) Others

C. Using autologous marrow or PBSCs is not feasible for patients who have a deficiency of their functional bone marrow, as with aplastic anemia, inborn errors of metabolism, and immunodeficiency states.[1]

D. In certain circumstances, using autologous marrow or PBSCs may be preferable to using an allogeneic source of stem cells, for example, to avoid graft-versus-host disease (GVHD) in situations when marrow contamination with malignant cells is likely, and there is no evidence of an immunologic antitumor effect ("graft versus leukemia" or something similar) with allogeneic transplant.

E. In older patients (> 50 years of age), autografting may also be considered more desirable because of the high morbidity and mortality associated with allografting and GVHD.

F. Autografting is most frequently used in the setting of high-risk solid tumors in which the chance for cure is relatively low with standard or conventional doses of chemotherapy. In this case, autografting is considered a marrow or stem cell "rescue."

G. In some autografting situations, it is questioned whether a low (undetectable) level of tumor cells persisting in the infused cells may promote relapse. However, routine purging, even in diseases that involve the marrow, is unproved. Research in this area continues.

H. PBSCs are used as an autografting source in cases of prior pelvic irradiation, marrow fibrosis, unacceptable anesthesia risk, or when early engraftment is desired.[2]

III. When should marrow or blood cell transplantation be considered?

A. Acute myelogenous leukemia (AML)[1,3]

1. The classification of AML can be divided into seven main categories based on morphology and cytochemistry as proposed by the French American and British (FAB) group[4] (Table I.1). Some of these subtypes, such as M5, are associated with poor outcomes after chemotherapy alone. Other subtypes, such as M3, are associated with more favorable outcomes. Overall, the FAB classification has not been found to be significantly useful as a predictive factor for outcome after chemotherapy alone.

Table I.1 FAB Morphologic Classification of AML

Disease class	Morphology
M0	AML with minimal evidence of myeloid differentiation
M1	AML without maturation
M2	AML with maturation
M3	Acute hypergranular promyelocytic leukemia
M4	Acute myelomonocytic leukemia
M5	Acute monocytic/monoblastic leukemia
M6	Erythroleukemia
M7	Acute megakaryoblastic leukemia

2. Allogeneic bone marrow transplantation (BMT) for AML
   a) Patients with AML who have an HLA-identical donor have the best prognosis when transplanted in first remission (40% to 60% probability of long-term survival).
   b) It may be preferable for patients with AML to be transplanted in first relapse rather than second remission, since the additional chemotherapy may increase transplant-related complications. The probability of long-term survival of the two groups appears to be about the same, approximately 25% to 35%.
   c) Transplant results using family members who are one-antigen HLA-mismatched with the patient do not differ from those in patients with genotypically or phenotypically HLA-identical donors.
   d) Results obtained using related donors who are more severely mismatched (two- or three-antigen disparity) are inferior (< 20%) to using chemotherapy alone and are usually only considered after first or subsequent relapse(s) or in patients who do not achieve first remission (refractory AML).

e) Matched unrelated donor transplants are considered for AML patients in first remission who are considered very high risk for relapse, patients with refractory disease, or as salvage therapy in second or later remission.

3. Autologous BMT for AML
a) May be performed in first or second remission.
b) Autologous BMT is most often considered for patients over age 50 in order to eliminate the morbidity and mortality associated with GVHD.
c) Major drawbacks include the presence of minimal residual disease at the time of marrow harvest, and the absence of the "graft versus leukemia" effect associated with allogeneic BMT.
d) To date, no statistically significant difference in disease-free survival has been demonstrated for autologous marrow purged of tumor cells compared to unpurged marrow.
e) The use of PBSCs may circumvent the problem of minimal residual marrow disease, but this is still under investigation.

B. Acute lymphoblastic leukemia (ALL)[1,3]
1. In adults, ALL carries a much poorer prognosis than does childhood ALL, with only approximately 20% of patients remaining disease-free after five years with chemotherapy alone. Adult patients should probably undergo allogeneic BMT in first remission. Patients with newly diagnosed ALL can be subdivided into high and low-risk groups. Assignment to the high-risk group is based on the following criteria:
a) White blood cell (WBC) count greater than 30 x 10^9/L at diagnosis
b) Phenotype of blast cells: B or null
c) Slow to achieve first complete remission
d) Age of patient

e) Presence of a mediastinal mass at diagnosis
f) Central nervous system

2. With children, the position is less clear. Overall, the disease carries a good prognosis (80% disease-free survival) with chemotherapy alone, if the following risk factors are not present at diagnosis:
   a) WBC count greater than 100×10^9/L
   b) Infants
   c) Males with high WBC count at presentation
   d) Some chromosomal translocations (t[9;22] and t[4;11])
   e) Cell phenotype (ß-cell ALL)
   f) Presence of extramedullary disease
   g) Relapsed disease

3. Allogeneic BMT for ALL
   a) Patients who belong to "high-risk" groups should receive an allogeneic BMT in first remission if an HLA-identical or one-antigen mismatched related donor is available.
   b) Patients lacking an HLA-identical or one-antigen mismatched related donor should be considered for a matched unrelated donor transplant (using marrow or UCB as source).
   c) Patients with a two- or three-antigen mismatched donor may be considered for BMT in second or subsequent remission if they are less than 20 years old.
   d) "Low-risk" patients are generally considered for allogeneic BMT on achieving a second remission, using a matched related donor, matched unrelated donor, or partially matched donor if they are less than 20 years old.

4. Autologous BMT for ALL
   a) Preferred for patients who are more than 50 years old or who lack a matched related or matched unrelated donor.

b) The bone marrow or PBSCs of such patients may be harvested and stored after achieving a first remission. Autologous BMT is then carried out in second or subsequent remission.

c) Relapse rates remain high using autologous versus allogeneic BMT for ALL (52% vs. 9%).

d) Use of purged marrow for ALL remains controversial and is still under investigation.

C. Chronic myelogenous leukemia (CML)[1,3]

1. CML is characterized by the presence of the Philadelphia (Ph') chromosome; chromosome 22 is shortened, secondary to a reciprocal translocation between chromosomes 9 and 22. CML usually follows a prolonged chronic phase (three to five years) that eventually proceeds through an accelerated phase and a blastic transformation (blast crisis) to acute leukemia, which may be myeloid or lymphoid type. With CML, no conventional chemotherapy is curative; hydroxyurea, busulfan, and interferon-α offer only temporary control.

2. Allogeneic BMT for CML

a) CML patients with an HLA-identical, one-antigen mismatched, or matched unrelated donor should be transplanted in chronic phase.

b) Patients transplanted in blast transformation have a very poor prognosis.

c) Patients who achieve a second chronic phase following blast transformation, using conventional chemotherapy, have a better prognosis than if transplanted in blast transformation.

3. Autologous BMT for CML

a) Overall, autologous BMT for CML has met with little success, since autologous BMT fails to ablate the Ph' chromosome.

b) Autologous BMT after in vitro long-term culture of the bone marrow is under investigation to evaluate if the Ph[1] cells die early in the culture, thus leaving only normal marrow cells.[5]

   c) Studies treating marrow with interferon-α before autologous marrow reinfusion are also under way.

   d) Patients who achieve a cytogenetic remission with interferon-α may also be considered for autologous BMT.

D. Myelodysplastic syndromes (MDS)[1,3]

1. MDS are morphologically classified as follows:
   a) Refractory anemia
   b) Refractory anemia with ring sideroblasts (RARS)
   c) Refractory anemia with excess blasts (RAEB)
   d) Chronic myelomonocytic leukemia
   e) Refractory anemia with excess blasts in transformation (RAEBIT)

2. All of these syndromes eventually metamorphose into acute myeloid leukemia, and treatment with chemotherapy alone is usually less satisfactory than with de novo AML. These syndromes are referred to as preleukemia.

3. Allogeneic BMT for MDS
   a) Most patients should be transplanted shortly after diagnosis if an HLA-matched related or partially-matched related, or matched unrelated donor is found.
   b) Since marrow morphology cannot always clearly distinguish between MDS and aplastic anemia, cytogenetic analysis should be performed prior to transplant.
   c) Patients who have extensive marrow fibrosis do poorly secondary to graft failure.
   d) Patients with secondary MDS after previous anticancer treatment also have a less favorable prognosis.

4. Autologous BMT for MDS is not an option for this patient population.

E. Severe aplastic anemia (SAA) and Fanconi's anemia (FA)[1,3]

1. Allogeneic marrow transplantation is the treament of choice for patients with SAA. Aplastic anemia is considered severe when anemia is associated with a corrected reticulocyte count of less than 1%, a neutrophil count of less than 500/mL, and a platelet count of less than 20,000/µL associated with a hypocellular marrow.

2. Several known etiologies exist for SAA:
   a) Acquired
      (1) Idiopathic
      (2) Secondary to drugs and chemical agents, radiation, and viral infections
      (3) Paroxysmal nocturnal hemoglobinuria
   b) Constitutional
      (1) Dyskeratosis congenita
      (2) Familial aplastic anemia

3. Allogeneic BMT for SAA
   a) Complete recovery of hematopoiesis occurs and long-term event-free survival is experienced in 60% of patients when a fully-matched HLA-identical sibling is utilized.
   b) Should be performed soon after diagnosis if an HLA-matched related donor is found.
   c) Best results are observed in patients who have had a short duration of disease, have had few prior transfusions, and are conditioned with cyclophosphamide alone.[6]
   d) Graft rejection occurs most commonly in patients who have received multiple transfusions; such patients should be conditioned with a total body irradiation regimen.

e) In untransfused patients, the probability of long-term survival following allogeneic BMT is about 80% to 90%, while transfused patients have a probability of survival of about 60%.

f) Since finding a donor can be time-consuming, platelet transfusions should be given only in the case of bleeding. Family members should not be used as platelet donors pre-BMT.

g) Survival rates are low using matched unrelated donors or partially-matched related donors for patients with SAA (< 20%). Such transplants are only considered for patients who fail immunosuppressive therapy, hematopoietic growth factors, and/or androgens.

h) Patients older than 30 years have more complications with BMT. End results with BMT versus immunosuppressive treatment alone are similar.[7]

4. Autologous BMT for SAA is not an option for this patient population.

5. Allogeneic BMT for FA

a) FA is an autosomal recessive disorder characterized by bone marrow hypoplasia, microcephaly, genital hypoplasia, strabismus, skin hyperpigmentation, abnormalities of the skeleton, heart, and kidneys, and growth and mental retardation.

b) Marrow cells of FA patients show high chromosomal breakage and failure of DNA repair.

c) Marrow aplasia may not be evident until adulthood but is almost always fatal. Timing of BMT is appropriate when progressive pancytopenia develops, associated with transfusions or multiple infections.

d) FA patients are commonly conditioned with reduced doses of alkylating agents and radiation because of extremely high incidence of transplant-related morbidity and mortality (due to ineffective DNA repair and chromosomal breakage).

  e) Mucositis, skin toxicity, hemorrhagic cystitis, and GVHD are often severe in these patients.

6. Autologous BMT for FA is not an option for this patient population.

F. Primary immunodeficiency diseases[1,8]

  1. Various congenital immunodeficiency disorders may be corrected by BMT[8]:

    a) Combined immunodeficiencies
      (1) Severe combined immunodeficiencies (SCID)
      (2) X-linked SCID
      (3) Autosomal recessive agammaglobulinemia
      (4) Adenosine deaminase deficiency
      (5) Purine nucleoside phosphorylase deficiency
      (6) Major histocompatibility complex Class II deficiency
      (7) Reticular dysgenesis
      (8) Omenn's syndrome

    b) Syndromes associated with immunodeficiency
      (1) Chromosome abnormalities
      (2) X-linked lymphoproliferative disorder

    c) Defects of phagocytic function
      (1) Chronic granulomatous disease
      (2) Leukocyte adhesion defect
      (3) Chédiak-Higashi syndrome

    d) Predominate antibody defects
      (1) X-linked agammaglobulinemia
      (2) Common variable immunodeficiency

    e) Other well-defined immunodeficiency syndromes
      (1) Wiskott-Aldrich syndrome
      (2) Ataxia-telangiectasia
      (3) DiGeorge syndrome

2. Several disorders of the myeloid and monocyte-macrophage system have been corrected by allogeneic bone marrow transplantation:
   a) Infantile genetic agranulocytosis (Kostmann's syndrome)
   b) Neutrophil actin deficiency
   c) Neutrophil membrane gp 180 deficiency
   d) Familial hemophagocytic lymphohistiocytosis
   e) Osteopetrosis
3. Allogeneic BMT for primary immunodeficiency and disorders of the myeloid and monocyte-macrophage system
   a) Such patients are generally transplanted soon after diagnosis to avoid further recurrent, and often fatal, infections pretransplantation.
   b) Alternative sources of stem cells are often used, since healthy sibling donors are often not available.
   c) Haploidentical parents are often used as donors, along with other histoincompatible family donors, matched unrelated donors, fetal tissues, and UCB.
   d) Patients who have profound immunodeficiency and who lack signs of maternal GVHD may not require pretransplant conditioning. Engraftment in such patients is often delayed (up to six months to one year).
   e) Complete engraftment of the donor marrow (i.e., lymphoid as well as myeloid lineage) is not essential in all cases. Type and extent of engraftment required to correct the clinical manifestations of the disease depend on the nature of the underlying defect.
   f) About 30% of immunodeficiency patients with T-depleted histoincompatible transplants will develop Epstein-Barr-associated polyclonal

B-lymphoproliferative disease, which is
usually donor in origin.[9]
4. Autologous BMT for primary immunodeficiency
diseases is not an option for this patient population.

G. Inborn errors of metabolism[10]

Table I.2 Inborn Errors of Metabolism Treated with Allogeneic BMT

Lysosomal storage diseases	Nonlysosomal diseases
Mucopolysaccharidoses (MPS)	Lesch-Nyhan syndrome
Hurler's syndrome (MPSI H)	Adrenoleukodystrophy
Scheie's syndrome (MPSI S)	
Wolman's disease	
Hunter's syndrome (MPSII)	
Sanfilippo A (MPSII A)	
Sanfilippo B (MPS III B)	
Morquio's syndrome (MPSIV)	
Maroteaux-Lamy syndrome (MPSVI)	
Leukodystrophies	
Metachromatic leukodystrophy	
Krabbe's disease	
Sphingolipidoses	
GM1 gangliosidosis	
Niemann-Pick disease	
Other lipidoses	
Gaucher's disease	
Pompe's disease	
Others	
Farber's disease	
Mucolipidosis II	
α-mannosidosis	
Fucosidosis	

Adapted from Hoogerbrugge, Vellodi, and Pasquini.[10]

1. Allogeneic BMT has been used since about 1980 to treat infants, children, and young adults suffering from lysosomal enzyme deficiencies (Table 1.11).
2. At least four different mechanisms may explain why allogeneic BMT is effective in the treatment of lysosomal storage disorders:
   a) Allogeneic BMT replaces the enzymatically deficient macrophages in the liver, spleen, skin, and lung tissues, particularly in those diseases in which the mononuclear phagocytic cell system is primarily affected (e.g., Gaucher's disease).
   b) Allogeneic BMT is effective in the transfer of enzymes from the enzymatically normal, bone marrow-derived cells to deficient cells by direct cell-to-cell contact.
   c) BMT may be effective through the release of enzymes into plasma, as may occur with the disintegration of donor-derived WBCs. Subsequently, the circulating enzymes may be taken up by enzymatically deficient cells.
   d) The presence of a concentration gradient of storage product between the tissues and the plasma compartment may result from the break-down of circulating substrate by the lysosomal enzymes present in WBCs and tissue macrophages of donor origin and give rise to clearance of the storage product.
3. It is still unclear whether allogeneic BMT offers an overall survival advantage. What has been reported is that allogeneic BMT[11]
   a) Reduced storage materials in the liver and spleen of patients, suggesting replacement of storage product-laden host macrophages by enzymatically competent donor-derived cells

b) Had little effect on skeletal deformities seen in these diseases

c) May diminish neurologic symptoms

4. Autologous BMT for inborn errors of metabolism is not an option for this patient population.

H. Inherited defects of red cell production.[12]

1. Allogeneic BMT for thalassemia

a) Thalassemia is an autosomal recessive disease characterized by abnormal synthesis of one or more globin chains. In its homozygous form, the absence or reduced synthesis of the ß chain is responsible for the serious clinical condition known as Thalassemia major or Cooley's anemia.

b) Thalassemia major results in ineffective erythropoiesis and hemolysis, and thus severe anemia.

c) BMT is generally performed in patients who do not have a large iron load, prior to growth retardation, and in patients who have little or no liver damage.

d) Matched sibling or parental donors who carry the ß-thalassemia trait can be used as donors.

e) These patients require complete marrow ablation and immunosuppression; preparative regimens may be modified for patients with underlying liver disease to reduce the risk of veno-occlusive disease.

f) Graft rejection and graft failure are high in these patients (13%).[12]

g) Autologous BMT for thalassemia is not an option for this patient population.

3. Allogeneic BMT for sickle cell anemia (SCA)

a) SCA is an autosomal recessive disease characterized by deoxygenation of the hemoglobin variant, thus permitting the formation of rigid hemoglobin S (HbS) polymers that give the red cells their typical sickle shape and make their progression through the microcirculation difficult.

   b) Common symptoms include infections, veno-occlusive events, sequestration, and hemolytic and aplastic episodes.

   c) Since 85% of patients with SCA live longer than 20 years, the decision for BMT is a difficult one.

   d) Nagel[13] recommends BMT for children who are complication-prone, such as those with high levels of HbS, coexistence of α-thalassemia, Central African Republic haplotype, frequent or early central nervous system insult(s), or repetitive acute chest syndrome.

   e) Graft rejection and graft failure are problems with these patients.

   f) Autologous BMT for SCA is not an option for this patient population.

I. Hodgkin's disease and non-Hodgkin's lymphoma (NHL)[14]

   1. Autologous BMT for Hodgkin's disease

      a) Table I.3 outlines the Costwold staging for Hodgkin's disease. Hodgkin's disease is a malignant condition characterized by lymphadenopathy, usually a large mediastinal mass, and of constitutional symptoms (fevers, night sweats, weight loss). Histopathologically, Reed-Sternberg cells are the malignant cell in Hodgkin's disease and is derived from specialized reticular cells found in the paracortex of lymph nodes.

Table I.3 Costwold Staging of Hodgkin's Disease

Stage	Extent of disease
Stage I	Involvement of a single lymph node region or structure
Stage II	Involvement of > 2 lymph node regions on the same side of the diaphragm (the mediastinum is considered a single site, whereas hilar lymph nodes are considered bilaterally)
Stage III	Involvement of lymph node regions or structures on both sides of the diaphragm
Stage III.1	With or without involvement of splenic, hilar, colic, or portal nodes
Stage III.2	With involvement of para-aortic, iliac, and mesenteric nodes
Stage IV	Involvement of one or more extranodal sites in addition to a site for which the designation "E" has been used

Designations Applicable to Any Disease Stage

Designation	Characteristic
A	No symptoms
B	Fever, night sweats, weight loss (> 10% within the preceding six months)
X	Bulky disease (a widening mediastinum by > 1/3, or presence of a nodal mass > 10 cm)
E	Involvement of a single extranodal site that is contiguous or proximal to the known nodal site
CS	Clinical stage
PS	Pathologic stage as determined by laparotomy

b) Hodgkin's patients considered for transplant are those who are primarily resistant to chemotherapy or radiation therapy or who have relapsed early after initial treatment.

c) Since many of these patients have received mantle radiation therapy in the past, high-dose chemotherapy only, containing conditioning regimens, is generally used.

d) Total body irradiation may be used in patients who have demonstrated previous chemoresistance.

e) PBSCs are often used as the stem cell source of choice, since these patients often experience delayed hematopoietic recovery with autologous marrow.

f) Allogeneic BMT for Hodgkin's disease is generally reserved for patients with known marrow involvement who have an HLA-matched sibling donor.

3. Autologous BMT for NHL

a) Table I.4 outlines the working formula for NHL. Non-Hodgkin's lymphomas are a diverse collection of malignant neoplasms of lympho reticular cell origin including all of the malignant lymphomas that are not classified as Hodgkin's disease.

Table I.4 Non-Hodgkin's Lymphoma Working Formula Classification

Classification	Cell type
Low grade	Small lymphocytic
	Follicular predominately small cleaved cell
	Follicular mixed small cleaved and large cell
Intermediate grade	Follicular predominately large cell
	Diffuse small cleaved cell
	Diffuse mixed small cleaved and large cell
High grade	Large cell, immunoblastic
	Lymphoblastic
	Small noncleaved; Burkitt's

b) Problems encountered with BMT for NHL include:

(1) Long natural history of indolent NHL

(2) High frequency of bone marrow involvement at diagnosis

(3) Decreased marrow reserve

(4) Potential prolonged engraftment time due to previous therapy

(5) Resistance to therapy following multiple relapses

c) BMT is most commonly used in NHL patients with a conversion to a more aggressive form of the disease who are still responsive to salvage therapy.

d) Fifty percent of patients with high- or intermediate-grade NHL will relapse conventional therapy. Thus, such patients with disease retaining chemosensitivity are commonly salvaged with chemotherapy to achieve a state of minimal disease prior to BMT.

e) Patients with small noncleaved cell lymphoma, lymphoblastic, and peripheral T-cell lymphoma should be considered for autologous or allogeneic BMT as consolidation treatment in first remission.

4. Allogeneic BMT for NHL is generally reserved for patients with known marrow involvement or lymphoblastic lymphoma cell type who have an HLA-matched sibling or matched unrelated donor.

J. BMT for multiple myeloma (MM)[3]

1. Autologous BMT for MM

a) The majority of patients diagnosed with MM are more than 60 years of age and are therefore inappropriate candidates for BMT.

b) Transplant-related toxicity is higher than that seen with the leukemias and is most likely related to increased patient age, a high incidence of active disease, subclinical renal impairment, and increased susceptibility to infection.

c) Because of such toxicity, autologous BMT or the use of PBSCs is preferred, although the incidence of long-term remission is higher with allogeneic BMT.

d) Bone marrow in MM patients is usually contaminated with plasma cells even after response to treatment. Such cells can be used because they contain healthy progenitor cells. However, it is unknown whether infusion of autologous marrow may increase the patient's risk of relapse.

e) MM patients with high-risk factors of high β^2-microglobulin and non-IgG isotype are generally considered poor candidates for autologous BMT due to their high risk of relapse.

f) Autologous BMT is now carried out earlier in the patient's disease, after achieving a response to initial therapy, to reduce the amount of myeloma in the harvested marrow.

g) PBSCs are a viable option for patients who do not achieve a reduction of plasma cells in the bone marrow.

h) Granulocyte-macrophage colony-stimulating factor is generally not used to mobilize PBSCs, since it is known to be a growth factor for myeloma cells.

2. Allogeneic BMT for MM

a) Transplant-related toxicity is high in this group. However, long-term remission rates are higher than with autologous BMT/PBSC patients.

b) Is reserved for younger MM patients with poor prognostic factors (ß-microglobulin and non-IgG isotype) who have an HLA-identical matched sibling donor.

c) MM patients should be carefully screened for underlying renal dysfunction, prior thoracic radiation, infection, and degree of active disease.

K. Autologous BMT for solid tumors [3,15]

1. Overall purpose of autologous BMT/PBSC rescue in solid tumors is to accelerate hematopoietic recovery following high-dose chemotherapy or radiation therapy.

2. No "graft versus tumor" effect has been demonstrated in patients with solid tumors, thereby lending no advantage to allogeneic BMT following high-dose therapy.

3. In order for high-dose therapy to be a tenable strategy in patients with solid tumors, the following conditions should exist:
   a) The tumor should be inherently drug sensitive at standard doses.
   b) There should be in vitro, in vivo, or clinical evidence supporting a dose-response treatment effect.
   c) Hematologic toxicity should be the dose-limiting toxic effect of the drugs to be employed in the conditioning regimen.[15]
4. High-dose chemotherapy and autologous BMT/PBSC rescue for breast cancer[15, 16]
   a) Controversy exists regarding selection of subgroups of breast cancer patients who will benefit from autologous BMT/PBSC rescue.
   b) Early trials have demonstrated benefit for patients with limited stage IV disease who have not received previous therapy for metastatic disease.
   c) Certain high-risk groups may also benefit, such as those patients with 10 or more positive lymph nodes at diagnosis, stage III disease, or inflammatory breast cancer. Clinical trials are currently under way.
   d) Early trials in stage IV disease have demonstrated improved tumor response rates but have failed to demonstrate superior long-term survival when compared to conventional chemotherapy or hormonal therapy.
   e) When comparing both clinical and financial considerations for stage IV disease, high-dose chemotherapy with autologous BMT, or PBSC rescue has been determined to be of modest efficacy in improving survival, but at an untenable cost.[2, 15]
   f) Results are encouraging enough to warrant further investigation.

5. High-dose chemotherapy with autologous BMT/PBSC rescue for ovarian cancer[15]
   a) Median survival of women with ovarian cancer is about two years with conventional therapy.
   b) Ovarian cancer is known to be drug sensitive and has demonstrated a dose-response relationship, thereby making high-dose chemotherapy, autologous BMT or PBSC rescue a reasonable strategy.
   c) High-dose chemotherapy with autologous BMT or PBSC rescue has been used as both salvage therapy and consolidation therapy in patients who have demonstrated a response to cisplatin-based chemotherapy.
   d) Several studies indicate that the administration of high-dose alkylating agents plus autologous BMT in patients with advanced ovarian cancer who respond to cisplatin-based chemotherapy is safe and feasible.[17]
   e) Only patients with nonbulky disease appear to benefit from high-dose chemotherapy with autologous BMT or PBSC rescue.
   f) Clinical trials are ongoing.
6. High-dose chemotherapy with autologous BMT/PBSC rescue for melanoma.[15]
   a) Advanced melanoma is considered a relatively chemotherapy-resistant disease. However, dose escalation of alkylating agents plus autologous BMT demonstrated higher response rates than those seen with conventional chemotherapy.
   b) Despite such responses, remissions have been only partial and short in duration.
   c) Clinical trials are ongoing.

7. High-dose chemotherapy with autologous BMT/PBSC rescue for germ cell tumors[15]
   a) Autologous BMT/PBSC rescue for germ cell tumors is generally utilized in patients who have resistant or relapsed disease since the majority of patients are cured by conventional therapy alone.
   b) Recent studies have demonstrated a survival advantage in such patients when compared to conventional salvage therapy.
   c) Clinical trials are ongoing.
8. High-dose chemotherapy with autologous BMT/PBSC rescue for brain tumors[15]
   a) Dose-intense carmustine is the primary drug of choice for conditioning regimens with autologous BMT/PBSC rescue in patients with brain tumors.
   b) High-dose chemotherapy with autologous BMT/PBSC rescue combined with whole-brain irradiation appears to be capable of producing sustained progression-free survival in patients with malignant gliomas and other cerebral tumors that have progressed after primary therapy.
   c) Early studies also suggest that such an approach is feasible for certain patients as primary therapy, particularly those below age 50 who have a good performance status.
   d) Clinical trials are ongoing.
9. High-dose chemotherapy with autologous BMT for neuroblastoma[5,8]
   a) Despite recent advances, 80% of children over 1 year of age who have neuroblastoma will die.
   b) Studies suggest that children with stage III or stage IV disease benefit most when high-dose chemotherapy, radiotherapy, and autologous BMT are used as consolidation therapy.

c) When used as salvage therapy, prognosis remains poor.

d) Since children are affected by neuroblastoma, little data regarding the use of PBSCs is available. However, studies are currently under way.

e) Purging techniques are currently being evaluated since occult tumor contamination with neuroblastoma is common.

f) Clinical trials are ongoing.

References

1. Treleaven J, Wiernik P, eds. *Bone Marrow Transplantation.* London, England: Mosby-Wolfe; 1995.

2. Hillner BE, Smith TJ, Desch CE. Efficacy and cost effectiveness of autologous bone marrow transplantation in metastatic breast cancer: estimates using decision analysis while awaiting clinical trial results. *JAMA.* 1992;267:2055–2061.

3. Deeg HJ, Klingemann HG, Phillips GL, eds. *A Guide to Bone Marrow Transplantation: When Should Marrow Transplantation Be Considered?* New York: Springer-Verlag; 1988.

4. Bennett JM, Catovsky D, Daniel MT, et al. Proposed revised criteria for the classification of acute myeloid leukemia (AML). *Bone Marrow Transplantation.* 1991;7 (suppl 2):59–61.

5. Butterini A, Goldman J, Keiting A, et al. Auto-transplants in chronic myelogenous leukemia: strategies and results. *Lancet.* 1990;1:255–1258.

6. Champlin RE, Ho WG, Nimer SD, et al. Bone marrow transplantation for severe aplastic anemia: recent advances and comparisons with alternative therapies. Presented at the UCLA Symposium on Molecular and Cellular Biology; Keystone, Colo; 1990;185–199.

7. Bacigalupo A. Bone marrow transplantation versus immunosuppression for the treatment of severe aplastic anemia (SAA): a report of the EBMT SAA working party. *Br J Haematol.* 1988;70:177–182.

8. Mehta J. Primary immunodeficiency diseases. In: Treleaven J, Wiernik P. *Bone Marrow Transplantation.* London, England: Mosby-Wolfe; 1995:55–62.

9. Shapiro RS, McLain K, Frizzera G. et al. Epstein-Barr virus associated B cell lymphoproliferative disorders following bone marrow transplantation. *Blood.* 1988;71:1234–1243.

10. Hoogerbrugge P, Vellodi A, Pasquini R. Inborn errors of metabolism. In: Treleaven J, Wiernik P, eds. *Bone Marrow Transplantation*. London, England: Mosby-Wolfe; 1995:19–35.

11. Krivit W, Whitley CB, Chang P, et al. Lysosomal storage diseases treated by bone marrow transplantation. In: Gale RP, Champlin R, eds. *Bone Marrow Transplantation: Current Controversies*. New York: Alan R Liss; 1989:367–378.

12. Borgna-Pignatti C. Inherited defects in red cell production. In: Treleaven J, Wiernik P, eds. *Bone Marrow Transplantation*. London, England: Mosby-Wolfe; 1995:37–47.

13. Nagel RL. The dilemma of marrow transplantation in sickle cell anemia. *Seminars in Hematology*. 1991;29:180–201.

14. Luckit J, Treleaven J. Leukemias and lymphomas. In: Treleaven J, Wiernik P, eds. *Bone Marrow Transplantation*. London, England: Mosby-Wolfe; 1995:63–76.

15. Sparano JA, Ciobanu N, Gucalp R. Solid tumors. In: Treleaven J, Wiernik P, eds. *Bone Marrow Transplantation*. London, England: Mosby-Wolfe; 1995:77–100.

16. Engelking C, Kalinowski B, eds. *A Comprehensive Guide to Breast Cancer Treatment: Current Issues and Controversies*. New York: Triclinica Communications; 1995.

17. Herzig R. Phase I-II studies with high dose thiotepa and autologous marrow transplantation in patients with refractory malignancies. Presented at the Proceedings from the American Society of Clinical Oncology; 1988:74.

18. Graham-Pole J, Casper J, Elfenbein G, et al. High-dose chemotherapy supported by marrow infusion for advanced neuroblastoma: a pediatric oncology group study. *J Clin Oncol*. 1991;9:152–158.

Pretransplant Evaluation

Comprehensive pretransplant evaluation of the patient is essential both to determine the patient's ability to withstand the rigors of transplantation and to establish parameters that will provide a valuable basis for post-transplant evaluation. In the setting of allogeneic transplantation, thorough evaluation of a potential bone marrow/peripheral blood stem cell donor is performed to determine donor suitability.

I. Patient evaluation[1,2]

A. Although much of the pretransplant work-up of the patient is standard among transplant centers, the evaluation of any individual patient must also include testing appropriate to the patient's diagnosis and disease staging.

B. From the standpoint of the patient, the pretransplant work-up is essentially the same for allogeneic, autologous, and peripheral blood stem cell transplants.

C. A complete medical history must be obtained with attention to previous treatment, chemotherapeutic regimens, response to chemotherapy, duration of remissions, and current status of disease.

D. In premenopausal female patients, status of menses and method of contraception should be determined.

E. A thorough physical examination should be performed with special attention to any measurable disease, pulmonary status, cardiovascular status, neurologic function, and skin integrity.

F. Laboratory studies
   1. Complete blood count (CBC) with differential
   2. Platelet count
   3. Reticulocyte count
   4. Chemistry panel
   5. Prothrombin time (PT) and activated partial thromboplastin time (APTT)
   6. Immunoglobulin levels
   7. Type and screen
   8. Direct Coombs' test
   9. Reactive protein reagent (RPR)
   10. Hepatitis screen
   11. Viral titers: human immunodeficiency virus (HIV), cytomegalovirus (CMV), herpes simplex virus (HSV), varicella-zoster virus (VZV), Epstein-Barr virus (EBV)
   12. Toxoplasmosis titer
   13. Antinuclear antibodies (ANA)
   14. Copper and zinc levels
   15. Sickle cell studies, if indicated
   16. Fetal hemoglobin (juvenile chronic myelogenous leukemia [CML])
   17. Serum follicle-stimulating hormone (FSH), luteinizing hormone (LH), human chorionic gonadotropin (HcG) and estradiol (female of childbearing age)
   18. Serum markers of disease (e.g., carcinoembryonic antigen [CEA], CA-125)

G. Marrow studies
   1. Aspirate and biopsy for morphology
   2. Additional testing as indicated: cytogenetics
   3. Flow cytometry
   4. Break point cluster region for Philadelphia chromosome (BCR-abl)
   5. Polymerase chain reaction (PCR)

H. Diagnostic studies
   1. Chest x-ray
   2. Panorex
   3. Electrocardiogram (ECG)
   4. Cardiac ejection studies
   5. Pulmonary function testing including DLCO
   6. Disease staging scans, as indicated
   7. Diagnostic lumbar puncture (LP) in patients at risk for central nervous system (CNS) disease

I. Additional studies
   1. Dental evaluation
   2. Nutritional evaluation
   3. Neuropsychiatric evaluation
   4. Social work evaluation
   5. Gynecologic evaluation (female patients)

II. Donor identification/HLA system

A. The primary focus of donor identification for allogeneic transplant is the determination of human leukocyte antigen (HLA) compatibility.

B. HLAs are proteins found on the surface of many cells. These proteins have the ability to distinguish foreign tissue from self.

C. Each individual expresses a group of antigens that differentiates that individual from others. The set of genes that determines an individual's HLA type is known as the major histocompatibility complex (MHC) and is found on chromosome 6 (Figure 1.1).

D. The MHC is divided into three classes of antigens: HLA class I, HLA class II, and HLA class III.

E. HLA class I antigens include HLA*A, HLA*B, and HLA*C genes and are found on all nucleated cells in the body.

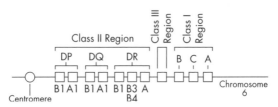

Figure 1.1 Depicts the organization of the HLA/MHC complex. (Reprinted with permission from Whedon, *Bone Marrow Transplantation*, 1997.)

F. HLA class II antigens include HLA*DRB1, *DRB3, *DRB4, *DRB5, *DQA1, *DQB1, *DPA1, and *DPB1 genes. These antigens are found mainly on B lymphocytes, macrophages, monocytes, and dendritic cells. In transplantation, the DR molecule is the most important of the class II antigens.[3]

G. HLA class III antigens are involved in immune function, especially with the serum complement system. The role of class III antigens in transplantation is not well understood.

H. For the purpose of allogeneic transplantation, the HLA genes considered to be most significant are HLA*A, HLA*B, and HLA*DRB1.

III. Inheritance of HLA type

A. The term *phenotype* refers to the HLAs observed in any individual. The phenotype is composed of two sets of antigens, one inherited from each parent.

B. A haplotype is the set of antigens inherited from one parent. These genes/antigens are tightly linked and inherited in blocks. Each individual's phenotype is composed of two haplotypes.

C. There are four possible haplotype combinations within any biologic family.[3] Figure 1.2 demonstrates an inheritance pattern. Each sibling has a 25% chance of matching any other sibling.

	Father (male)		Mother (female)	
	F1	F2	M1	M2
HLA-A	1	2	3	24
HLA-B	8	7	63	12
HLA-DR	3	7	6	2

	F1	M1	F2	M2	F1	M2	F2	M1
HLA-A	1	3	2	24	1	24	2	3
HLA-B	8	63	7	12	8	12	7	63
HLA-DR	3	6	7	2	3	2	7	6
	Child		Child		Child		Child	

Figure 1.2 Outlines HLA inheritance. (Reprinted with permission from Whedon, *Bone Marrow Transplantation*, 1991.)

D. Identical twins are HLA-identical.

E. Certain HLA types and patterns are found more frequently among certain racial and ethnic groups.

IV. HLA typing

A. Several laboratory methods are available for determining an individual's HLA type.

B. Serologic typing identifies HLA type on the surface of white blood cells (WBCs). Because this typing utilizes the WBC, success of the typing depends on adequate numbers of viable WBCs.

C. Cellular typing involves the use of mixed lymphocyte culture. Lymphocytes from two HLA-identical individuals will remain inactive when placed together in culture. Conversely, lymphocytes from two HLA-mismatched individuals will stimulate each other when placed in culture. Traditionally, this test has been used to determine HLA class II compatibility but is now becoming less widely used.

D. DNA typing directly determines the HLA alleles of an individual. Typing is generally accomplished by the polymerase chain reaction technique. Restriction fragment length polymorphism may be used adjunctively to provide higher-resolution testing.

E. Advantages of HLA typing
   1. Provides a higher level of accuracy than other methods
   2. Does not require live cells
   3. Uses manufactured reagents (increased availability)

F. Compatibility between donor and recipient is essential to minimize the potential of graft-versus-host disease (GVHD), graft rejection, and graft failure. Risk increases significantly as the number of mismatched antigens increases (i.e., one-antigen mismatch, two-antigen mismatch, and so on).

G. Most transplant centers will not attempt allogeneic transplantation with anything less than a five out of six HLA match. Even in related HLA-identical transplantation, 10% to 20% of recipients experience clinically significant GVHD.[3] This percentage is increased in unrelated HLA-identical transplants.

H. With the advent of cell selection technology, studies are being conducted to consider the use of mismatched donors, such as haplotype matches, for allogeneic transplantation.

V. Donor evaluation

A. There are numerous physiologic and psychological risks involved with bone marrow/peripheral blood stem cell donation. Donors must be screened carefully to identify potential problems and to minimize risk.

B. Donor evaluation also provides valuable information that may impact the recipient's post-transplant course (e.g., positive viral titers, GVHD risk factors).

C. Medical evaluation
   1. Complete medical history
   2. Attention to chronic medical problems
   3. Medications
   4. Pregnancy history (female)
   5. Anesthesia history
   6. Transfusion history
   7. History of blood donation
   8. Comprehensive physical examination

D. Laboratory studies
   1. CBC with differential
   2. Platelet count
   3. Reticulocyte count
   4. Chemistry panel
   5. Urinalysis
   6. Antinuclear antibodies (ANA)
   7. Immunoglobulin levels
   8. Type and screen
   9. Red blood cell antigens
   10. Hepatitis screen
   11. RPR
   12. Viral titers: HIV, CMV, HSV, VZV, EBV
   13. Toxoplasmosis titer
   14. Serum HcG (female of childbearing age)
   15. Sickle cell studies, if indicated

E. Diagnostic studies
1. Chest x-ray
2. ECG, if indicated by donor age
3. May consider diagnostic bone marrow aspirate

F. Additional studies: psychosocial evaluation

G. In addition to the evaluation process, the donor will also receive extensive instruction regarding the donation (harvesting) process.

H. In the event that more than one donor is identified to be HLA identical, the following factors may be considered in donor selection:
1. Gender compatibility with patient
2. ABO compatibility with patient
3. Donor state of health
4. Negative viral titers
5. Minimal donor exposure to blood products
6. Nulliparity (or fewer pregnancies than other potential donors)

I. Potential donors with active hepatitis or HIV are excluded from donation.[2]

References

1. Malmberg C, Wilson MW. Pretransplant care. In: Buschel PC, Whedon MB, eds. *Bone Marrow Transplantation: Administrative and Clinical Strategies*. Boston: Jones and Bartlett; 1995.

2. Buckner CD, Petersen FB, Bolonesi BA. Bone marrow donors. In: Forman SJ, Blume KG, Thomas ED, eds. *Bone Marrow Transplantation*. Boston: Blackwell Scientific Publications; 1994.

3. Benjamin S. Tissue typing: the human leukocyte antigen (HLA) system. In: Trealeaven J, Wiernik P, eds. *Bone Marrow Transplantation*. London: Mosby-Wolfe; 1995.

Bibliography

Begovich AB, Erlich HA. HLA typing for bone marrow transplantation. *JAMA*. 1995;273: 586–591.

Brostoff J, Scadding GK, Male D, Roitt IM. *Clinical Immunology*. London: Gower Medical Publishing; 1991.

Dupont B, Yang SY. Histocompatibility. In: Forman SJ, Blume KG, Thomas ED, eds. *Bone Marrow Transplantation*. Boston: Blackwell Scientific Publications; 1994.

Flowers MED, Pepe MS, Longton G, et al. Previous donor pregnancy as a risk factor for acute graft-versus-host disease in patients with aplastic anemia treated by allogeneic marrow transplantation. *Br J Haematol*. 1990; 74:492–496.

Martin P. Overview of transplant immunology. In: Forman SJ, Blume KG, Thomas ED, eds. *Bone Marrow Transplantation*. Boston: Blackwell Scientific Publications; 1994.

Weinberg PA. Transplant immunology: HLA and issues of stem cell donation. In: Whedon MB, ed. *Bone Marrow Transplantation: Principles, Practice, and Nursing Insights*. Boston: Jones and Bartlett; 1997.

Conditioning Regimens and Management of Common Toxicities

The conditioning phase of the bone marrow transplantation (BMT) process sets the stage for not only potential cure, but also a myriad of transplant-related toxicities and complications. This chapter outlines common conditioning regimens utilized in both autologous BMT/peripheral blood stem cell (PBSC) rescue and allogeneic BMT as well as practices common in the management of acute conditioning-related toxicities.

I. Combination chemotherapy conditioning and immunosuppressive regimens

A. The ideal chemotherapy conditioning regimen for BMT should be capable of eradicating malignant disease and have tolerable side effects. Large numbers of different preparative regimens are currently in use (Table 2.1).

Table 2.1 Common Preparative Regimens

Preparative regimen	Acronym	Diseases
Busulfan/cyclophosphamide	BU/CY	Hematologic malignancies
Busulfan/cyclophosphamide/etoposide	BU/CY/VP, BCP	Hematologic malignancies
Busulfan/cyclophosphamide/ total body irradiation	BU/CY/TBI	Hematologic malignancies
Busulfan/melphalan	BU/MEL	Hematologic malignancies
Carmustine/etoposide/cytarabine/ cyclophosphamide	BEAC	Non-Hodgkin's lymphoma

(continued)

Table 2.1 (continued)

Preparative regimen	Acronym	Diseases
Etoposide/total body irradiation	VP/TBI	Hematologic malignancies
Cytarabine/total body irradiation	Ara-C/TBI	Acute leukemias
Ifosfamide/carboplatin/etoposide	ICE	Solid tumors
Mitoxantrone/etoposide/thiotepa	MVT	Breast
Melphalan/total body irradiation	Mel/TBI	Multiple myeloma
Carmustine/etoposide/cytarabine/melphalan	BEAM	Hodgkin's and non-Hodgkin's lymphoma
Cyclophosphamide/carmustine/cisplatin	CBP	Breast and solid tumors
Cyclophosphamide/carmustine/etoposide	CBV	Hodgkin's and non-Hodgkin's lymphoma
Cyclophosphamide/etoposide/cisplatin	CVP, CPE	Breast, testicular, and solid tumors
Cyclophosphamide/etoposide/total body irradiation	CY/VP/TBI	Acute leukemias, non-Hodgkin's lymphoma
Cyclophosphamide/total body irradiation	CY/TBI	Hematologic malignancies
Cyclophosphamide/thiotepa/carboplatin	CTC, STAMP-5	Breast and solid tumors
Cyclophosphamide/thiotepa/cisplatin	CTP	Breast and solid tumors
Cyclophosphamide/cytarabine/total body irradiation	TCC	Acute leukemias

B. Conditioning regimens using single-agent chemotherapy combined with total body irradiation (TBI)

1. Early preparative regimens contained TBI as the only primary method used in patients undergoing BMT for hematologic malignancies.[1]

2. This approach was based on the initial findings demonstrating that BMTs could salvage animals that were accidentally exposed to lethal doses of radiation.

3. Radiation therapy is used as a cell cycle specific antitumor therapy.

4. Cyclophosphamide was added to radiation therapy because it was found to be an effective cytotoxic approach and appeared to have few nonhematopoietic toxicities that overlapped with TBI. It was noted that

when cyclophosphamide preceded a single dose of TBI, it reduced the risk of tumor lysis in patients undergoing BMT for relapsed leukemia.[2]

5. Clinical trials were aimed at increasing the effectiveness of TBI and also replacing cyclophosphamide with an alternative cytotoxic drug in combination with TBI. Cytarabine (ara-C), etoposide (VP-16), and melphalan each could be successfully used as a single drug in place of cyclophosphamide.[3-5]

6. Other areas of clinical research focused on changing the sequencing of cytotoxic drugs in relation to TBI.[3,6] The changes were made to minimize some of the toxicity-related symptoms that patients experienced.

C. Dose escalation and TBI

1. Dose escalation trials of TBI, preceded by the standard cyclophosphamide dose of 60 mg/kg for 4 days, have shown that the maximum tolerated dose of TBI is 10 Gy when given in a single dose, 14.4 Gy when given in 1.2-Gy fractions tid, 16 Gy when given in 2-Gy fractions bid, and 15.75 Gy when given in 2.25-Gy fractions qd.[7,8]

2. In these studies, interstitial pneumonitis was found to be the dose-limiting toxicity. In dose escalation studies of etoposide combined with 12- or 13.2-Gy fractionated TBI, 60 mg/kg of etoposide was found to be the maximum tolerated dose; stomatitis and hepatic tolerance were the dose-limiting toxicities.[3]

3. It was also shown that 110 to 180 mg/m^2 of melphalan could be combined with 9.5- to 14.85-Gy TBI[5,9] and that 36 g/m^2 of cytarabine could be combined with 10- to 12-Gy TBI.[4,6,7,10]

4. Dose-limiting toxicities that patients experienced were mucositis and veno-occlusive disease with melphalan plus TBI and central nervous system (CNS) and skin toxicity with the cytarabine plus TBI regimen.

5. Common TBI-containing conditioning regimens.

Regimen	Dose	Type of Transplant
CY/TBI		
Cyclophosphamide	120 mg/kg	Autologous & allogeneic
Total body irradiation	8 to 16 Gy	
VP-16 /TBI		
Etoposide	60 mg/kg	Allogeneic
Total body irradiation	12–13.2 Gy	
Ara-C/TBI		
Cytarabine	36 g/m^2	Autologous & allogeneic
Total body irradiation	10–12 Gy	
Melphalan/TBI		
Melphalan	110 mg/m^2	Autologous & allogeneic
Total body irradiation	9.5–14.85 Gy	

D. Conditioning regimens using two cytotoxic drugs and TBI
   1. Conditioning regimens combining a single
      chemotherapy agent with TBI were shown to
      result in long-term survival in a majority of patients
      undergoing transplant for acute myelogenous leukemia
      (AML) in first remission or chronic-phase-chronic
      myelogenous leukemia (CML).
   2. Disease recurrence remained a major reason for
      treatment failure when used in patients undergoing
      transplantation for advanced-stage disease. This
      finding led to clinical trials of conditioning regimens
      using several chemotherapy drugs along with TBI.
   3. The rationale for this approach derived from settings
      other than BMT, where combinations of cytotoxic
      drugs had been shown to be more effective than
      single agents.
   4. The use of a combination of agents allowed for dose
      escalation without significant overlap in toxicity.

5. The development of new conditioning regimens was explored with the use of two chemotherapy drugs, busulfan and cyclophosphamide. They were given with standard 12-Gy fractionated TBI. It was found that 50 mg/kg of cyclophosphamide combined with 7 mg/kg of busulfan or 103 mg/kg of cyclophosphamide combined with 44 mg/kg of etoposide was the maximum tolerated dose level that could be given with 12-Gy fractionated TBI.[7,11]

6. Clinical trials have determined the maximum tolerated dose levels of combined cyclophosphamide cytarabine, cyclophosphamide and busulfan, and cyclophosphamide and etoposide, all in combination with TBI:[7, 10, 12, 13]

Regimen	Dose	Type of Transplant
CY/Ara-C/TBI		
Cyclophosphamide	60–120 mg/kg	Autologous & allogeneic
Cytarabine	3 g/m^2	
Total body irradiation	5–12 Gy	
CY/BU/TBI		
Cyclophosphamide	50 mg/kg	Autologous & allogeneic
Busulfan	7 mg/kg	
Total body irradiation	12 Gy	
CY/VP=16/TBI		
Cyclophosphamide	80–100 mg/kg	Autologous
Etoposide	40–60 mg/kg	
Total body irradiation	12 Gy	

E. Combination conditioning regimens without TBI

1. Conditioning regimens without TBI are used for several reasons:

a) Transplant centers may lack adequate access to a radiation therapy facility.[14]

b) Some patients in need of a transplant may have already received maximum tolerated doses of radiation to critical organs.[15]

2. Initial trials with combinations of carmustine (BCNU), cytarabine, cyclophosphamide, and 6-thioguanine evolved into regimens that combined cyclophosphamide, carmustine, and etoposide with or without cytarabine. The BEAM and BCV conditioning regimens (see section 6) are mostly used in patients undergoing BMT for lymphoid diseases, such as lymphoma or acute lymphoblastic leukemia.[16–19]

3. The TCC, TC, BCC, MVT, and ICE regimens (see section 6) are mostly used in BMT for patients with breast cancer and other solid tumors.[20–27]

4. Clinical use of busulfan plus cyclophosphamide (BU/CY) was introduced by Santos.

   a) The initial clinical trials used 16 mg/kg of busulfan plus 200 mg/kg of cyclophosphamide. This regimen was known as big BU/CY. This was found to be the maximum tolerated dose, with VOD being the dose-limiting toxicity of this regimen.

   b) Later clinical trials led to the development of a lower dose of cyclophosphamide, 120 mg/kg, which was known as small or little BU/CY.[28] The lower-dose regimen was noted to have less treatment-related side effects and had the same antileukemic effect. Patient survival appeared to be similar to that for patients who received CY/TBI.[14]

   c) BU/CY gained wide acceptance as a conditioning regimen mainly due to the fact that TBI can be avoided. Data suggest that BU/CY is as effective as TBI-containing regimens in the treatment of patients with AML and CML.[28–30]

   d) Clinical trials are investigating the possibility of reducing the dose of busulfan in patients who are at high risk for treatment-related toxicity.

5. TBI is known to be associated with a significant risk of long-term side effects, such as chronic pulmonary disease, leukoencephalopathy, cataracts, secondary malignancies, and hormonal impairment.

   a) The search for a similar conditioning regimen without TBI would avoid the long-term effects that alter quality of life.

   b) Preliminary results of the long-term consequences of BU/CY are not encouraging, suggesting that the incidence of long-term effects is similar to those of CY/TBI.[31, 32]

6. Common high-dose chemoptherapy-only conditioning regimens

Regimen	Dose	Type of Transplant
BU/CY		
Busulfan	14–16 mg/kg	Autologous & allogeneic
Cyclophosphamide	120–200 mg/kg	
BCV		
Carmustine (BCNU)	300–600 mg/m^2	Autologous & allogeneic
Cyclophosphamide	6.0–7.2 g/m^2	
Etoposide (VP-16)	600–2400 mg/m^2	
BEAM		
Carmustine (BCNU)	300 mg/m^2	Autologous
Etoposide	400–800 mg/m^2	
Cytarabine (Ara-C)	800–1600 mg/m^2	
Melphalan	140 mg/m^2	
TCC		
Thiotepa	800 mg/m^2	Autologous
Cyclophosphamide	6000 mg/m^2	
Carboplatin (Paraplatin)	800 mg/m^2	
TC		
Thiotepa	800 mg/m^2	Autologous
Cyclophosphamide	6000 mg/m^2	

Regimen	Dose	Type of Transplant
BCC		
Carmustine (BCNU)	600 mg/m^2	Autologous
Cisplatin	165 mg/m^2	
Cyclophosphamide	5625 mg/m^2	
MVT		
Mitoxantrone	30 mg/m^2	Autologous
Etoposide (VP-16)	1200 mg/m^2	
Thiotepa	750 mg/m^2	
ICE		
Ifosfamide	1500 mg/m^2	Autologous
Carboplatin	1000 mg/m^2	
Etoposide	1250 mg/m^2	

II. Management of conditioning regimen-related toxicities

A. There are many combinations of agents used in the various preparatory regimens. The success of BMT as a curative therapy for patients is limited, in part, by the preparatory toxicities (Table 2.2).

B. Drugs and radiation therapy combinations, their doses, and their schedules of administration are limitless, making the evaluation of treatment-related toxicity a challenge.

Table 2.2 Conditioning Regimen-Related Toxicities

Toxicity	Drug/treatment
Cutaneous	
Hyperpigmentation	Busulfan, carmustine, cyclophosphamide, TBI, thiotepa
Rash	Carmustine, cyclophosphamide, cytarabine, etoposide, melphalan, TBI
Cardiotoxicity	Busulfan, cyclophosphamide, cytarabine, TBI
Gastrointestinal	
Constipation	Etoposide
Diarrhea	Cisplatin, cyclophosphamide, cytarabine, etoposide, melphalan, TBI

Table 2.2 *(continued)*

Toxicity	Drug/treatment
Hepatotoxicity	Carboplatin, carmustine, cyclophosphamide, cytarabine, etoposide, TBI
Nausea & vomiting	Busulfan, carboplatin, carmustine, cisplatin, cyclophosphamide, cytarabine, etoposide, melphalan, TBI, thiotepa
Stomatitis	Cisplatin, cyclophosphamide, cytarabine, etoposide, melphalan, TBI
Genitourinary	
Hemorrhagic cystitis	Cyclophosphamide
Nephrotoxicity	Carboplatin, carmustine, cisplatin, cytarabine
Ocular	
Cataracts	Busulfan, TBI
Conjunctivitis	Carmustine, cytarabine
Nasal congestion	Cyclophosphamide
Ototoxicity	Carboplatin, cisplatin
Hematologic	
Anemia	Busulfan, carboplatin, carmustine, cisplatin, cyclophosphamide, cytarabine, etoposide, melphalan, TBI, thiotepa
Thrombocytopenia	Busulfan, carboplatin, carmustine, cisplatin, cyclophosphamide, cytarabine, etoposide, melphalan, TBI, thiotepa
Hypersensitivity	Busulfan, carboplatin, cisplatin, cytarabine, etoposide, thiotepa
Metabolic	
Hyperuricemia	Busulfan, cisplatin, etoposide
Hypocalcemia	Carboplatin, cisplatin
Hypokalemia	Carboplatin, cisplatin
Hypomagnesemia	Carboplatin, cisplatin
Hyponatremia	Carboplatin, cisplatin
Hypophosphatemia	Carboplatin, cisplatin, cyclophosphamide
Syndrome of inappropriate antidiuretic hormone	Carboplatin, cyclophosphamide
Arthalgias	Carboplatin, cytarabine
Pulmonary fibrosis	Busulfan, carmusitne, cyclophosphamide, cytarabine, melphalan, TBI
Neurologic	
Headache	Cyclophosphamide, thiotepa
Neuropathy (peripheral)	Carboplatin, cisplatin, etoposide
Seizures	Busulfan, carmustine

Source: Data from King,[16] Tennebaum,[17] Whedon,[18] and Whedon.[19]

C. Hematopoietic toxicity

1. Conditioning regimens in BMT destroy normal cells as well as neoplastic cells, resulting in myelosuppression. The result after transplant is the development of cytopenias during, and sometimes beyond, the normal period of engraftment.

2. Initially after transplant, this may be merely a delay in engraftment, but if myelosuppression is persistent, it represents a serious disorder of hematopoietic function. Secondly, a hemostatic disturbance can occur, usually due to thrombocytopenia, although other alterations leading to both a bleeding tendency and thrombotic tendency have been reported.

3. Factors associated with reversible cytopenia after transplantation
   a) Drug therapy: ganciclovir, methotrexate
   b) Bacterial and viral infection
   c) Septicemia
   d) Graft-versus-host disease (GVHD)

4. Factors that influence the duration of cytopenias:
   a) Dose of stem cells that have been infused
   b) Source of stem cells
   c) Underlying disease (particularly in autologous BMT)
   d) Post-transplant immunosuppression therapy
   e) Splenomegaly

5. There are three initial hematopoietic toxicities that are seen in the immediate period after conditioning therapy and transplant BMT: anemia, thrombocytopenia, and leukopenia.

6. Anemia
   a) Anemia can result from inadequate marrow production and supply of red cells. This results in inadequate tissue oxygenation.
   b) Seven to 10 days after the ablative conditioning chemotherapy or radiation therapy, circulating

nucleated red cells will be evident in the
buffy coat.
   c) Circulating reticulocytes are often not evident until
about two to three weeks after marrow infusion.
   d) Return of normal erythropoiesis is evident by the
appearance of the reticulocyte in the circulation.
   e) Etiology
      (1) Excessive loss of red cells caused by bleeding
and hemolysis
      (2) Alloimmune immune hemolytic anemia caused
by red cell ABO antigen mismatch between the
marrow donor and the recipient
      (3) Autoimmune
      (4) Microangiopathic (e.g., thrombotic
thrombocytopenic purpura, hemolytic-
uremic syndrome)
      (5) Red cell aplasia caused by ABO
incompatibility
      (6) Inadequate production of red cells due to an
insufficiency of marrow stem cells
      (7) Impaired erythropoietin production in the
kidneys, leading to insufficient stimulus of
red cell production (seen in allogeneic BMT)
      (8) Marrow suppression related to drug therapy
(e.g., antibiotics)
      (9) Enlarged spleen
   f) The clinical presentation
      (1) Pallor
      (2) Fatigue
      (3) Shortness of breath
   g) Management
      (1) Transfusion support with irradiated packed
red blood cells
      (2) Administration of erythropoietin

7. Thrombocytopenia
   a) Megakaryocytes are usually the last cell line to engraft. Most allogeneic patients are platelet transfusion dependent beyond the first two weeks following BMT. Normal platelet counts are not evident until one to three months after BMT.
   b) Thrombocytopenia can be transient or prolonged; however, persistent and prolonged thrombocytopenia can indicate a worse overall prognosis.
   c) Thrombocytopenia after BMT can result from inadequate platelet production or transient benign thrombocytopenia. Patients usually achieve a normal platelet count; however, it tends to fall. Influencing factors include drug therapy (e.g., trimethroprim-sulfamethoxazole, ganciclovir), delayed megakaryocyte engraftment, and GVHD.
   d) Thrombocytopenia after BMT can also result from excessive loss of platelets or chronic persistent thrombocytopenia. A normal platelet count is usually not achieved despite normal granulocyte and reticulocyte counts. Influencing factors include:
      (1) Hypersplenism
      (2) Autoimmune destruction
      (3) Disseminated intravascular coagulation
      (4) GVHD
      (5) Thrombotic thrombocytopenic purpura
      (6) Autologous transplant in leukemia
      (7) Cyclosporin A prophylaxis
      (8) Purged marrow
   e) Management consists of platelet transfusions.
8. Leukopenia
   a) Profound neutropenia usually lasts for two to four weeks after the conditioning regimen. After this time, neutrophils begin to appear and steadily increase in number.

b) Peripheral white blood cells reach a normal count in several weeks. However, normal immune function often does not return until months or up to a year after transplant.

c) In an uncomplicated transplant, the recovery is a gradual process. The effect of drugs on granulocytes is primarily an alteration in the function of the mature cells and the number of cells in the blood.

d) The number of neutrophils can be influenced by inadequate production or increased peripheral destruction.

e) Older patients experience more severe myelosuppression than younger patients because of decreased cellularity or smaller total marrow mass.

f) Patients who are malnourished prior to the conditioning regimen generally have more severe myelosuppression.

g) Previous chemotherapy and radiation therapy prior to BMT are risk factors for leukopenia.

h) Renal function and hepatic dysfunction may prolong leukopenia post-BMT.

i) TBI and cyclophosphamide cause profound immune dysfunction that persists for months.

j) Busulfan has a less myelosuppressive effect.

k) Antimetabolites (e.g., cytarabine) in the conditioning regimen may prolong the leukopenia period post-BMT.

l) Defects in cellular immunity where there is a reversal in the helper-suppressor ratio, due to the reduction in helper cell numbers, is seen post-transplant.

m) Defect in humoral immunity leading to decreased antibody production is also seen post-BMT.

n) Pathogens associated with infections post-BMT:

Causes of infection	Type of infections
Cellular defects	**Fungi**
	Candida
	Aspergillus
	Protozoa
	Pneumocystis carinii
	Toxoplasma
	Virus
	Herpes simplex
	Varicella zoster
	Cytomegalovirus
Humoral defects	**Pyrogenic organisms**
	Streptococcus
Phagocytotic disorder	**Low-virulence bacteria**
	Escherichia coli
	Pseudomonas

o) The clinical presentation of infection includes temperature greater than 38°C (100.4°F), rigors, malaise, headache, inflammation, erythema, rash, skin tenderness, tachypnea, cough, dyspnea, dysuria, and urinary frequency and hesitancy.

p) Management includes treating the underlying cause with empiric antibiotics, monitoring peak and trough drug levels if appropriate, preserving the skin and mucous membrane integrity (e.g., avoid or minimize peripheral venous access for IV access or blood specimen acquisition), stressing the importance of good personal hygiene (e.g., perineal or rectal care), and instructing the patient regarding the signs and symptoms of infection to report.

D. Fever and chills

1. The development of fever in a neutropenic BMT patient must be regarded as infection until proved otherwise and the condition immediately treated.

The main predisposing factors to bacterial infection post-transplant are neutropenia and defects in humoral immunity.

2. As normal neutrophil counts recover after transplant, neutrophil function including chemotaxis and killing of intracellular organisms may remain normal.

3. B-cell humoral immunity remains low even when serum immunoglobulin levels recover to normal at three months post-transplant.

4. Etiology
   a) Fever occurs when bacteria, viruses, toxins, or other agents are phagocytosed by leukocytes.
   b) Interleukin-1 and other chemical mediators (endogenous pyrogens) are produced and activate the production of prostaglandins.
   c) Prostaglandins act on the regulatory mechanism in the hypothalamus and subsequently readjust the body's thermostat.
   d) Raising the hypothalamic set point initiates the process of heat production by increasing metabolism, triggering peripheral vasoconstriction, and less frequently triggering shivering or rigors, which increase heat production to the muscles.

5. Clinical presentation
   a) Abscesses may be difficult to detect.
   b) Absence of neutrophilic exudate in infected tissue
   c) Pulmonary infections may present without cough, sputum, or x-ray abnormalities.
   d) Common sites of infection are the oropharynx, lung, perirectal area, and skin.
   e) Malaise, myalgias, fatigue, tachycardia (pulse rate up 10 to 15 beats per minute)
   f) Common infections during the first 30 days post-transplant include fever of unknown origin (presumed to be bacterial), gram-positive septicemia, and central venous catheter site infections.

g) Common infections 31 to 90 days post-transplant include fever of unknown origin, gram-positive and gram-negative septicemia, and bronchopulmonary infection.

6. History and physical examination
    a) A careful history should be taken to search for symptoms suggestive of infection in a specific organ.
    b) A complete physical examination should pay special attention to localized infection such as of the pharynx, skin, ocular fundus, CNS, pelvis, and rectum.
    c) Assess vital signs.
    d) Assess for signs of dehydration.
    e) Check for lymphadenopathy.

7. Laboratory studies
    a) Complete blood count, serum electrolytes, and creatinine levels
    b) Urinalysis
    c) Sputum culture and sensitivity
    d) Blood cultures: peripheral venipuncture site and central venous catheter lumens and exit site
    e) Chest x-ray
    f) Surveillance cultures of the skin, throat, and feces have questionable value in a neutropenic BMT patient. They may be useful in identifying possible resistant organisms the transplant recipient may colonize. Individual BMT programs should decide on the cost-effectiveness and usefulness of such cultures.

8. Management
    a) Aminoglycosides (gentamicin, tobramycin, amikacin) are used because of their broad-spectrum coverage of gram-negative bacteria. All of these drugs are nephrotoxic, and dosage modifications may be required in patients with

renal insufficiency. Serum creatinine levels should be monitored at least every other day. Initially, drug levels should be measured to establish effective dose and to avoid toxic levels.

b) Antipseudomonal penicillins (i.e., piperacillin, 4 g IV q6h; ticarcillin) are added to aminoglycosides to provide bactericidal activity against highly lethal *Pseudomonas* infections.

c) Cephalosporins can be first-line therapy in the management of the granulocytopenic patients. These drugs have the advantage of low toxicity as compared to the aminoglycosides, and newer agents have good penetration into the CNS. These agents are synergistic for nephrotoxicity with aminoglycosides, and several cause platelet or clotting abnormalities. Platelet counts and prothrombin times should be routinely followed. Third-generation cephalosporins, such as ceftriaxone, have long half-lives and can be administered every 12 hours. Ceftazidime has broad aerobic and anaerobic coverage as well as special coverage for bacteria such as *Pseudomonas*. Aztreonam is a cephalosporin-like drug that can be used with minimal caution in BMT patients who are allergic to cephalosporins. The spectrum of this unique drug is almost identical to that of aminoglycosides. Imipenem is the broadest spectrum of the third-generation cephalosporins and has been used as a single drug for granulocytopenic and febrile BMT patients. In all cases of culture-proven infection, sensitivities should be checked with these agents and resistance followed.

d) Initial therapy: An aminoglycoside plus an antipseudomonal penicillin may be immediately given to a neutropenic BMT patient with fever.

Other drugs may be added in certain clinical situations. The majority of fevers will resolve within 48 hours to 72 hours.

e) Nafcillin, oxacillin, or vancomycin is added if there is evidence of staphylococcal infection.

f) Erythromycin is added until the diagnosis is established if there are pulmonary infiltrates.

g) Intrathecal therapy: Third-generation cephalosporins, such as cefotaxime and ceftriaxone, cross the blood-brain barrier well, particularly in the presence of inflammation.

h) Amphotericin B is added if there is presumed or objective evidence of a fungal infection. Nephrotoxicity is a significant side effect of amphotercin therapy.

i) Quinolone antibiotics: Ciprofloxacin has broad-spectrum effectiveness, although it has poor anaerobe coverage. It provides excellent coverage for both gram-negative and gram-positive organisms. The quinolones have little toxicity and are available in oral form.

j) If a patient improves on empiric antibiotic therapy, it should be continued for 9 to 10 days, despite negative cultures.

k) If the fever persists 48 to 72 hours after the initiation of primary antibiotic therapy, a strategy should be in place for further management, such as the addition of an antifungal agent (e.g., amphotericin or fluconazole), depending on the local microbacteria flora that exists.

l) If the fever persists after 7 to 14 days of antibiotic therapy, neutropenic BMT patients will benefit from amphotericin B therapy. This therapy is clearly indicated when fungal colonization has been demonstrated.

m) If the patient does not improve on empiric
   therapy after 4 days, antibiotics should be stopped,
   and cultures should be repeated. The patient
   probably is either on the wrong antibiotics or has
   a condition for which antibiotics are ineffective
   (i.e., viral or fungal infection). The antibiotics
   should be resumed if the patient becomes worse
   or if fever persists.
n) For management of specific infections,
   see Table 2.3.

Table 2.3 Management of Specific Infections (None of the Following Supersede the Demonstrated Antibiotic Sensitivity)

Organism	First-choice therapy	Second-choice therapy
Campylobacter jejuni	Fluoroquinolones	Erythromycin
Chlamydia trachomatis	Tetracycline	Erythromycin
Clostridium difficile	Metronidazole PO	Vancomycin PO
Enterobacter species	Aminoglycoside	Antipseudomonal penicillin
Enterococci group D streptococci	Penicillin or ampicillin & gentamicin	Vancomycin & gentamicin
Haemophilus influenzae	Amoxicillin	Co-trimoxazole, third-generation cephalosporin
Mycoplasma pneumoniae	Erythromycin	Tetracycline
Pseudomonas aeruginosa	Aminoglycoside and antipseudomonal penicillin	Aztreonam or imipenem
Methicillin-resistant Staphylococcus epidermidis	Vancomycin	Rifampin

9. Prevention of infection (see Chapter 3)
   a) Handwashing by the staff before touching the
      patient is the most important prevention technique
      for nosocomial infections.
   b) Skin care is important in preventing infections
      with *Staphylococcus* and other pathogens.
   c) Diet: Avoiding foods that have a high bacterial
      content is a common practice in the BMT patient:

however, this is controversial in the literature.

    d) Oral care should be compulsively performed by the BMT patient.

    e) Invasive procedures such as taking rectal temperatures and subcutaneous injections should be avoided to protect the integrity of the mucous membrane.

E. Nausea, vomiting, and anorexia

    1. This protective mechanism is activated by the vomiting or emetic center located in the dorsal lateral reticular formation of the medulla. The reflex is stimulated by several pathways: chemoreceptor trigger zone, vagal viscera afferents, labyrinth of the inner ear, cerebral cortex, and the limbic system.[33]

    2. Neurotransmitters such as dopamine, acetylcholine, 5-hydroxytryptamine (serotonin), histamine, norepinephrine, enkephalins, and glutamine are also responsible for inducing vomiting.

    3. Drugs induce vomiting by a variety of neurotransmitters, causing different patterns of nausea.

       a) The incidence of acute nausea is related to: emetic potential, dose, route of administration, schedule, infusion rate, time of day, and combination of drugs.

       b) Delayed and persistent nausea: vomiting occurs 24 hours after the completion of conditioning regimens containing cisplatin or cyclophosphamide. The duration of nausea can be from two to three weeks after the completion of the conditioning regimen, reaching a peak at 10 to 14 days after BMT. Persistent nausea is more common than vomiting once the conditioning regimen has been finished and appears to be less responsive to antiemetic therapy.

c) Anticipatory nausea and vomiting is a learned response to the previous effects of receiving chemotherapy treatment. It is a conditioned or learned response to previous effects from therapy and environmental stimuli. Predictors for the development of these symptoms are increased anxiety levels, younger-age patients, odors, and the actual treatment setting.

4. Etiology
   a) High emetic potential of conditioning chemotherapy drugs. The intensity of the vomiting tends to be worse with high-dose regimens.
   b) Support medications, particularly nystatin, oral amphotericin, clotrimazole, and cyclosporine
   c) GVHD of the upper gastrointestinal tract
   d) Hepatic disease including GVHD
   e) Infections involving the esophagus, stomach, or intestine

5. Clinical presentation
   a) Epigastric and/or abdominal pain
   b) Retching that can be characterized as prolonged or intractable
   c) Vomiting that can be refractory to antiemetics
   d) Onset of nausea and vomiting occurring several days prior to the BMT and reaching a peak 10 to 14 days after BMT
   e) Watery diarrhea
   f) Hiccuping

6. History
   a) Question the patient about the onset, duration, quantity, and quality of vomitus (undigested food, medication, or blood).
   b) Question the patient about the timing of vomiting with respect to the administration of chemotherapy, TBI, and meals.

7. Physical examination
   a) Assess hydration status; checking for dry mucous membranes, decreased skin turgor, tachycardia, and oliguria.
   b) Assess cardiovascular status (i.e., pulse, blood pressure), and check for postural hypotension.
   c) Examine abdomen for tenderness, rigidity, abnormal tympany, and bowel sounds.
8. Laboratory studies
   a) If there are no other systemic symptoms and duration is less than 24 hours, no laboratory studies are indicated.
   b) If vomiting persists for longer than 24 hours, consider serum chemistry screening for acid-base and electrolyte status and glucose screening.
9. Management
   a) Identification of the most likely cause
   b) Supportive measures: fluids, electrolyte replacement
   c) Limit solid foods.
   d) Clear liquids only until no vomiting is present. Start with 15 mL every 10 minutes.
   e) If vomiting **does not occur,** double the amount of fluid each hour.
   f) If vomiting **does occur,** allow the gut to rest.
   g) The vomiting should be minimized for symptomatic relief and to minimize the risk of an esophageal tear or gastric mucosal hemorrhage, especially during the thrombocytopenic phase during early transplant.
   h) For pharmacologic interventions, see Table 2.4.

Table 2.4 Pharmacologic Management of Nausea and Vomiting

Medications	Dosing schedule	Administration guidelines
Antihistamine		
Diphenhydramine (Benadryl)	30 mg/m^2 IV 30 min before each metoclopramide dose Continue for q4h X 6 doses after last dose of chemotherapy	Prevents extrapyramidal side effects of dopamine receptor antagonists and has sedative properties. Can be used alone in some infants and children. Not a potent antiemetic
Benzodiazepine		
Lorazepam (Ativan)	1–2 mg IV q6h	Useful adjunct to ondansetron, especially for anticipatory nausea and vomiting, because of its sedative and anxiolytic effects
Corticosteroids		
Dexamethasone (Decadron)	10–20 mg IV q6h	Useful adjunct to ondansetron, especially for regimens that contain cisplatin. Side effects include hyperglycemia and mental status changes.
Dopamine blocking agents		
Droperidol (Inapsine)	625–2.5 mg IV q4-6h	Extrapyramidal side effects may occur. Use with caution in children.
Metoclopramide (Reglan)	40 mg/m^2 IV q4h X times 6 doses for each chemotherapy infusion	Extrapyramidal side effects seen with this drug. Use cautiously with children.
Serotonin Receptor Antagonist		
Granisetron (Kytril)	10µg/kg IV over 5 min 30 min prior to chemotherapy 1 mg bid PO 1 h prior to chemotherapy and 12 h after chemotherapy	Doses may become less effective over time.
Ondansetron (Zofran)	0.15–0.18 mg/kg IV 4 h for 3 doses given 15 min prior to chemotherapy and 4 and 8 h after chemotherapy. 32 mg dose IV 15 min prior to chemotherapy. 8 mg bid PO 30 min prior to chemotherapy and 8 h after chemotherapy	Doses may become less effective over time. Therapy is not effective for refractory nausea

F. Mucositis/stomatitis
1. Mucositis and xerostomia usually develop during the administration of the conditioning regimen, with ulceration of the mucosal lesions developing around the time of the marrow infusion.
2. Resolution of symptoms usually occurs two to three weeks after the completion of therapy, once engraftment occurs and the patient demonstrates neutrophil recovery. It may persist longer, with pain affecting swallowing, and can lead to aspiration.
3. Direct damage to the proliferating cells of the oral epithelium causes mucosal atrophy, with subsequent damage to the connective tissue.
4. Patients receiving single-agent chemotherapy conditioning regimens tend to have mild to moderate oropharyngeal mucositis. TBI added to the conditioning regimen significantly increases mucositis due to increased mucosal damage and xerostomia.
5. The development and severity of oral mucositis are dependent on the conditioning regimen used. Conditioning regimens containing the following drugs or types of radiation therapy lead to more severe mucositis.
   a) Radiation therapy
      (1) TBI greater than 15.75 Gy
      (2) Total lymphoid irradiation
      (3) Hyper-fractionated TBI
   b) Chemotherapy
      (1) Busulfan
      (2) Etoposide
      (3) Thiotepa
      (4) Cyclophosphamide
      (5) Cisplatin
      (6) BCNU
      (7) GVHD prophylaxis with methotrexate

6. Clinical presentation
   a) Sensitivity to acid foods or hot foods
   b) Xerostomia secondary to salivary gland edema and dysfunction
   c) Erythema followed by mucosal ulceration
   d) Patchy mucosal atrophy
   e) Mucositis progressing to extensive ulceration as damage to the mucosal epithelium becomes more pronounced
   f) Severe pain
7. Differential diagnosis
   a) Xerostomia
   b) Oral infections
   c) GVHD
8. History
   a) Question the patient regarding the presence of burning sensation.
   b) Ask how long the burning sensation has been present.
   c) Determine if the patient is experiencing dysphagia, algophagia, or xerostomia.
   d) Ask if the patient is experiencing sensitivity or pain when drinking or eating hot or cold fluids or foods.
9. Physical examination
   a) Examine the buccal mucosa and tongue for areas of pallor and/or erythema.
   b) Examine mucous membranes for dryness.
   c) Examine pharynx for mucous membrane changes.
10. Management
   a) Until healing occurs, the symptomatic approach to mucositis management is used. The success of management depends on the frequency use of all supportive care approaches.

b) Encourage daily oral care routines, such as frequent rinsing with 0.9% normal saline. The frequency of oral mouth care should increase as the severity of mucositis increases (i.e., for moderate mucositis, every two to four hours; for severe mucositis, every one to two hours).

c) Topical anesthetics or a mucosal coating agent can be used if the patient is experiencing significant xerostomia or moderate to severe mucositis. Preparations such as:

   (1) artificial salvia

   (2 water-soluble lubricants

   (3) kaolin preparation (Kaopectate®)

   (4) antacids

   (5) lidocaine preparations: Xylocaine viscous solution 2%, Xylocaine 10% spray, Xylocaine 5% ointment can be taken alone or in combination with an antacid, and diphenhydramine hydrochloride (Benadryl elixir), 15mL q2-4h.

d) Prevention and treatment of infection with topical or systemic antiviral, antibacterial, and antifungal therapy may be required. Common agents that are used depending on culture results are listed in Table 2.5.

Table 2.5 Agents Used for Prophylaxis and Treatment of Infectious Mucositis/stomatitis

Topical antibacterial	Topical antifungal	Antiviral
Chlorhexidine	Clotrimazole	Acyclovir
Povidone-iodine	Nystatin	Ganciclovir
Tobramycin rinses	Amphotericin	
Vancomycin rinses		

  e) Minimize trauma to mucous membranes by using a soft tooth-brush or toothette. While brushing may be uncomfortable, it is necessary.

  f) Daily oral debridement with diluted hydrogen peroxide can be helpful to debride mouth ulcers. Mix hydrogen peroxide with water or saline 1:4 or 1:2 immediately before using so that the solution does not lose its oxidizing ability. Swish for several minutes, expectorate, and rinse.

G. Diarrhea

 1. Diarrhea in the BMT patient can result from a direct toxic effect to the mucosa of the intestinal tract caused by the conditioning regimen. This leads to mucous membrane damage.

 2. Secondary causes contributing to diarrhea are GHVD, intestinal infections, and side effects from support medications.

 3. Diarrhea is noted within 10 days of the administration of high-dose chemotherapy. Diffuse mucosal changes can occur along the intestinal tract leading to flattening or necrosis of the intestinal crypt cells and damage to the intestinal villi.

 4. As further damage occurs to the intestinal villi, the patient will have difficulty with malabsorption of drugs and nutrients.

 5. Etiology

  a) Chemotherapy conditioning regimens containing the following drugs: busulfan, melphalan, cytarabine, methotrexate, etoposide, thiotepa

  b) Support medications: antacids, metoclopramide, antibiotics, magnesium

  c) TBI-containing preparative regimens

  d) Thrombocytopenia can occur concomitantly, exacerbating the problem.

  e) Infections (i.e., bacterial, fungal, viral, or parasitic). The use of antibiotics predisposes

the patient to an overgrowth of gram-negative
bacteria and fungal organisms.
f) GVHD
6. Clinical presentation: Symptoms can persist for
2 to 3 weeks after the conditioning regimen has
been administered. The patient experiences symptoms
such as:
a) abdominal cramps
b) pain
c) anorexia
d) watery diarrhea
7. Physical examination
a) Assess hydration status, checking mucous
membranes, skin turgor, tachycardia, and oliguria.
b) Assess for postural hypotension.
c) Examine abdomen for tenderness, rigidity,
abnormal tympany, and bowel sounds.
d) Consider rectal examination for tenderness.
8. Laboratory studies include stool for occult blood,
for ova and paracites, clostridium difficile, and enteric
pathogens if the following are present:
a) Blood-tinged mucous diarrhea
b) Fever over 24 hours
c) Wet preparation shows white blood cells.
9. Management
a) Treat the underlying cause.
b) Antidiarrheal agents are generally not helpful
in this setting.
c) Control any fluid and/or electrolyte imbalance.
d) Provide any symptomatic relief.
e) Consider irritants in the diet, carefully selecting
food choices, and avoiding dairy products.
H. Hemorrhagic cystitis
1. Hemorrhagic cystitis can occur in patients receiving
high-dose cyclophosphamide and ifosfamide in conditioning regimens for BMT preparation.

2. The final active metabolite, acrolein, when exposed to the urothelium, causes mucosal hyperemia and ulceration with hemorrhage and focal necrosis.
3. Hemorrhagic cystitis can occur several weeks after the last dose of cyclophosphamide and can remain a clinical problem for months after transplant.
4. The incidence of hemorrhagic cystitis in patients receiving cyclophosphamide post-transplantation can be as high as 50% to 70%.[35]
5. Conditioning regimens containing the following drugs can cause hemorrhagic cystitis:
   a) Cyclophosphamide
   b) Ifosfamide
   c) Busulfan combined with cyclophosphamide causes an increased incidence.
6. Clinical presentation
   a) Hematuria may be macroscopic (visible to the naked eye) or microscopic (detected on dipstick or microscopic examination).
   b) Hematuria may be reported as early as the termination of the first cyclophosphamide dose or as late as three months post-transplant.
   c) Dysuria, which may progress to flank pain
   d) Hematuria with clots
7. Urinalysis may reveal the presence of more than five red blood cells per high-power field on microscopic examination of the urine. Protenuira may also be present.
8. Management
   a) Continuous bladder irrigations can be used to dilute the urine and minimize exposure of acrolein to the urothelium. The results of clinical trials have been mixed as to the effectiveness of continuous bladder irrigations on preventing hemorrhagic cystitis. The following approaches can be used: three-way bladder irrigations at 100 to 500

mL/hour of continuous irrigation, which can be initiated at the start of the first chemotherapy dose and continued until 24 hours after the last dose or until the urine demonstrates no evidence of blood; or aggressive hydration with fluids at twice the usual maintenance rate.

b) Forced diuresis with hydration and diuretics, monitoring the patient to prevent a prerenal state

c) In patients receiving continuous bladder irrigations, monitor the patient to prevent fluid overload.

d) The use of uroprotective agents such as N-acetyl-cysteine and sodium 2-mercaptoethane sulfonate (mesna) has been shown to reduce the incidence of hemorrhagic cystitis. Several dosing methods have been used, and doses vary significantly. Mesna doses range between 60% and 160% of the cyclophosphamide or ifosfamide dose. Mesna can be administered prior to the initiation of the chemotherapy (cyclophosphamide or ifosfamide) and every 4 hours thereafter. Mesna by continuous infusion has also been used. Dosing should continue for 12 to 24 hours longer than either cyclophosphamide or ifosfamide, due to the short half-life of mesna.[35]

e) If bleeding persists, cystoscopy and cautery of bleeding may be required.

f) Identify parameters for platelet transfusion requirements to prevent thrombocytopenia.

I. Skin breakdown

1. TBI and most of the chemotherapy agents used in preparative regimens can cause cutaneous manifestations.

2. Cutaneous presentations can occur during the infusion of chemotherapy and continue to develop

until weeks later.

3. Chemotherapy drugs that have been reported to cause skin toxicity include:
   a) Carmustine
   b) Etoposide
   c) Busulfan
   d) Thiotepa
   e) Cytosine arabinoside
   f) Cytarabine

4. The metabolites of thiotepa are concentrated in perspiration and can accumulate on dressings and in skin folds. Consequently, irritation occurs, resulting in skin toxicity.

5. Clinical presentation
   a) Maculopapular rash
   b) Painful and nonpruritic erythema
   c) Bullae formation or fluid-filled vesicle (blister)
   d) Acral erythema or dermatitis is a condition that is characterized by demarcated, painful, and dusky erythematous patches involving the palms and soles. This condition is particularly seen with cytarabine-, busulfan-, and daunorubicin-containing conditioning regimens.
   e) Flexural erythema localized to the axillary, inguinal folds and the scrotum can be associated with busulfan.
   f) Skin desquamation: Dry desquamation can cause skin peeling. Moist desquamation refers to skin weeping. This presentation is especially seen in patients receiving carmustine, etoposide, and thiotepa.
   g) Hyperpigmentation can develop from desquamation-type presentations.
   h) Permanent alopecia has been reported in combination busulfan and cyclophosphamide conditioning regimens.

i) Diffuse erythema is a transient response to TBI.

j) Radiation recall has been reported in patients receiving carmustine.

k) Stevens-Johnson syndrome has been reported with etoposide, characterized by macules or papules that can progress to bullae involving the mucous membrane of the mouth, pharynx, and conjunctiva.

6. Differential diagnosis
   a) GVHD
   b) Drug allergy
   c) Folliculitis

7. Skin biopsy may be of benefit.

8. Management
   a) Showering after the completion of thiotepa infusion is recommended for patients receiving doses of thiotepa of 700 mg/m^2.

   b) Frequent dressing changes and not using tape due to the damage caused to the epidermal layer are recommended.

   c) Avoid local irritants such as antiperspirants and lotions containing alcohol.

   d) Medications for pruritus may be used (e.g., hydroxyzine, 25 to 50 mg tid prn).

   e) Antibiotic therapy may be required, with therapy changes based on culture results and clinical response.

   f) If blistering has occurred, after the blistering stages, hydrocortisone cream 2.5% may be applied thinly qid. Topical steroids will penetrate blisters.

References

1. Thomas ED, Strob R, Buckner CD. Total body irradiation in preparation for marrow engraftment. *Transplant Proc.* 1976;8:591–594.

2. Buckner CD, Rudolp RH, Fefer A, et al. High dose cyclophosphamide therapy for malignant disease. *Cancer.* 1972;29:357–365.

3. Blume KG, Forman SJ, O'Donnell MR, et al. Total body irradiation and high-dose etoposide: a new preparatory regimen for bone marrow transplantation in patients with advanced hematologic malignancies. *Blood.* 1987;69:1015–1020.

4. Coccia PF, Strandjord SE, Warkentin PI, et al. High dose cytosine arabinoside and fractionated total body irradiation: an improved reparative regimen for bone marrow transplantation of children with acute lymphoblastic leukemia in remission. *Blood.* 1988;71:888–893.

5. Powles RL, Milliken S, Helenglass G. The use of melphalan in conjunction with total body irradiation as a treatment for leukemia. *Transplant Proc.* 1989;21:2955–2957.

6. Woods WE, Ramsay NK, Weisdorf DJ, et al. Bone marrow transplantation for acute lymphocytic leukemia utilizing total body irradiation followed by high doses of cytosine arabinoside: lack of superiority over cyclophosphamide-containing conditioning regimens. *Bone Marrow Transplant.* 1990;6:9–16.

7. Petersen FB, Appelbaum FR, Bigelow CL, et al. High dose cytosine arabinoside, total body irradiation and marrow transplantation for advanced malignant lymphoma. *Bone Marrow Transplant.* 1989;4:483–488.

8. Clift RA, Buckner CD, Thomas ED, et al. Allogeneic marrow transplantation using fractionated total body irradiation in patients with acute lymphoblastic leukemia in relapse. *Leuk Res.* 1982;6:407–410.

9. Gandola L, Lombardi F, Siena S, et al. Total body irradiation and high dose melphalan with bone marrow transplantation at Isituto Nazionale Turmori, Milan Italy. *Radiother Oncol*. 1990;18(suppl):105–109.

10. Ridell S, Appelbaum FR, Buckner CD, et al. High-dose cytarabine and total body irradiation with or without cyclophosphamide as a reparative regimen for marrow transplantation for acute leukemia. *J Clin Oncol*. 1988;6:576–582.

11. Petersen FB, Buckner CD, Appelbaum FR, et al. Etoposide, cyclophosphamide and fractionated total body irradiation as a preparatory regimen for marrow transplantation in patients with advanced hematological malignancies: a phase I study. *Bone Marrow Transplant*. 1992;10:83–88.

12. Horning SJ, Chao NJ, Negrin RS, et al. Preliminary analysis of high dose etoposide cytoreductive regimens and autologous bone marrow transplantation in intermediate and high grade non-Hodgkin's lymphoma. In: Dicke KA, Armitage JO, Dickie MJ, eds. *Autologous Bone Marrow Transplantation*. Houston: Proceedings of the Fifth International Symposium; 1990:445–452.

13. Bostrom B, Weisdorf DJ, Kim T, et al. Bone marrow transplantation for advanced acute leukemia: a pilot study of high energy total body irradiation, cyclophosphamide and continuous-infusion etoposide. *Bone Marrow Transplant*. 1990;5:83–89.

14. Santos GW, Tutschka PJ, Brookmeyer R, et al. Marrow transplantation for acute nonlymphocytic leukemia after treatment with busulfan and cyclophosphamide regimen. *Blood*. 1983;70:1347–1353.

15. Appelbaum FR, Sullivan KM, Buckner CD, et al.: Treatment of malignant lymphoma in 100 patients with chemotherapy, total body irradiation, and marrow transplantation. *J Clin Oncol*. 1987; 5:1340–1347.

16. Gaspard MH, Maraninchi D, Stopps AM, et al. Intensive chemotherapy with high doses of BCNU, etoposide, cytosine arabinoside, and melphalan (BEAM) followed by autologous bone marrow transplantation: toxicity and antitumor activity in 26 patients with poor risk malignancies. *Cancer Chemother Pharmacol.* 1988;22:256–262.

17. Reece DE, Barnett MJ, Connors JM, et al. Intensive chemotherapy with cyclophosphamide, carmustine, and etoposide followed by autologous bone marrow transplantation for relapsed Hodgkin's disease. *J Clin Oncol.* 1991;9:1871–1879.

18. Zander AR, Culbert S, Jagannath S, et al. High dose cyclophosphamide, BCNU, and VP 16 (CBV) as a conditioning regimen for allogeneic bone marrow transplantation for patients with acute leukemia. *Cancer.* 1987;59:1083–1086.

19. Wheeler C, Antin JH, Churchill WH, et al. Cyclophos-phamide, carmustine, and etoposide with autologous bone marrow transplantation in refractory Hodgkin's disease and non-Hodgkin's lymphoma: a dose-finding study. *J Clin Oncol.* 1990;8:648–656.

20. Peters WP, Shpall EJ, Jones RB. High dose combination alkylating agents with bone marrow support as initial treatment for metastatic breast cancer. *J Clin Oncol.* 1990;6:1368–1376.

21. Eder JP, Elias A, Shea TC, et al. A phase I-II study of cyclophosphamide, thiotepa, and carboplatin with autologous bone marrow transplantation in solid tumor patients. *J Clin Oncol.* 1990;8:1239–1245.

22. Antman K, Ayash L, Elais A, et al. A phase II study of high dose cyclophosphamide, thiotepa, and carboplatin with autologous marrow support in women with measurable advanced breast cancer responding to standard-dose therapy. *J Clin Oncol.* 1992;10:102–110.

23. Eder JP, Antman L, Elais A, et al. Cyclophosphamide and thiotepa with autologous bone marrow transplantation in patients with solid tumors. *J Natl Cancer Inst.* 1988;80:1221–1226.

24. Wallerstein R Jr, Spitzer G, Dunphy F, et al. A phase II study of mitoxantrone, etoposide, and thiotepa with autologous marrow support for patients with relapsed breast cancer. *J Clin Oncol*. 1990;8:1782–1788.

25. Ellis ED, Williams SF, Moormier JAA, et al. A phase I-II study of high-dose cyclophosphamide, thiotepa and escalating doses of mitoxantrone with autologous stem cell rescue in patients with refractory malignancies. *Bone Marrow Transplant*. 1990;6:439–442.

26. Lotz JP, Machover D, Malassagne B, et al. Phase I-II study of two consecutive courses of high dose epipodophylloxin, ifosfamide, and carboplatin with autologous bone marrow transplantation for treatment of adult patients with solid tumors. *J Clin Oncol*. 1991;9:1860–1870.

27. Rosenfeld CS, Przeppiorka D, Schwinghammer TL, et al. Autologous bone marrow transplantation following high dose busulfan and VP 16 for advanced non-Hodgkin's lymphoma and Hodgkin's disease. *Exp Hematol*. 1991;19:317–321.

28. Tutschka PJ, Kapoor N, Copelean EA, et al. Early experience with 16 mg/kg of busulfan and low dose cyclophosphamide of 90 mg/kg as conditioning for allogeneic marrow grafting in leukemia. *Exp Hematol*. 1991;19:570.

29. Petersen FB, Appelbaum FR, Hill R, et al. Busulfan and cyclophosphamide as a preparative regimen for bone marrow transplantation in patients with prior chest radiotherapy. *Bone Marrow Transplant*. 1991;8:211–215.

30. Copelan EA, Kapoor N, Gibbins B, et al. Allogeneic marrow transplantation in non-Hodgkin's lymphoma: a report of 100 cases from Seattle. *J Clin Oncol*. 1990;8:638–647.

31. Sanders J, Sullivan K, Witherspoon R, et al. Long term effects and quality of life in children and adults after marrow transplantation. *Bone Marrow Transplant*. 1989;4(suppl 4):27–29.

32. Wingard JR, Plontnick LP, Freemer CS, et al. Growth in children after bone marrow transplantation: busulfan plus cyclophosphamide plus total body irradiation. *Blood*. 1992;79:1068–1073.

33. Rhodes, VA. Nausea, vomiting and retching. *Nurs Clin North Am*. 1990;25:885–899.

34. Efros M, Ahmed T, Choudhury M. Cyclophosphamide induced hemorrhagic pyelitis and ureteritis associated with cystitis in marrow transplantation. *J Urol*. 1990;144:1231–1232.

35. King CR. Peripheral stem cell transplantation: past present and future. In: *Bone Marrow Transplantation: Administrative and Clinical Strategies*. Buschel P, Whedon M, eds. Boston: Jones & Bartlett; 1995:187–212.

36. Tennebaum L. Chemotherapeutic agents used in the treatment of cancer. In: Tennebaum L, ed. *Cancer Chemotherapy and Biotherapy: A Reference Guide*. 2nd ed. Philadelphia: Saunders; 1994:69–150.

37. Whedon MB. Allogeneic bone marrow transplantation: clinical indications, treatment process and outcomes. In: Whedon MB, ed. *Bone Marrow Transplantation: Principles, Practice and Nursing Insights*. Boston: Jones & Bartlett; 1991:20–48.

38. Whedon MB. Autologous bone marrow transplantation: clinical indications, treatment process and outcomes. In: Whedon MB, ed. *Bone Marrow Transplantation: Principles, Practice and Nursing Insights*. Boston: Jones & Bartlett; 1991:49–69.

Bibliography

Anemia

Bosi A, Vannucchi AM, Grossi A. Serum erythropoietin levels in patients undergoing autologous bone marrow transplantation. *Bone Marrow Transplant.* 1991;7:421–425.

Ireland RM, Atkinson K, Conconnon AJ. Serum erythropoietin changes in autologous and allogeneic bone marrow transplant patients. *Br Hematol.* 1990;76:128–134.

Klumpp TR. Immunohematologic complications of bone marrow transplantation. *Bone Marrow Transplant.* 1991;8:159–170.

Thrombocytopenia

Adams JA, Gordon AA, Jiang YZ, MacDonald D. Thrombocytopenia after bone marrow transplantation for leukemia; changes in megakaryocyte growth and growth promoting activity. *Br J Hematol.* 1990;75:195–201.

Anastate A, Vannucchi AM, Grossi A. Graft versus host disease is associated with autoimmune like thrombocytopenia. *Blood.* 1989;73:1054–1058.

Ball ED. Autologous bone marrow transplantation in acute myeloid leukemia using monoclonal body purged marrow. *Blood.* 1990;75:1199–1206.

First LR, Smith BR, Lipton J. Isolated thrombocytopenia after allogeneic bone marrow transplantation: existence of transient and chronic thrombocytopenic syndromes. *Blood.* 1985;65:368–374.

Leukopenia

Atkinson K. Reconstruction of the hematopoietic and immune systems after marrow transplantation. *BMT.* 1990;5:209–226.

Lum LG. Immune recovery after bone marrow transplantation. *Hematol Oncol Clin North Am.* 1992;4:659–675.

Fever and Chills

Atkinson K. Bacterial infection. In: Atkinson K, ed. *Clinical Bone Marrow Transplantation: A Reference Textbook.* Cambridge, England: Cambridge University Press; 1994:325–336.

Gluckman E, Roudet C, Hirsch I. Prophylaxis of bacterial infections after bone marrow transplantation: a randomized prospective study comparing oral broad spectrum nonabsorbable antibiotics to absorbable antibiotics. *Chemotherapy*. 1991;37(suppl 1):33–38.

Lew MA, Kehoe K, Ritz J. Prophylaxis of bacterial infections with ciprofloxacin in patients undergoing bone marrow transplantation. *Transplantation*. 1991;5:630–635.

Or R, Mehta J, Nagler A, Cvacium I. Neutropenia enterocolitis associated with autologous bone marrow transplantation. *Bone Marrow Transplant*. 1992;9:383–385.

Petersen FB, Clift RA, Hickman R. Hickman catheter complications in marrow transplant recipients. *J Parenter Enter Nutr*. 1986;10:58–62.

Russell JA, Poon MC, Jones AR. Allogeneic bone marrow transplantation without protective isolation in adults with malignant disease. *Lancet*. 1992;339:38–40.

Villablanca JG, Steiner M, Kersey J. The clinical spectrum of infections with viridans streptococci in bone marrow transplant patients. *Bone Marrow Transplant*. 1990;5:387–393.

Hemorrhage

Atkinson K, Biggs JC, Golovsky D. Bladder irrigation does not prevent haemorrhagic cystitis in bone marrow transplant recipients. *Bone Marrow Transplant*. 1991;7: 351–354.

DeVries CR, Freiha FS. Hemorrhagic cystitis: a review. *Journal of Urology*. 1990;143;1–9.

Elias AD, Eder JP, Shea T, et.al. High dose ifosfamide with mesna uroprotection: a phase I study. *J Clin Oncol*. 1990;8:93–100.

Hows JM, Mehta A, Ward L. Comparison of mesna with forced diuresis to prevent cyclophosphamide induced hemorrhagic cystitis in marrow transplantation: a prospective randomized study. *Br J Cancer*. 1984;50:753–756.

Shepard JD, Pringle LE, Barren MJ. Mesna versus hyperhydration for the prevention of cyclophosphamide induced haemorrhagic cystitis in bone marrow transplantation. *J Clin Oncol.* 1991;16:2016–2020.

Skin Breakdown

Baack BR, Burgdorf WHC. Chemotherapy induced acral erythema. *J Am Acad Dermatol.* 1991;24:457–461.

Baker BW, Wilson CL, Davis AL. Busulfan/cyclophosphamide conditioning for bone marrow transplantation may lead to failure of hair regrowth. *Bone Marrow Transplant.* 1991;7: 43–47.

Hartmann O, Beaujean F, Pico JL. High dose bulsulfan and cyclophosphamide in advanced childhood cancers: phase II study of 30 patients. In: Dickie KA, Spitzer G, Jagannath S, eds. *Autologous Bone Marrow Transplantation.* Houston: Proceedings of the Third International Symposium; 1986:581–588.

Herzig RH, Fay JW, Herzig GP, et al. Phase I-II studies with high-dose thiotepa and autologous marrow transplantation in patients with refractory malignancies. In: Herzig GP, ed. *High-Dose Thiotepa and Autologous Marrow Transplantation.* Dallas: Proceeding Advances in Cancer Chemotherapy Symposium; 1986:17–23.

Kerker BJ, Hood A. Chemotherapy induced cutaneous reactions. *Semin Dermatol.* 1989;8:173–181.

Linassier C, Colombat P, Reisenkeiter M, et al. Cutaneous toxicity of autologous bone marrow transplantation in nonseminomatous germ cell tumors. *Cancer.* 1990;665:1143–1145.

Riddell S, Appelbaum FR, Buckner CD. High dose cytarabine and total body irradiation with or without cyclophosphamide induced preparative regimen for marrow transplantation for acute leukemia. *J Clin Oncol.* 1988;6:576–582.

Nausea and Vomiting

Chapko MK, Syrjala KL, Schilter I, et al. Chemotherapy toxicity during bone marrow transplantation: time courses and variation in pain and nausea. *Bone Marrow Transplant.* 1989;4:181–186.

Hewett M, Cornish D, Pamphilon D, Oakhill A. Effective emetic control during conditioning of children for bone marrow transplantation using ondansetron, a 5HT[3] antagonist. *Bone Marrow Transplant.* 1991;7:431–433.

Hunter AE, Prentice HG, Pothecary K. Granisetron, a selective 5 HT3 receptor antagonist for the prevention of radiation induced emesis during total body irradiation. *Bone Marrow Transplant.* 1991;7:439–441.

Sonis ST, Clark J. Prevention and management of oral mucositis induced by antineoplastic therapy. *Oncology.* 1991;5:11–22.

Squire CA. Mucosal alterations. *NCI Monogr.* 1990;9:169–172.

Stroncek DF, Fautsch SK, Lasky LC, et al. Adverse reactions in patients transfused with cryopreserved marrow. *Transfusion.* 1991;31:521–526.

Wingard JR. Infectious and noninfectious systemic consequences. *NCI Monogr.* 1990:21–26.

Mucositis

Carnel SB, Blakeslee DB, Oswald SG, Barnes M. Treatment of radiation and chemotherapy induced stomatitis. *Otolaryngol, Head Neck Surg.* 1990;102:326–330.

Chapko MK, Syrjala KL, Schilter L, et al. Chemoradiotherapy toxicity during bone marrow transplantation: time course and variation in pain and nausea. *Bone Marrow Transplant.* 1989;4:181–186.

Epstein JB. Infections prevention in bone marrow transplantation and radiation patients. *NCI Monogr.* 1990;9:73–85.

Kolbinson DK, Schubert MM, Flournoy N, Truelove EL. Early oral changes following bone marrow transplantation. *Oral Surg Oral Med Oral Pathol.* 1988;66:130–138.

Peterson DE. Pretreatment strategies for infection prevention in chemotherapy patients. *NCI Monogr.* 1990;9:61–71.

Saral R. Management of acute viral infections. *NCI Monogr.* 1990;9:107–110.

Schubert M, Williams BE, Lliod ME, et al. Clinical assessment scale for the rating of oral mucosal changes following bone marrow transplantation. *Cancer.* 1992;69:2469–2477.

Diarrhea

Bearman SI, Appelbaum FR, Back A. Regimen related toxicity and early post transplant survival in patients undergoing bone marrow transplantation for lymphoma. *J Clin Oncol.* 1989;6:1562–1568.

Jones B. Gastrointestinal inflammation after bonez marrow transplantation: graft-versus-host disease or opportunistic infection? *AJR.* 1988;150:277–281.

Lotz PJ, Machover D, Malassagne B. Phase I-II study of two consecutive courses of high dose epipodophylloxin, ifosfamide, and carboplatin with autologous bone marrow transplantation for treatment of adults with solid tumors. *J Clin Oncol.* 1991;9:1860–1870.

Prophylactic Regimens

Due to the high-risk nature of bone marrow transplantation (BMT), prophylaxis of potentially lethal complications is crucial to the management of patients. This chapter outlines the essential elements for prevention of infection, graft-versus-host disease and veno-occlusive disease of the liver.

I. Infection in stem cell and bone marrow transplant patients

A. Risk factors for infection in stem cell and BMT patients[1]

1. Prolonged neutropenia
2. Graft-versus-host-disease (GVHD)
3. Infection prior to conditioning
4. Relapsed disease
5. Colonization early post-BMT
6. Allogeneic transplant recipient
7. Defects in T- and B-cell immunity
8. Older age
9. Hematologic malignancy
10. Extensive antibiotic use
11. Higher radiation dose

B. Figure 3.1 displays the time sequence of infection following BMT.

C. Table 3.1 outlines infectious complications in BMT recipients.[2]

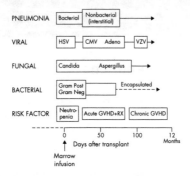

Figure 3.1 outlines the time sequence of infection following BMT.

D. Methods to prevent infection
1. Mechanisms to prevent exogenous organisms from reaching the patient (isolation)
2. Mechanisms to diminish the patient's potentially pathogenic endogenous microorganisms (oral nonabsorbable antibiotics, prophylactic antimicrobials)
3. Reduction of invasive procedures known to predispose to infection (e.g., indwelling catheters, rectal temperature, enemas, suppositories)
4. Augmentation of host defenses (growth factors, remission of disease before transplant)

Table 3.1 Infectious Complications and Occurrence in BMT Recipients

Organism	Common site
First Month Post-Transplant	
Viral	
Herpes simplex virus (HSV)	Oral, esophageal, skin, gastrointestinal (GI) tract, genital
Respiratory syncytial virus (RSV)	Sinopulmonary
Epstein-Barr virus (EBV)	Oral, esophageal, skin, GI tract
Bacterial	
Gram-positive (*Staphylococcus epidermidis, Staphylococcus aureus,* streptococci)	Skin, blood, sinopulmonary
Gram-negative (*Escherichia coli, Pseudomonas aeruginosa, Klebsiella*)	GI, blood, oral, perirectal
Fungal	
Candida (*C. albicans, C. glabratta krusei*)	Oral, esophageal, skin
Aspergillus (*A. fumigatus, A. flavus*)	Sinopulmonary
1–4 Months Post-Transplant	
Viral	
Cytomegalovirus (CMV)	Pulmonary, hepatic, GI
Enteric viruses (rotavirus, coxsackievirus, adenovirus)	Pulmonary, urinary, GI, hepatic
RSV	Sinopulmonary
Parainfluenza virus	Pulmonary
Bacterial	
Gram-positive	Sinopulmonary, skin
Fungal	
Candida	Oral, hepatosplenic, integument
Aspergillus	Sinopulmonary, central nervous system (CNS)
Mucormycosis	Sinopulmonary
Coccidioidomycosis	Sinopulmonary
Cryptococcus neoformans	Pulmonary, CNS
Protozoa	
Pneumocystis carinii	Pulmonary
Toxoplasma gondii	Pulmonary, CNS

(continued)

Table 3.1 (*continued*)

Organism	Common site
4–12 Months Post-Transplant	
Viral	
CMV, echoviruses, RSV, varicella zoster virus (VZV)	Integument, pulmonary, hepatic
Bacterial	
Gram-positive (*Streptococcus pneumoniae, Haemophilus influenzae*, pneumococci)	Sinopulmonary, blood
Fungal	
Aspergillus	Sinopulmonary
Coccidioidomycosis	Sinopulmonary
Protozoa	
P. carinii	Pulmonary
T. gondii	Pulmonary, CNS
Greater than 12 Months Post-Transplant	
Viral	
VZV	Integument
Bacterial	
Gram-positive (*streptococci, H. influenzae,* encapsulated bacteria	Sinopulmonary, blood

Reprinted with permission from Ezzone and Camp-Sorrell, 1994

II. Antimicrobial prophylaxis

A. Table 3.2 outlines common BMT infection control practices.[2]

Table 3.2 Common Infection Control Practices

Type of isolation	Room preparation	Nursing management	Proper attire	Diet
Laminar air flow room (LAFR): Sterile or clean	1. Housekeeping practices per institutional protocol 2. Weekly air and water cultures 3. Private room 4. Sterile patient zone separated from an anteroom by a transparent curtain 5. High efficiency particle air (HEPA) filtration with continuous horizontal or positive pressure air flow 6. Sterile supplies (sterile LAFR)	1. Meticulous hand washing prior to entering the unit, upon entering the patient room, and after leaving the patient room 2. Indirect care: Nursing care performed from anteroom through the curtain (e.g., infusion of IV solutions and blood, oral medication, diet) 3. Direct care: Physical assessment, treatments, and vital signs performed in patient zone	1. May include masks, head covers, gowns, gloves, and shoe covers; varies among BMT centers	1. Sterile food (sterile LAFR) 2. Low-bacterial diet (clean LAFR)
Strict protective isolation	1. Housekeeping practices per institutional protocol 2. Routine air and water cultures 3. Private room	1. Meticulous hand washing prior to entering the unit, upon entering the patient room, and after leaving the patient room	1. May include masks, head covers, gowns, gloves, and shoe covers; varies among BMT centers	1. Sterile or low-bacterial diet

Table 3.2 (continued)

Type of isolation	Room preparation	Nursing management	Proper attire	Diet
	4. HEPA and/or positive air pressure	2. Direct and indirect nursing care provided at the bedside		1. Low-bacterial diet
Simple protective isolation	1. Housekeeping practices per institutional protocol	1. Meticulous hand washing prior to entering the unit, upon entering the patient room, and after leaving the patient room	1. With or without masks, gowns, or gloves; varies among BMT centers	
	2. Routine air and water cultures	2. Direct and indirect nursing care provided at the bedside		
	3. Private room			
	4. HEPA and/or positive air pressure			

Decontamination	Surveillance cultures	Visitor restrictions
1. Skin: Daily bath/shower with an anti-microbial soap such as chlorhexidine	1. Institutional protocol for cultures of stool, urine, blood, sputum, wound, skin, throat, nares, vaginal area, perirectal area, and catheter exit site	1. Screen visitors for cold/flu/viral symptoms or transmissible diseases such as chicken pox, herpes, or influenza.
2. Application of topical antibacterial and/or antifungal powders and/or ointments to axilla, groin, vaginal, and perirectal area		2. Restrict visitation by children younger than age 12.
3. Gastrointestinal, nonabsorbable oral antibiotics		3. Follow hand washing and isolation procedures.
4. Vaginal: Daily antimicrobial douche		4. Restrict visitors who have recently received live or attenuated virus vaccine for at least 48-72 hours.
5. Recontamination with nonpathogenic normal flora		5. Discourage visitors from bringing coats, hats, or purses into the patient's room.

Reprinted with permission from Ezzone and Camp-Sorrell, 1994.

B. Isolation: Filtered air to 0.3 μm is indicated
   for BMT patients. Options include
   1. Laminar airflow room (LAF)
      a) LAF with sterile environment, bacteriologic
         monitoring, skin cleansing, topical antibiotics,
         sterile diet, and oral nonabsorbable antibiotics
      b) LAF with a clean environment, fever surveillance,
         meticulous hygiene, low-microbial diet, and
         sometimes oral nonabsorbable antibiotics
   2. Hepafiltration in protective isolation rooms

C. Gut decontamination: 80% of acute transplant infections
   are caused by *Pseudomonas aeruginosa*, *Klebsiella
   pneumoniae*, *Escherichia coli*, *Staphylococcus aureus*,
   and *Candida* species, the incidence of which may be
   diminished by gut decontamination.
   1. Combination therapy for bacterial and fungal gut
      decontamination using oral nonabsorbable antibiotics
      is most often used. Table 3.3 outlines agents used
      most often in combination with one another.

Table 3.3 Oral Nonabsorbable Antibiotics Used in
Gut Decontamination

Agent	Preparation	Dosage*
Vancomycin caps	125 mg/cap	1–4 caps PO tid
Polymyxin caps	62.5 mg/cap	1–4 caps PO tid
Gentamicin	IV preparation	200–250 mg PO qd
Ciprofloxacin	250-, 500-, 750-mg tabs	1 tabs PO bid
Co-trimoxazole (trimethoprim-sulfamethoxazole)	80 mg/400 mg/tab or 10-mL suspension 160 mg/800 mg/tab	1 PO bid
Nystatin suspension	100,000 U/mL	5–10mL tid–qid/ 1–3 million U/d
Clotrimazole	10 mg/troche	1 PO 4–5 times/d
Nystatin tabs	500,000 U/tab	1 PO qid
Fluconazole	50-, 100-, 200-mg tabs	> 50 kg, 200–400 mg/d
Peridex oral rinse		5–15mL PO 3–5 times/d

*See Chapter 7 for specific pediatric dosage adjustments.

2. Therapy is initiated pretransplant and continued until engraftment is achieved.
3. These agents are emetogenic. Ciprofloxacin and fluconazole in combination may be used in patients who do not tolerate other agents.

D. Antibacterial prophylaxis (see Chapter 7 for further dosage and toxicity information)
1. Gut decontamination and sterile or low-microbial diet. The following foods are excluded on a typical low-microbial diet:
   a) Fresh fruit and vegetables
   b) Hand-squeezed juices
   c) Shellfish
   d) Buffet foods
   e) Microwaved foods from scratch (reheating OK)
   f) Yogurt
   g) Raw fish (sushi)
   h) Cheeses with live culture
   i) Stir-fried foods (e.g., Chinese)
   j) Restaurant foods (some centers)
2. Meticulous oral and perineal care
3. Skin decontamination with antibacterial soap
4. Meticulous central venous catheter site care
5. Avoidance of procedures that risk hematogenous spread of bacteria from the gastrointestinal and genitourinary tracts, especially while neutropenic
6. Ciprofloxacin (Cipro)
   a) Dosage: 750 mg PO bid
   b) Duration: Started with pretransplant conditioning and continued while neutropenic until onset of first fever.
   c) Found to reduce fever duration, antibiotic days, and number of antibiotics needed while neutropenic.[3]
7. Co-trimoxazole (trimethoprim-sulfamethoxazole; Bactrim, Septra)

     a) Dosage:
       (1) Adults: double-strength tablet PO bid
       (2) Children: 8 to 10 mg/kg bid
     b) Duration: Stopped just prior to transplant day.
     c) Its use in antimicrobial prophylaxis is declining, since it self-selects for overgrowth of some gram-positive and gram-negative organisms.

8. Intravenous immune globulin
     a) Dosage: 150 to 500 mg/kg/dose IV.
     b) Duration
       (1) Autologous: Dose generally given 1 to 2 times pretransplant, then once a month for 2 to 3 doses. Dose may be given based on IgG less than 500 mg/dL.
       (2) Allogeneic: If patient and donor are cytomegalovirus (CMV) negative, dose generally given 1 to 2 times pretransplant, then once a month for 2 to 3 doses. Dose may be given based on IgG less than 500 mg/dL. If patient and/or donor is CMV positive, 1 to 2 doses pretransplant, and once a week thereafter until day +100 to +120 post-transplant. Dose then may be given monthly thereafter if patient develops chronic GVHD or by institution standard.
     c) May prevent or modify infections other than CMV, such as bacteremias.[4,5]

9. Colony-stimulating factors[6,7]
     a) Granulocyte-macrophage colony-stimulating factor (GM-CSF); Leukine (Prokine) is a multilineage colony-stimulating factor glycoprotein used to stimulate early progenitor cells of all three cell lineages (red cells, platelets, and white cells). Decreases period of neutropenia and thus decreases the number of neutropenia-associated infections. Dosage: 250 µg/m^{2}d IV over at least

2 hours. Infusion generally started two to four hours after marrow/peripheral blood stem cell (PBSC) infusion. Continued until absolute neutrophil count is greater than 7000 to 10,000/μL.

b) Granulocyte colony-stimulating factor (G-CSF; Neupogen) is a lineage-specific colony-stimulating factor used to stimulate neutrophil progenitor cells. Decreases period of neutropenia and thus decreases the number of neutropenia-associated infections. Dosage: 5 to 10 μg/d IV. Infusion generally started the evening or day following marrow/PBSC infusion; may also be started around day +7 to +8 post-transplant.

c) Interleukin-3 (IL-3) is used to stimulate the earliest progenitor cells of all cell lineages (red cell, platelets, and white cells). May decrease the period of neutropenia and thus decrease the number of neutropenia-associated infections. Currently used in clinical trials focusing on the combination use of IL-3 and GM-CSF. Dosage: 2.5 to 5.0 μg/kg/day SQ or IV. Generally given prior to GM-CSF administration.

10. Chronic GVHD on immunosuppressives
    a) Adults: Penicillin, ampicillin, or amoxicillin, 250 mg PO bid
    b) Children (< 40 kg): 20 to 40 mg/kg PO bid

E. Antifungal prophylactic medications (see Chapter 7 for further dosage and toxicity information)
1. Topical antifungals are generally used pretransplant for gut decontamination. Are discontinued when systemic antifungals are started. Used post-transplant when systemic antifungals are discontinued (autologous or PBSC rescue patients).
    a) Nystatin Suspension: 100,000 U/mL
        (1) Adults: 5 to 10 mL qid or 1.3 million U/d (divided qid)

        (2) Children: 4 to 6 mL qid

        (3) Tablets: 500,000 U/tablet

        (4) Troches/pastilles: 200,000 U/dose

        (5) Adults and children: 400,000 to 600,000 U qid

    b) Clotrimazole

        (1) Oral: 10 mg/troche; Adults: 1 troche PO 4 to 5 times/d; Children: 1 troche PO 4 to 5 times/d

        (2) Vaginal: 100–500-mg tablets; 1% vaginal cream 1 tablet or applicator dose (5g)/24 h

2. Systemic antifungals are generally used post-transplant to prevent serious systemic fungal infection, especially fungal septicemia and invasive aspergillosis. Systemic antifungal therapy is common practice in the allogeneic BMT setting, especially throughout the first 100 days post-transplant.

    a) Amphotericin B (Fungizone)[8,9]

        (1) Prophylaxis (low-dose): Covers most every species of *Candida* and may help prevent aspergillosis infection. Dosage: 0.1 to 0.25 mg/kg/d IV over 2 to 4 hours. Continued until patient is no longer neutropenic and is afebrile.

        (2) Empiric: Used in febrile patients with suspected fungal infection and those who remain febrile on broad-spectrum antibacterials. Dosage: 0.5 to 1.5 mg/kg/d over 2 to 4 hours. Continued until patient is no longer neutropenic and is afebrile with negative cultures for fungus.

    b) Liposomal-encapsulated amphotericin B (Abelcet) may be used empirically in patients with poor renal function. Generally used in the setting of documented fungal infections requiring long-term antifungal therapy. Dosage: 5 mg/kg/d over 2 to 4 hours.

c) Fluconazole (Diflucan) is commonly used prophylactically; however, its use has resulted in an increase in infection rates of *Torulopsis glabrata* and *Candida krusei*. Lacks fungicidal activity against *Aspergillus* species. Generally given IV early post-transplant and continued for 30 to 40 days in autologous or PBSC transplant patients and through day +100 in allogeneic BMT patients. Treatment may be continued longer for allogeneic patients on immunosuppression for GVHD. Dosage:

    (1) Adults (> 50 kg): 200 to 400 mg qd IV/PO

    (2) 20 to 40 kg: 200 mg qd IV/PO

    (3) < 20 kg: 3 to 8 mg/kg qd IV/PO

d) Itraconazole has similar fungicidal activity as amphotericin B against *Aspergillus* species. Less *Candida* species resistance is seen versus fluconazole. Is expensive and therefore its use is generally limited to allogeneic BMT patients. Generally started post-transplant when patient can tolerate oral medication. Prophylaxis continued through day +100 in allogeneic BMT patients. Treatment may be continued longer for allogeneic patients on immunosuppression for GVHD. Dosage:

    (1) Adults: 200 mg PO bid

    (2) Children: Dosage information not yet available

e) Ketoconazole: Most *Candida* species are sensitive. Has significant hepatic toxicity, and its use is therefore limited in the BMT setting. Dosage:

    (1) Adults: 200 mg PO qd

    (2) < 20 kg: 50 mg PO daily

    (3) 20 to 40 kg: 100 mg PO daily

    (4) > 40 kg: 200 mg PO daily

F. Antiprotozoan prophylactic medications (see Chapter 7 for further dosage and toxicity information).

1. *Pneumocystis carinii* pneumonia (PCP) prophylaxis
   a) PCP is relatively rare due to successful prophylaxis.
   b) Prophylaxis in autologous or PBSC patient population is controversial.
   c) Co-trimoxazole (trimethoprim-sulfamethoxazole; Bactrim, Septra, Sulfatrim) is inexpensive and most effective prophylaxis available. Incidence of PCP is less than 1% in patients on effective prophylaxis. Can be myelosuppressive. Folinic acid is sometimes used to prevent or treat associated myelosuppression. Generally given one to two weeks pretransplant, stopped around day 0, and resumed around day +30 or when absolute neutrophil count is greater than 1000/µFL. Autologous BMT patients generally remain on PCP prophylaxis for 60 to 100 days post-BMT. Allogeneic BMT patients generally remain on PCP prophylaxis for six months to one year post-BMT. May continue longer if on immunosuppressive therapy for GVHD. Dosage:
      (1) Adults: 1 double-strength tablet qd or bid PO 3 times/wk
      (2) Children: 5 to 10 mg/kg (trimethoprim)/d or 150 mg/m² qd or bid PO 3 times/wk
   d) Dapsone (Avlosulfon) provides effective PCP prophylaxis in BMT patients who cannot take co-trimoxazole due to myelosuppression (platelet count < 100,000 µL or absolute neutrophil count < 1000/µL). Patients who are hypersensitive to co-trimoxazole will also be hypersensitive to dapsone. Should not be used in patients with glucose-6 phosphate dehydrogenase deficiency. Generally started around day +30 in patients whose platelet count is less than 100,000 µL or absolute neutrophil count is less than 1000/µL

(and therefore co-trimoxazole cannot be started due to low blood counts. Patients may be switched back to co-trimoxazole when counts recover further. Autologous BMT patients generally remain on PCP prophylaxis for 60 to 100 days post-BMT. Allogeneic BMT patients generally remain on PCP prophylaxis for six months to one year post-BMT. May continue longer if on immunosuppressive therapy for GVHD. Dosage:

   (1) Adults: 100 mg PO qd or 3 times/wk
   (2) Children: 1 mg/kg PO qd or 3 times/wk

e) Pentamidine (Pentam 300) is generally used in patients who cannot tolerate co-trimoxazole or dapsone due to hypersensitivity, hemolysis, or myelosuppression. Efficacy in preventing PCP is not yet known in BMT. Autologous BMT patients generally remain on PCP prophylaxis for 60 to 100 days post BMT. Allogeneic BMT patients generally remain on PCP prophylaxis for six months to one year post-BMT. May continue longer if on immunosuppressive therapy for GVHD. Dosage:

   (1) Adult: 4 mg/kg/dose IV q2wk or 300 mg inhaled q2–4 wk
   (2) Children: 4 mg/kg/dose IV q2wk (inhaled doses difficult to administer to younger children)

2. *Toxoplasma gondii prophylaxis*

   a) Incidence of infection is approximately 0.8% to 5% in allogeneic BMT population; therefore, the necessity of prophylaxis has not been established.[10]

   b) Oral dapsone and IV or inhaled pentamidine may provide some protection against *T. gondii* when given as PCP prophylaxis.

   c) Pyrimethamine-sulfadoxine (Fansidar) may also

provide effective prophylaxis, but its use for prophylaxis has been limited to clinical trials. Dosage for both adults and children is 1 tablet/ 20 kg (1 tablet contains 25 mg of pyrimethamine and 500 mg of sulfadoxine) on day 1, with folinic acid, 50 mg on day 2, then qd following engraftment (absolute neutrophil count > 1000/μL). Generally given for first 100 days after allogeneic BMT. Therapy may be stopped due to myelosuppression. Conventional PCP prophylaxis should be instituted in such cases.

G. Antiviral prophylaxis (see Chapter 7 for further dosage and toxicity information)

    1. Herpes simplex virus (HSV) prophylaxis[11,12]

        a) Generally provided for autologous and allogeneic BMT patients who are seropositive for HSV or have a donor who is seropositive for HSV. Some centers provide prophylaxis regardless of the patient's serologic status.

        b) Most cases are associated with viral reactivation (oral or genital).

        c) Acyclovir (Zovirax) is the antiviral of choice for HSV prophylaxis. Inhibits DNA synthesis needed for viral replication. Prophylaxis generally continues for six months post-transplant. Patients on ganciclovir for CMV prophylaxis do not also need to be on acyclovir for HSV prophylaxis. Dosage: (switch to oral dosing when tolerated post-BMT)

            (1) IV: 250 mg/m^2 q8–12h starting around day -3 through day +5

            (2) PO (adults): 400 mg tid or 200 mg 5 times/d

            (3) PO (children): 200 mg tid

        d) Foscarnet may be used in patients with known HSV-acyclovir resistance. It should be used with caution in patients with impaired renal function or those on other nephrotoxins. Dosage: 40 to 60 mg/kg IV q8h. Maintenance dose: 90 mg/kg/day.

2. Varicella-zoster virus (VZV)/herpes zoster prophylaxis
   a) Infection caused by reactivation of VZV.
   b) May be disseminated or isolated to one dermatome (shingles).
   c) Patients with Hodgkin's disease are at increased risk of VZV infection.
   d) Acyclovir is the antiviral of choice for VZV prophylaxis. Dosages for prophylaxis are the same as those used for HSV prophylaxis (see p.00). Patients who develop more than one episode of VZV reactivation should be placed on long-term prophylaxis.

3. Cytomegalovirus (CMV) prophylaxis [5,13-15]: CMV infection can be caused by endogenous viral reactivation or primary infection through the transfusion of blood products or bone marrow. Incidence is approximately 20% to 25% in allogeneic BMT patients who are seropositive for CMV and who receive prophylaxis.[13] CMV infection in autologous transplant and PBSC patients is rare (< 1%).
   a) Donor screening: If patient is seronegative for CMV, a seronegative donor should be used when feasible.
   b) Transfusion screening for allogeneic patients: If patient is CMV negative and donor is CMV negative, patient should receive blood products that are seronegative for CMV. If patient is CMV negative and donor is CMV positive, it is not known if patient should receive blood products that are seronegative for CMV. If patient is CMV positive and donor is CMV positive, patient can receive blood products that are CMV positive or

unscreened for CMV.

c) Transfusion screening for autologous transplant and PBSC rescue patients: Most centers do not transfuse CMV seronegative blood products to autologous BMT patients who are CMV negative due to the low probability of CMV infection in this population.

d) Leukopoor filtering of blood products removes the buffy-coated cells and thus virtually renders the product CMV negative. This method is sometimes used when CMV-negative products are not available or for all blood products administered to allogeneic and autologous BMT patients.

e) Acyclovir (Zovirax), when used at higher doses early post-transplant, has been associated with decreased incidence of CMV infection. Dosage: 500 mg/m^2 IV q8h starting around day -3 through day +5. Generally continued until the patient starts other CMV prophylaxis (ganciclovir or foscarnet).

f) Ganciclovir (Cytovene) is the drug of choice for prophylaxis against CMV infection. It inhibits viral replication. Generally administered to allogeneic BMT patients who are CMV positive or have a CMV-positive donor. May also be administered to patients with grade II or greater GVHD. Not used in autologous BMT population. Usually used in combination with intravenous immune globulin or CMV immune globulin. Dosage: 5 to 6 mg/kg/dose 3 to 5 times/wk starting around day +30 or when patient has engrafted (absolute neutrophil count > 1000/µL). May be poorly tolerated due to myelosuppression or impaired renal function. May require discontinuation or dose reduction (3 mg/kg/dose). Prophylaxis generally continues until day +100 to +120.

g) Foscarnet (Foscavir) may be used in allogeneic patients who cannot tolerate ganciclovir due to myleosuppression or renal function. Dosage: 90 to 120 mg/kg/day IV. Prophylaxis generally continues until day +100 to +120.

h) Intravenous immune globulin provides passive immunity by providing concentration of antibodies against CMV. Dosage: 250 to 500 mg/kg IV once a week. Generally allogeneic patients are dosed 1 to 2 times pretransplant and then weekly until day +100 to +120. Allogeneic patients who are CMV negative and who have a CMV-negative donor as well as autologous patients may be dosed q2–3 wk as needed to maintain a quantitative IgG above 500 mg/dL.

i) CMV immune globulin provides higher antibody titer against CMV than regular intravenous immune globulin. Dosage: 100 to 150 mg/kg IV once a week. Generally allogeneic patients are dosed 1 to 2 times pretransplant and then weekly until day +100 to +120.

III. Graft-versus-host disease (GVHD) prophylaxis[16–19]

A. Incidence

1. GVHD occurs in approximately 45% of patients receiving HLA-identical allogeneic transplants from a matched sibling donor.
2. Incidence is as high as 75% in allogeneic patients receiving marrow from a matched unrelated donor.
3. Mean onset is 25 days post-transplant, with a range of 10 to 100 days.

B. Risk factors for acute GVHD[2,19]

1. HLA-mismatched transplant

2. Increased age of donor and recipient
3. Prior donor pregnancy
4. Viral infection
5. No GVHD prophylaxis
6. Unrelated donor transplant
7. Gender mismatch
8. Relapse at time of transplant
9. Microorganism colonization
10. Low Karnofsky score

C. Pharmacologic prophylaxis of acute GVHD[20] (see Chapter 7 for further dosage and toxicity information)

1. Methotrexate (MTX); Mexate is an antimetabolite chemotherapeutic agent that blocks folate synthesis. Generally used in combination with cyclosporine or corticosteroids to prevent acute GVHD. Folinic acid (leucovorin) "rescue" has been used for amelioration of toxicities (mucositis/marrow suppression), which may or may not show positive benefit without compromise of GVHD prevention. Dosage of MTX:

   a) Short course
      (1) Day +1: 15 mg/m²
      (2) Days +3, +6, +11: 10 mg/m²
      (3) Day +11 dose may be eliminated.

   b) Long course
      (1) Day +1: 15 mg/m²
      (2) Days +3, +6, +11: 10 mg/m²
      (3) Weekly until day +100: 10 mg/m²

   c) Day +11 dose may be eliminated due to oropharyngeal mucositis, fever and neutropenia, or hyperbilirubinemia. This does not seem to affect the incidence of grade II to IV acute GVHD.[21]

2. Cyclophosphamide (Cytoxan) is an alkylating agent with potent immunosuppressive activity. The incidence of acute GVHD is similar to that seen with MTX, although the severity (e.g., GVHD mortality) may be somewhat higher. Cyclophosphamide is

no longer commonly used as GVHD prophylaxis.
Dosage: 7.5 mg/kg on days +1, +3, +5, +7, +9,
and then weekly to day +100.

3. Cyclosporin A (CsA, Sandimmune, Neoral)
   a) Induces tolerance by inhibiting the development
      of regulatory antigen–specific T cells.[22]
   b) Often used in combination with MTX or
      corticosteroids for GVHD prophylaxis. Is
      also used in the treatment of chronic GVHD.
   c) Dosage is 2 to 3 mg/kg/d IV divided q12h or by
      24-hour continuous infusion starting 1 to 3 days
      prior to marrow infusion; q12h infusion may
      be infused over 1 to 6 hours. When patients are
      able to tolerate oral medications and no active
      gastrointestinal disease is present, may switch to
      oral CA at 6 mg/kg divided bid for 3 to 6 months
      unless active GVHD is present.
   d) Blood or serum levels should be monitored and
      doses adjusted appropriately. Dose should be
      adjusted based on whole-blood radioimmunoassay
      levels between 325 and 375 ng/mL or by fluores-
      cence immunoassay levels between 450 and 520
      ng/mL. Serum levels should be maintained at a
      level of 150 to 250 ng/mL. Table 3.4 lists drugs
      that are known to affect CsA levels.

Table 3.4 Drug Interactions with Cyclosporin A

Drug	Effect
Potentiate CsA (increase serum concentration)	
Ketoconazole	Increase nephrotoxicity
Fluconazole	
Erythromycin	
Methylprednisolone	Increase seizure risk
Verapamil	
Cimetidine	
Metoclopramide	
Inhibit CsA (decrease serum concentration)	
Rifampin	Decrease immunosuppression
Phenobarbital	Increase risk of rejection
Co-trimoxazole	Increase risk of GVHD
Phenytoin	
Oral contraceptives	
Additive with CsA	
Amphotericin	Additive renal toxicity
Aminoglycoside	
Acyclovir	
Ganciclovir	
Digoxin	Digoxin toxicity

    e) Nephrotoxicity is the major dose-limiting toxicity of CsA. Causes a decrease in GFR and acute tubular necrosis. Dosages should also be adjusted for changes in renal function:

Creatinine	CsA dose adjustment (adult ranges)
> 1.5 mg/dL	25%
> 1.75 mg/dL	75%
> 2.0 mg/dL	Hold until creatinine < 2.0 mg/dL then resume at 25% of prior dose.

    f) Since CsA causes afferent arteriole vasoconstriction, hypertension is a common toxicity frequently requiring antihypertenive therapy. Calcium channel blockers are the drug class of choice. ß-Blockers are also commonly used. Angiotensin-converting enzyme inhibitors should be avoided, since they are known to decrease renal blood flow.

g) CsA can cause a number of neurologic symptoms, including tremors, muscle weakness and myalgias, headaches, burning in the hands and feet, ataxia, confusion, seizures, encephalopathy, and cortical blindness. Such symptoms are not necessarily related to serum concentrations of the drug. An association has been identified between CsA neurotoxicity and hypomagnesemia. Thus, magnesium supplements (IV or PO) are recommended to maintain serum magnesium levels as near normal as possible.

h) CsA is metabolized in the liver and excreted through the biliary channels. Liver toxicity is manifested as a rise in the serum bilirubin levels. Such toxicity may result in delayed metabolism and elimination, thus increasing the risk of renal toxicity.

i) CsA can cause a microangiopathic hemolytic-uremic syndrome manifested by a drop in the hematocrit, elevated serum bilirubin, elevated blood urea nitrogen and creatinine, proteinuria, and heme-positive urine. Such toxicity usually resolves with withdrawal of CsA. Such toxicity may not occur when switching over to FK-506.

4. Tacrolimus (FK-506, Prograf)[23]

a) Inhibits T-cell activation by forming a complex with the FK binding protein-12, thus preventing interleukin-2 (IL-2) transcription. The net result is the inhibition of T-lymphocyte activation.

b) Often used in combination with MTX or corticosteroids for GVHD prophylaxis. However, it has been used as effective monotherapy in the prevention of acute GVHD.[24] Is also used in the treatment of chronic GVHD.

c) IV dosage:
  (1) Adult IV starting dose: 0.05 to 0.10 mg/kg/d as continuous IV infusion
  (2) Pediatric IV starting dose: 0.10 mg/kg/d as continuous IV infusion
d) When patients are able to tolerate oral medications and no active gastrointestinal disease is present, may switch to oral tacrolimus. First oral dose should be given 8 to 12 hours after discontinuing IV drug.
  (1) Adult oral dose: 0.15 to 0.30 mg/kg/d divided bid
  (2) Pediatric oral dose: 0.3 mg/kg/d divided Bid for 3 to 6 months unless active GVHD is present.
e) Blood or serum levels should be monitored and doses adjusted appropriately. Dose should be adjusted based on whole-blood concentration levels between 2.0 ng/mL (by ELISA).
  Table 3.5 lists drugs that are known to affect tacrolimus levels.
f) Renal function should be monitored closely, since nephrotoxicity is the most significant adverse effect. Accurate renal dosing is still unknown, since most toxicity studies are recent or still under way.
g) Mild to severe hyperkalemia can occur. Serum potassium levels should be regularly monitored and potassium-sparing diuretics should not be used in patients receiving tacrolimus.

Table 3.5 Drug Interactions with Tacrolimus

Drug	Effect
Potentiate tacrolimus (increase serum concentration)	
Ketoconazole	Increase nephrotoxicity
Fluconazole	
Erythromycin	
Clarithromycin	
Methylprednisolone	Increase seizure risk
Danazol	
Verapamil	
Diltiazem	
Nicardipine	
Bromocriptine	
Cimetidine	
Metoclopramide	
Inhibit tacrolimus (decrease serum concentration)	
Rifampin	Decrease immunosuppression
Rifabutin	
Phenobarbital	Increase risk of rejection
Carbamazepine	Increase risk of GVHD
Phenytoin	

   h) Neurotoxicity has been noted in more than half of
      patients receiving tacrolimus. Tremor, headache,
      seizure, coma, and delirium have been associated
      with high whole-blood concentrations.
   i) Tacrolimus has been used effectively in patients
      who cannot tolerate CsA due to microangiopathic
      hemolytic-uremic syndrome.[25]
5. Corticosteroids (steroids: methylprednisolone,
   prednisone)[26]
   a) Potent anti-inflammatory drugs that suppress
      migration of polymorphonuclear leukocytes
   b) Are effective in the treatment of established acute
      and chronic GVHD and are occasionally used in
      combination with MTX, CsA, or tacrolimus for
      prophylaxis against acute GVHD.

    c) Dosage: Prophylaxis is generally started at
0.5 to 1 mg/kg/d divided q8–12h IV as
methylprednisolone starting day +7. Dose is
generally reduced or tapered around day +22
through day +35 if no signs of acute GVHD
are present. May be switched to oral prednisone
at an equivalent dose when patient is tolerating
oral medications.

    d) May be used alone for GVHD prophylaxis
in patients who do not tolerate MTX or CsA.

D. Ex vivo T-cell depletion[27]

1. Numerous studies involving ex vivo removal of
T lymphocytes from donor marrow prior to infusion
have shown this method to be the most effective in
the prevention of acute GVHD.

2. Methods of ex vivo T-cell depletion
    a) Monoclonal antibodies
    b) Counterflow centrifugation
    c) Soybean agglutinin and E-rosetting
    d) Immunotoxins

3. It is unclear which method is the most effective.

4. The efficacy of T-cell depletion has been offset
by the two major complications of graft rejection
and increased probability of leukemic relapse.

5. Patients with aplastic anemia, matched unrelated
donors, and non–HLA-identical marrow experience
problems with graft failure and sustained engraftment
when receiving ex vivo T-cell–depleted marrow.

6. Attempts to overcome these problems have included
increased immunosuppression, selective depletion of
T-cell subsets, and adding back a specified number
of T-cells to the infused marrow graft.

E. In vivo T-cell depletion[27]

1. Antilymphocyte globulin (antithymocyte globulin)
has been used in the treatment of steroid-resistant
GVHD with some effectiveness. Two trials have

studied its usefulness when used in addition to post-BMT methotrexate for the prevention of GVHD.[28,29] No benefit was demonstrated in either trial; therefore its use in preventing GVHD is generally no longer practiced.

2. Anti–T-cell monoclonal antibodies (anti-CD3 antibodies) are monoclonal antibodies to the CD3 antigen of human T-cells, which functions as an immunosuppressant.

   a) OKT3 (Orthoclone), an anti-CD3 antibody, has been used with limited success in the treatment of resistant GVHD and is associated with moderate to severe toxicity. OKT3 side effects include cytokine release syndrome (high fever, dyspnea, nausea, vomiting, chest pain, diarrhea, wheezing, headache, tachycardia, rigors, hypertension) and hypersensitivity reactions (fevers/chills, bradycardia/cardiac arrest, respiratory arrest, adult respiratory distress syndrome, rash/urticaria, pancytopenia, elevated liver transaminases, arthalgias/myalgias).

   b) Another anti-CD3 antibody, BC3, has recently been described. This antibody shows little interaction with the Fc receptor on cell activation and consequent toxicities. Studies evaluating its efficacy in preventing GVHD can be anticipated.

F. Anticytokine agents[27]

   1. Anti–interleukin-2 receptor antibody (aIL-2-ra) is a monoclonal antibody directed against structures associated with the IL-2 receptor that abolish most of the in vitro proliferation responses of antigen-stimulated T-cells. Has been used in steroid-resistant GVHD with some success, leading to trials for GVHD prophylaxis. Results are inconclusive, in that aIL-2-ra may only delay the onset of GVHD.

2. Anti– tumor necrosis factor (TNF) agents
   a) TNF has been strongly implicated in the development of GVHD.
   b) Agents include monoclonal anti-TNF antibody, pentoxifylline, lysophylline, and others currently under development.
   c) All have been found to reduce the incidence of acute GVHD while on therapy; however, most patients will develop acute GVHD or chronic GVHD once therapy is stopped.
   d) A number of studies evaluating the efficacy of anti-TNF agents in preventing GVHD are currently under way.

IV. Veno-occlusive disease (VOD) prophylaxis[30]

A. Endothelial injury leading to deposition of coagulation factors within the terminal hepatic venules is believed to be the pathogenesis of VOD.

B. Continuous low-dose heparin infusion has been found to be effective in preventing VOD, especially in patients with underlying liver dysfunction at the time of pretransplant conditioning.
   1. Administration (see Chapter 7 for more specific side effects and toxicity): 100–150 U/kg/d by continuous infusion starting just prior to conditioning until approximately day +30.
   2. Heparin infusion should be adjusted to keep the partial prothrombin time within normal range.
   3. Should not increase the patient's need for red cell or platelet transfusions.

References

1. Ford R, Ballard, B. Acute complications after bone marrow transplantation. *Sem Oncol Nurs*. 1988;4:15–24.

2. Ezzone S, Camp-Sorrell D, eds. *Manual for Bone Marrow Transplant Nursing: Recommendations for Practice and Education*: Pittsburgh: Oncology Nursing Press, Inc; 1994.

3. Lew MA. Prophylaxis of bacterial infections with ciprofloxacin in patients undergoing bone marrow transplantation. *Transplantation*. 1991;51:630–635.

4. Petersen FB, Bowden RA, Thornquest M, et al. The effect of prophylactic intravenous immune globulin on the incidence of septicemia in marrow transplant recipients. *Bone Marrow Transplant*. 1987;2:141–148.

5. Gale RP, Winston D. Intravenous immunoglobulin in bone marrow transplantation. *Cancer*. 1991;68 (suppl):1451–1453.

6. Cunningham R. *Prevention of Infection in Patients Receiving Myelosuppressive Chemotherapy*. New York: Triclinica Communications; 1992.

7. Wujcik D. Overview of colony-stimulating factors: focus on the neutrophil. In: Carroll-Johnson RM, ed. *A Case Management Approach to Patients Receiving G-CSF*. Pittsburgh: Oncology Nursing Press, Inc.; 1994.

8. Perfect JR, Klotman ME, Gilbert CC, et al. Prophylactic intravenous amphotericin B in Neutropenic autologous bone marrow transplant recipients. *J of Infect Dis*. 1992;165:891–897.

9. Rousey SR, Russlen S, Gottlieb M, et al. Low-dose Amphotericin B prophylaxis against invasive *aspergillus* infections in allogeneic marrow transplantation. *Am J of Med*. 1991;484–491.

10. Foot ABM, Gann YJF, Rihaud P, et al. Prophylaxis of toxoplasmosis infection with pyrimethamine/sulfadoxine (Fansidar) in bone marrow transplant recipients. *Bone Marrow Transplant*. 1994;14:241–245.

11. Ljungman P, Wilczek H, Gahton G, et al. Long-term acyclovir prophylaxis in bone marrow transplant recipients and lymphocyte proliferation responses to herpes virus antigens in vitro. *Bone Marrow Transplant*. 1986;1:185–192.

12. Wade J, Newton B, Flourney N. Oral acyclovir for prevention of herpes virus reactivation after marrow transplantation. *Ann of Intern Med*. 1984;100:823–828.

13. Schmidt GM, Horak DA, Niland JC, et al. A randomized, controlled trial of prophylactic ganciclovir for cytomegalovirus pulmonary infection in recipients of allogeneic bone marrow transplants. *N Engl J Med*. 1991;15:1005–1011.

14. Bowden RA, Sayers M, Flournoy N. Cytomegalovirus immune globulin and seronegative blood products to prevent primary cytomegalovirus infection after marrow transplantation. *N Engl J Med*. 1996;314:1006–1010.

15. Thomas ED, Buckner W, Meyers J. et al. Prevention of cytomegalovirus infection by cytomegalovirus immune globulin after marrow transplantation. *Ann Intern Med*. 1983;98:442–446.

16. Beatty PG. The use of unrelated donors for bone marrow transplantation. *Marrow Transplant Rev*. 1991;1:1–7.

17. Bortin MM, Atkinson K, van Bekkum DW, et al. Factors influencing the risk of acute and chronic graft versus host disease in humans: A preliminary report from the IBMTR. *Bone Marrow Transplant*. 1989;4(suppl)222–224.

18. Mickelson EM, Hansen JA. HLA-matching in marrow transplantation. *Marrow Transplant Rev*. 1991;1:8–13.

19. Vogelsang GV. Acute graft versus host disease following marrow transplantation. *Marrow Transplant Rev*. 1993;2:49–53.

20. Kanfer E. Graft versus host disease. *Bone Marrow Transplantation*. In: Treleaven J, Wiernik P, eds. (London: Mosby-Wolfe; 1995:143–153.

21. Atkinson K, Downs K. Omission of day 11 methotrexate does not appear to influence the incidence or moderate to severe graft

versus host disease, chronic graft versus host disease, relapse rate or survival after HLA-identical sibling bone marrow transplantation. *Bone Marrow Transplant*. 1995;16:755–758.

22.   Holmes W. Cyclosporin immunosuppression: clinical practice issues. *Curr Issues Cancer Nurs Prac*. 1993;1:1–7.

23.   Etzioni R, Nash RA, Stor, R, et al. Tacrolimus (FK506) alone or in combination with methotrexate or methylprednisilone for the prevention of acute graft versus host disease after marrow transplantation for HLA-matched siblings: A single center study. *Blood*. 1995;85:3746–3753.

24.   Fay JW, Nash RA, Wing JR, et al. FK-506-based immunosuppression for prevention of graft versus host disease after unrelated donor marrow transplantation. *Transplant Proc*. 1995;56;1374.

25.   McCauley J, Bronsthon O, Fung J, et al. Treatment of cyclosporin-induced haemolytic uraemic syndrome with FK-506. *Lancet*. 1989:1516–1517.

26.   Storb R, Pepe M, Anisetti C, et al. What role for prednisone in prevention of acute graft versus host disease in patient undergoing marrow transplantation. *Blood*. 1990;76:1037–1045.

27.   Treleaven J, Wiernik P, eds. *Bone Marrow Transplantation*. London: Mosby-Wolfe; 1995.

28.   Doney KC, Weiden PL, Storb R, et al. Failure of early administration of antithymocyte globulin to lessen graft versus host disease in human allogeneic marrow transplant recipients. *Transplantation*. 1987;31:1412–1430.

29.   Weiden PL, Doney KC, Storb R, et al. Antihuman thymocyte globulin for prophylaxis of graft-versus-host disease: a randomized trial in patients with leukemia treated with HLA-identical sibling marrow grafts. *Transplantation*. 1979;27:227–230.

30. Attal M, Huguet F, Rubie H, et al. Prevention of hepatic veno-occlusive disease after bone marrow transplantation by continuous infusion of low-dose heparin: a prospective, randomized trial. *Blood.* 1992;79:2834–2840.

Bone Marrow, Peripheral Blood Stem Cell, and Umbilical Cord Blood Procurement and Infusion

The term *harvest* refers to the procurement of bone marrow, peripheral blood stem cells (PBSCs), or umbilical cord blood stem cells for the purpose of transplantation.

I. Allogeneic bone marrow harvest

A. Allogeneic bone marrow transplantation is generally performed on an outpatient basis, with the donor being admitted on the morning of the procedure. Most commonly, the harvest is scheduled to take place on the same day as the marrow will be infused into the recipient.

B. The harvest procedure is performed in the operating room under the same sterile surgical conditions as any other surgical procedure.

C. The mode of anesthesia is mutually determined by the donor and the anesthesiologist. General anesthesia, spinal anesthesia, or epidural anesthesia may be used.

D. Initially, marrow is harvested from the posterior iliac crest. An effort is made to minimize the number of skin punctures, but successful harvesting requires multiple punctures of the bone (often numbering in the hundreds). Aspirations may also be obtained from the anterior iliac crests, if insufficient volume is obtained from the posterior crests.

E. In allogeneic harvesting, the volume of each aspiration should be 10 to 15 mL or less to minimize the amount of hemodilution and blood contamination. Blood contamination leads to increased exposure to donor T cells, which increases the risk of graft-versus-host disease (GVHD).

F. The total volume of marrow harvested is dependent on the body mass of the recipient as well as the cellularity of the donor marrow. The target number of donor stem cells for allogeneic engraftment of unmanipulated marrow is 2 to 3×10^8 nucleated marrow cells per kilogram of recipient weight.[1]

G. As marrow is aspirated, it is placed in a collection device containing tissue culture medium and heparin. Each syringe used for aspiration is also primed with this solution to minimize clotting during the aspiration process.

H. Marrow aspiration may be collected in an open beaker or a closed system that incorporates in-line filters. In theory, the closed system should minimize the amount of airborne bacterial contamination.

I. When the target amount of marrow has been obtained, the marrow is filtered in the operating room either by means of passage through several stainless steel mesh filters or via gravity flow through the in-line filters of a manufactured closed system set.

J. Most donors will store 1 to 2 U of autologous blood in the weeks prior to the harvest. This autologous blood can be infused during or after the harvest. Additionally, oral iron replacement (usually ferrous sulfate) is prescribed for donor use to facilitate hematopoiesis both pre- and post-harvest.

K. At the conclusion of the harvest, the aspiration sites are cleaned and covered with pressure dressings. Sutures are not required. Aspiration sites may be packed with an antibacterial ointment.

L. The donor is usually stabilized in the recovery room and then transferred to the outpatient area or a standard hospital room. Most donors are discharged later in the same day, if they do not experience hypotension, severe pain, bleeding, or intractable nausea.

II. Autologous bone marrow harvest

A. The technique for autologous bone marrow harvest is identical to the allogeneic harvesting, with the same options for anesthesia available to the patient.

B. The autologous harvest is generally performed on the day of admission, prior to initiation of conditioning/ preparative therapy. Some patients, however, undergo harvesting for cryopreservation and storage of marrow if they do not require immediate treatment.

C. In most cases, the total volume of marrow aspirated is higher in autologous harvesting. This may be related to
   1. Decreased quality or cellularity of the marrow, resulting from previous chemotherapy or radiation therapy[2]
   2. Plans for purging malignant cells from the marrow by means of physical methods (such as immunoabsorption), pharmacologic methods, or monoclonal antibody therapy. Any purging process or marrow manipulation will reduce the progenitor cell count.

D. Autologous blood donation is contraindicated in patients prior to autologous marrow harvesting. During or following the harvest procedure, the patient will require transfusion of allogeneic blood.

E. Following filtration in the operating room, as with allogeneic bone marrow harvests, autologous marrow is cryopreserved for later use, either following conditioning therapy or at a remote date.

F. Autologous bone marrow harvest patients are stabilized in the recovery room and then usually admitted to begin conditioning therapy.

III. Complications of bone marrow harvesting

A. The potential complications of bone marrow harvesting are as follows:
1. Pain
2. Anemia
3. Hypovolemia
4. Hypotension
5. Hematoma at harvest site
6. Bleeding
7. Fever
8. Infection
9. Anesthesia-related complications

B. Pain is the most common complication of bone marrow harvesting and results from trauma to the iliac bones and, more importantly, the overlying soft tissue. Excessive pain may indicate the presence of a hematoma with associated pressure neuropathy. This will resolve gradually with reabsorption of the hematoma.

IV. Bone marrow processing

A. Both allogeneic and autologous marrow can be processed in a variety of ways to provide a more suitable product for the recipient. Processing of marrow is done using highly specialized laboratory techniques and may involve cryopreservation of marrow for later use.

B. In most situations, especially when cryopreservation is planned, volume reduction by removal of plasma and red blood cells is necessary. Volume reduction decreases the potential for infusion-related toxicity as well as allows use of less cryoprotectant for cryopreservation.[3]

C. In addition to volume reduction, marrow may be processed to remove red blood cells (in the case of ABO incompatibility) or purged to remove either T cells or malignant cells.

D. T-cell depletion involves removal of donor T cells prior to an infusion in an attempt to decrease the risk of GVHD. Because this also reduces graft-versus-leukemia effect, T-cell depletion should be reserved for situations with high risk of GVHD, such as matched unrelated donor transplants and antigen-mismatched transplants.

E. Purging of malignant cells may be necessary in certain autologous transplant situations. Malignant cells can be detected by means of monoclonal antibody technology and molecular techniques such as polymerase chain reaction.[4] Purging can be accomplished by chemical means using chemotherapeutic agents such as 4-hydroperoxycyclophosphamide or immunologic agents such as monoclonal antibodies. Purging of marrow may prolong the period of cytopenia after transplant.

F. Cell purging technology utilizing monoclonal antibodies has led to investigation of positive selection of cells by use of anti-CD34 monoclonal antibodies. This technique is currently under study for use with both autologous and allogeneic transplants.

G. When processing is complete, donor marrow may be infused to the recipient. In the setting of autologous transplantation, the marrow stem cells must undergo cryopreservation for later use.

H. Cryopreservation requires the use of a cryoprotectant to prevent cell destruction during freezing and thawing. The most common cryoprotectant for such use is imethylsulphoxide (dimethyl sulfoxide [DMSO]) or DMSO with 6-hydroxyethyl starch.

I. Freezing of marrow/stem cells can be accomplished with liquid nitrogen or in a mechanical freezer. In either instance, the rate of freeze is carefully controlled to minimize cell damage.

J. If long-term storage is planned, liquid nitrogen (either in liquid phase or in vapor phase) is necessary. Mechanical freezing at -80°C is used for short-term storage.

V. Mobilization and collection of peripheral blood stem cells (PBSCs)

A. The use of PBSCs for transplantation has, in most cases, replaced bone marrow for autologous transplantation. Most recently, PBSCs have been used in the setting of allogeneic transplantation. Advantages of PBSC transplantation over bone marrow transplantation are as follows:

1. Provides more rapid engraftment
2. Decreases risk of malignant contamination
3. Decreases collection-related discomfort
4. Eliminates anesthesia risk
5. Decreases cost

B. PBSCs are collected via outpatient apheresis procedures. A series of several procedures is generally required to obtain an adequate number of mononuclear cells to achieve a durable engraftment. The target number of mononuclear cells varies by transplant center, but usually ranges from 4 to 7 X 10^8 mononuclear cells per kilogram of recipient body weight.[4,5] CD34 cell count can also be used to assay PBSC content.

C. PBSCs may be collected in the steady state (without mobilization) or following mobilization with cytokine administration or with chemotherapy.

D. Collection in the steady state requires many apheresis procedures, since peripheral blood contains significantly lower numbers of progenitor cells than does bone marrow. Use of PBSCs collected in the steady state may result in delayed engraftment, especially delayed platelet recovery; thus, this method of stem cell collection and transplant is rarely used.

E. The number of PBSCs available for collection is greatly increased by mobilization. Mobilization with chemotherapy can be used in the autologous transplant setting. Early techniques for mobilization with chemotherapy used high-dose cyclophosphamide. More recently, mobilization has been accomplished with a wide variety of single-agent or combination chemotherapy. Following administration of chemotherapy, most patients receive growth factor support to minimize fever and potential for infection as well as to enhance the mobilization effect. Generally, stem cell apheresis is scheduled to begin as the peripheral white blood cell (WBC) count starts to recover, when the mobilization effect is most pronounced.[6]

F. Mobilization with hematopoietic growth factors is most often accomplished by using granulocyte colony-stimulating factor or granulocyte-macrophage colony-stimulating factor. More recently, interleukin-3 has also been used, and additional growth factors or combinations of growth factors are being studied for use in mobilization.[7] Mobilization by growth factor can be used in both the autologous and allogeneic transplant setting. Growth factor is administered daily or twice daily for 6 to 14 days, with stem cell apheresis being performed on the last several days of therapy.[5]

G. Stem cell apheresis usually takes place over several days. Each day's collection is analyzed to determine the number of CD34 progenitor cells. Additionally, in the setting of autologous transplantation, CD34 cell selection may be employed to decrease the amount of tumor cell contamination of the apheresis product.

H. As each apheresis product is obtained, it is cryopreserved as described for bone marrow, using either 10% DMSO alone or 5% DMSO in combination with 6-hydroxyethyl starch.

VI. Umbilical cord blood collection

A. Umbilical cord blood transplantation has been used in allogeneic transplantation for patients with a variety of disorders (e.g., malignancy, immunodeficiency disease, Fanconi's anemia). Advantages and disadvantages of umbilical cord blood transplantation are as follows:

    1. Advantages
        a) Immunologic naivete of cord blood may decrease potential for GVHD.
        b) Provides rich source of progenitor cells
        c) Harvesting poses no risk to mother or fetus.
    2. Disadvantages
        a) Low volume with uncertain, finite cell yield
        b) Potential for contamination with maternal cells
        c) Patients with a larger body mass may not receive the number of cells necessary to achieve engraftment.

B. Cord blood harvesting techniques continue to be studied and refined to optimize cell yield and minimize risk of maternal contamination.

C. Umbilical cord blood is harvested at the time of delivery. The umbilical cord is drained prior to placental delivery. The cord blood is collected in a tissue culture medium containing heparin[7] or ACD-A. Following delivery of the placenta, placental vessels can be aspirated to provide additional volume. An average of 100 mL of umbilical cord blood can be obtained.[8]

D. It is essential to avoid manipulation of the umbilical cord blood product because any amount of manipulation will reduce volume and cell count. Although hematopoietic engraftment has been achieved in young children, it remains unclear if umbilical cord blood will provide hematopoietic reconstitution in an adult. Studies continue in an effort to improve stem cell expansion techniques to allow transplantation in an older child or adult.

VII. Infusion of marrow stem cells

A. Marrow or stem cell infusion is planned to occur at least 24 hours after completion of the conditioning therapy to eliminate any cytotoxic effect of the chemotherapy on the marrow/stem cells.

B. Both bone marrow and PBSCs are infused intravenously either by infusion or IV push via syringe. In either case, the patient must have secure intravenous access. The patient must be prehydrated to ensure high urine output.

C. Products that have been cryopreserved must be thawed prior to administration. This is generally performed at the patient's bedside, as rapid infusion is essential after thawing. Each bag of marrow/PBSC is thawed and infused individually.[9]

D. In situations of cryopreservation with DMSO, the patient should be advised of the unpleasant odor associated with this compound. Patients receiving cryopreserved product may experience a temporary red coloration of the urine secondary to red cell lysis, which occurs during the thawing process.

E. As with infusion of any blood product, the patient may experience infusion-related reactions. These can occur both in the allogeneic and autologous transplant settings. Signs of infusion-related toxicity/reaction are as follows:

1. Headache
2. Flushing
3. Nausea/vomiting
4. Abdominal cramping/diarrhea
5. Fever
6. Chest tightness
7. Dyspnea
8. Bradycardia
9. Hypertension
10. Fluid overload
11. Pulmonary embolism
12. Adult respiratory distress syndrome
13. Anaphylaxis

F. Stem cells migrate to the marrow spaces following intravenous infusion. Engraftment of stem cells begins within one to two weeks after infusion in most patients.

References

1. Patterson K. Bone marrow harvesting. In: Treleaven J, Wiernik P, eds. *Bone Marrow Transplantation*. London: Mosby-Wolfe; 1995.

2. Whedon MB. *Bone Marrow Transplantation: Principles, Practice, and Nursing Insights*. Boston: Jones and Bartlett; 1991.

3. Szer J. Cryopreservation and functional assessment of harvested autologous bone marrow and blood stem cells. In: Atkinson K, ed. *Clinical Bone Marrow Transplantation: A Reference Textbook*. Cambridge, England: Cambridge University Press; 1994.

4. King CR. Peripheral stem cell transplantation: past, present, and future. In: Buschel PC, Whedon MB, eds. *Bone Marrow Transplantation: Administrative and Clinical Strategies*. Boston: Jones and Bartlett; 1995.

5. Shpall EJ, Jones RB. Mobilization and collection of peripheral blood progenitor cells for support of high-dose cancer therapy. In: Forman SJ, Blume KG, Thomas ED, eds. *Bone Marrow Transplantation*. Boston: Blackwell Scientific Publications; 1994.

6. Vose JM, Armitage JO, Kessinger A. High-dose chemotherapy and autologous transplant with peripheral-blood stem cells. *Oncology*. 1993;7:23–29.

7. Vowels MR, Lam Po Tang R. Cord blood and fetal tissue transplants. In: Atkinson K, ed. *Clinical Bone Marrow Transplantation: A Reference Textbook*. Cambridge, England: Cambridge University Press; 1994.

8. Wagner JE, Broxmeyer HE, Cooper S. Umbilical cord and placental blood hematopoietic stem cells: collection, cryopreservation, and storage. *J Hematother*. 1992;1:167–173.

9. Patterson K. Bone marrow processing. In: Treleaven J, Wiernik P, eds. *Bone Marrow Transplantation*. London: Mosby-Wolfe; 1995.

Bibliography

Buckner CD, Petersen FB, Bolonesi BA. Bone marrow donors. In: Froman SJ, Blume KG, Thomas ED, eds. *Bone Marrow Transplantation*. Boston: Blackwell Scientific Publications; 1994.

Crouch MA, Rise C. Post-induction autologous bone marrow transplantation. *Nurs Care Issues Adult Acute Leukemia*. 1995;2:6–12.

Wagner JE, Kernan NA, Steinbuch M et al. Allogeneic sibling umbilical cord blood transplantation in children with malignant and non-malignant disease. *Lancet*. 1995;346:214–219.

C H A P T E R 5

Management of Stem Cell/Bone Marrow Transplantation Complications

Complications of bone marrow transplantation (BMT) (Figure 5.1) are frequent. Astute management of these complications requires a methodical and systematic approach (Figure 5.2).

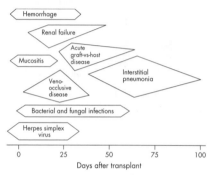

Figure 5.1 Outlines the time occurrence of acute complications after blood cell/marrow transplantation.[1]

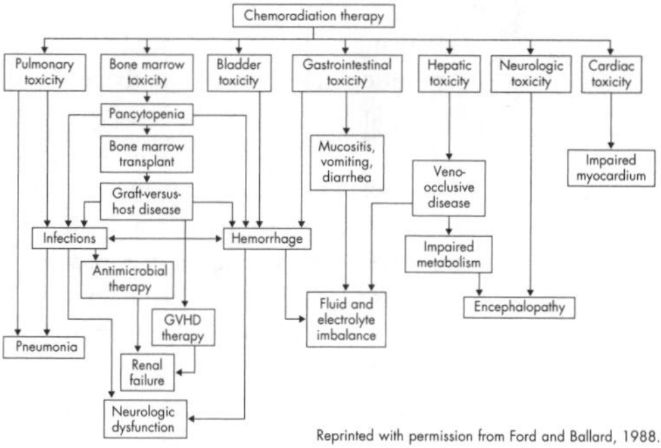

Figure 5.2 Depicts the interrelatedness between the major BMT complications, etiologies, and treatments.

Reprinted with permission from Ford and Ballard, 1988.

125

I. Hematopoietic complications[2-6]

A. Figure 5.3 outlines hematopoietic cellular development.[3]

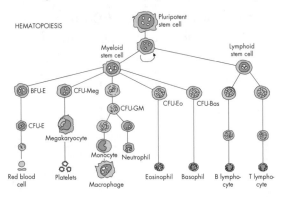

Figure 5.3 Provides a diagram of hematopoietic cellular development.

B. Bleeding/hemorrhage[1,2,7]

1. Definition: Any anticipated or unanticipated loss of blood. In the BMT setting, it is most likely secondary to thrombocytopenia or abnormal coagulation factors.

2. Etiology

a) Preparative regimen-induced myelosuppression resulting in profound thrombocytopenia and anemia. The megakaryocyte is the last cell to arrive in the myeloid engraftment process. Normal platelet counts are usually not evident until one to three months post-transplant.

b) Delayed platelet engraftment because of graft-versus-host disease (GVHD), cyclosporin A (CsA), infection, or marrow purging

c) Poor graft function related to bone marrow suppression from medication or infection (especially viral)

d) Coagulation abnormalities resulting from hepatotoxicity, GVHD, disseminated intravascular coagulation (DIC), or sepsis

e) Platelet autoantibodies

3. Risk factors

a) GVHD and use of CsA

b) Veno-occlusive disease (VOD) with impaired production of coagulation factors

c) Altered mucosal barriers

d) Failed or delayed engraftment

e) Viral infections

f) ABO-incompatible allogeneic BMT

g) Hypertension

4. Clinical features

a) Epistaxis, hematemesis, melana, hematuria, oral bleeding, guiac-positive stools

b) Sudden acute drop in hematocrit (> 4% in 8 hours)

c) Acute onset of abdominal pain

d) Central nervous system (CNS) bleed: acute change in mental status, headache, seizures, papilledema, focal neurologic findings

5. Differential diagnosis

a) Intra-abdominal infection, VOD

b) Acute hemolysis (decreased hematocrit, hematuria)

c) CNS infection or thrombosis

6. Diagnostic studies

a) Complete blood count (CBC) and platelet count at least daily during period of aplasia. Increase frequency if patient is actively bleeding or requires more than daily platelet transfusions.

b) One-hour post–platelet transfusion count

c) DIC screen: D-dimer, fibrinogen, prothrombin time (PT), partial thromboplastin time (PTT)

d) Hemolysis work-up: urinalysis, CBC with smear, haptoglobin, lactate dehydrogenase, direct and indirect Coombs' test, fractionated bilirubin

e) Guiac test for each stool and emesis; dipstick urine test for heme at least q8h.

7. Management[2,8]

a) See Table 5.1 for blood component therapy.

b) Avoid invasive procedures unless absolutely necessary. If necessary, transfuse platelets to 50,000/μL or higher if possible.

c) Avoid medications that inhibit platelet function acetylsalicylic acid (ASA), nonsteroidal anti-inflammatory drugs (NSAIDs).

d) Bleeding precautions if platelets are less than 20,000/μL

e) Transfuse platelets if less than 10,000 to 20,000/μ, if bleeding occurs, and prior to invasive procedures. All blood products must be irradiated to prevent GVHD. Leukocyte-reduction filters are used for packed red blood cells (PRBCs) and platelets to reduce exposure to HLA and cytomegalovirus (CMV). Give CMV-negative products to CMV-negative patients, since the virus is carried on granulocytes and may increase the risk of CMV infection. HLA-matched platelet products are indicated if the patient fails to respond to repeated transfusions of non-HLA-matched products. (Table 5.2 outlines degrees of platelet HLA antigen compatibility.) Pre-medicate with acetaminophen, diphenhydramine, or hydrocortisone (alone or in combination) if the patient has a history of transfusion reaction.

Table 5.1 Blood Component Therapy

Blood component	Composition	Approximate volume	Infusion time	Expected response	Indications	Special considerations
Red blood cells (RBCs)	RBCs, reduces plasma, white blood cells (WBCs), and platelets	250–300 mL	2–4 hrs	Increase hemoglobin (Hgb) to 1 g/dL per unit	Symptomatic anemia because of chronic or acute blood loss; myelosuppression	ABO compatibility is required; leukocyte-poor or filtered RBCs are given to patients at risk for febrile transfusion reactions.
Platelets from a single donor (pheresis)	Platelets, some RBCs, some WBCs, and plasma	200–300 mL per unit	20–60 min	Increase platelet count to 40,000 per unit	Bleeding because of thrombocytopenia; presence of antiplatelet antibodies; myelosuppression	Product may be human leukocyte antigen (HLA)- or random matched. ABO compatibility is not required. Bone marrow donor may be asked to donate platelets. Leukocyte-poor or filtered platelets are given in patients at risk for febrile transfusion reactions.

Table 5.1 (continued)

Blood component	Composition	Approximate volume	Infusion time	Expected response	Indications	Special considerations
Platelets from random donors	Platelets, some RBCs, some WBCs, and plasma	30–50 mL per unit	5–10 min per unit	Increase platelet count to 5000/µL per unit	Bleeding because of thrombocytopenia; myelosuppression	ABO compatibility is not required; usually not given to BMT recipients.
Fresh frozen plasma	Plasma, all coagulation factors, and complement	220 mL	10–15 min	Increase coagulation factors by 5%–10% per unit	Coagulation factor deficiency; disseminated intravascular coagulation (DIC)	ABO compatibility is required.
Cryoprecipitate	Plasma and stable clotting factors	200 mL	15–30 min	Increase factor VIII, factor XIII, and fibrinogen levels	Treatment of stable clotting factors deficiencies (II, VII, IX, X, XI); DIC	ABO compatibility is preferred.

Table 5.2 Degrees of Platelet HLA Antigen Compatibility

Match	Conditions of compatibility
A	All four donor antigens identical to recipient
B1U	3 donor antigens identical to recipient; 1 unknown
B2U	2 donor antigens identical to recipient; 2 unknown
B1X	3 donor antigens identical to recipient; one cross reactive
B2X	2 donor antigens identical to recipient; 2 cross reactive
B3X	One donor antigen identical to recipient; 3 cross reactive
B4X	4 cross reactive
C	One donor antigen major mismatch to recipient
D	2 donor antigens major mismatch to recipient

Reprinted with permission from Fuller, 1993.[7]

    f) Replace clotting factors as indicated
       (see Table 5.1 on pp. 130)[2]:
       (1) fresh frozen plasma (contains all
          clotting factors)
       (2) cryoprecipitate (contains factor VIII [5 to 10
          U/mL], von Willebrand's factor, fibrinogen)
    g) Replace vitamin K for elevated PT. Dosage:
       (1) Adults: 10 mg IV qd for 3 days. A total of
          30 mg should be given; includes total IV
          supplemental given in total parenteral
          nutrition solution.
       (2) Children: 1 to 5 mg/dose IV. Evaluate PT prior
          to redosing.
    h) Topical thrombin (see chapter 7 for further
       drug information): Apply 1000 to 2000 U/mL
       of solution where bleeding is profuse (operative
       sites); apply powder directly to the site of bleeding
       or on oozing surfaces; use 100 U/mL for bleeding
       from skin or mucosal surfaces.
    i) Aminocaproic acid (Amicar) is indicated for
       invasive procedures (central venous line place-
       ment, dental extraction) in the profoundly
       thrombocytopenic patient. It is also used as

bleeding prophylaxis in the profoundly
thrombocytopenic patient (chronic platelet
count < 5000 µL). It may also be used in patients
with chronic, profuse oral bleeding, gastrointestinal bleeding, or hemorrhagic cystitis. Dosage
(see chapter 7 for further drug information):

(1) Oral: 5 g during first hour, followed by 1.0 to
1.25 g/h for about 8 hours or until bleeding
stops. May swish and spit for oral oozing.
Total daily dose should not exceed 30 g.

(2) IV: 4 to 5 g in 250 mL of diluent during first
hour, followed by continuous infusion at the
rate of 1.0 to 1.25 g/h in 50 mL; continue for
8 hours or until bleeding stops.

(3) Children: Loading dose is 100 to 200 mg/kg
IV or PO; maintenance dose is 100 mg/kg/
dose q6h.

C. Anemia
1. Definition: decreased hemoglobin and hematocrit
levels resulting in potential alterations in body/
tissue oxygenation
2. Etiology
a) The bone marrow aplasia created by the
conditioning regimen creates a reduction in the
production and supply of RBCs. This results in a
potential reduction in adequate
tissue oxygentation.
b) About seven to 10 days after marrow ablative
chemotherapy and donor or autologous marrow
infusion, circulating nucleated red cells will be
evident in buffy coat preparations.
c) Reticulocytes, however, are not evident until two to
three weeks after stem cell or marrow reinfusion.

3. Risk factors
   a) All patients undergoing stem cell or marrow transplantation
   b) Patients with active bleeding
   c) Acute hemolysis due to CsA, FK–506, ABO-incompatible graft, infection, or hemolytic-uremic syndrome
4. Clinical features
   a) Hematocrit (HCT) less than 25% or hemoglobin (Hgb) less than 8 g/dL
   b) Fatigue, pallor, shortness of breath
   c) Hypotension (with acute drop in HCT, orthostasis
5. Differential diagnosis
   a) With acute drop in HCT: active bleeding versus acute hemolysis versus dilutional laboratory draw from central venous line
   b) Gradual drop in HCT is normal finding early post-transplant.
6. Diagnostic studies
   a) Hgb/HCT at least daily throughout period of aplasia. Increase frequency if patient is actively bleeding.
   b) Platelet count and PT/PTT for sudden acute drop in HCT
   c) Blood cell morphology
   d) Hemolysis work-up: urinalysis, CBC, haptoglobin, lactate dehydrogenase, direct and indirect Coombs' test, fractionated bilirubin
   e) Guiac test for each stool and emesis; dipstick urine test for heme at least q8h
   f) Blood urea nitrogen (BUN)/creatinine
   g) Reticulocyte count: May be helpful in evaluating red cell function following engraftment of myeloid cell line.

7. Management
   a) See Table 5.1 for blood component therapy.[2]
   b) Avoid invasive procedures that could result in additional blood loss, unless absolutely necessary.
   c) Transfuse packed red blood cells if HCT is less than 25% or Hgb is less than 8 g/dL, if active bleeding occurs, or prior to general anesthesia or invasive procedures where blood loss is anticipated (as clinically indicated).
      (1) All blood products must be irradiated to prevent GVHD.
      (2) Leukocyte-reduction filters are used for PRBCs and platelets to reduce exposure to HLAs and CMV.
      (3) Give CMV-negative products to CMV-negative patients, since the virus is carried on granulocytes and may increase the risk of CMV infection.
      (4) Premedicate with acetaminophen, diphenhydramine, or hydrocortisone (alone or in combination) if the patient has a history of transfusion reaction.
   d) Transfuse children more than 1 year of age with 10 to 15 mL/kg/transfusion.

D. Graft failure
   1. Definition: a complete absence of engraftment or a seemingly initial hematopoiesis post-transplant, with later decreasing blood counts and absence of normal hematopoiesis
   2. Etiology
      a) Thought to be a sensitization of the recipient to minor histocompatibilty antigens shared by the transfusion and the marrow/blood cell donor.
      b) May also be related to the persistence of host-derived cytotoxic T lymphocytes or natural killer cells.

   c) Graft rejection in the allogeneic matched sibling donor recipient is thought to result from marrow rejection by host T cells not eliminated during conditioning.[9]

   d) T-cell depletion of donor marrow to prevent GVHD also contributes to graft rejection.

   e) In the autologous BMT setting, graft failure is thought to be due to infusion of inadequate numbers of stem cells, ex vivo manipulation of marrow (purging), and cryopreservation.[3]

3. Risk factors

   a) Recipient of HLA-incompatible marrow graft

   b) Recipient of matched unrelated donor marrow graft

   c) Recipient of umbilical cord blood transplant

   d) Patients with severe aplastic anemia with history of multiple transfusions pretransplant

   e) Patients with thalassemia, immunodeficiency, or Fanconi's anemia

   f) Patients whose clinical condition necessitates limitation of pretransplant conditioning

   g) T-cell depletion of marrow graft or

   h) Ex vivo marrow manipulation (purging/cryopreservation)

4. Clinical features

   a) A complete absence of hematopoietic activity (rise in the WBC or platelet count) beyond the period expected. There is wide variation in mean day of engraftment between types of stem cell/marrow grafts; however, a sustained rise in the WBC count is expected before 30 to 40 days post-transplant.

   b) A loss of hematopoiesis after an initial rise in blood counts

   c) Little or no hematopoiesis noted on bone marrow analysis performed 30 to 40 days or greater post-transplant

5. Differential diagnosis
   a) Bone marrow suppression secondary to drugs (e.g., ganciclovir, co-trimoxazole, antithymocite globulin), infection, or GVHD
   b) Delayed engraftment
   c) Late engraftment with host cells (allogeneic)
   d) Relapse of underlying disease
6. Diagnostic studies
   a) CBC/differential/platelets daily to follow engraftment trends
   b) Bone marrow aspirate and biopsy (generally performed 30 to 40 days post-BMT in patients with little or no peripheral blood counts): analysis of cellularity, cytogenetics to evaluate chimerism, rule out relapse
7. Management
   a) Discontinuation of drugs known to be myelosuppressive (e.g., ganciclovir, co-trimoxazole, antithymocite globulin)
   b) Further immunosuppression is thought to be caused from an immune phenomenon.
   c) Reinfusion of allogeneic marrow with or without further conditioning (dependent on patient's clinical condition)
   d) Reinfusion of "backup" marrow or stem cells if available
   e) Attempted marrow stimulation with colony-stimulating factors: granulocyte-macrophage colony-stimulating factor (Leukine, Prokine), 250 μg/m^2/d IV, **or** granulocyte colony-stimulating factor (Neupogen): 5 to 10 μg/kg/d

II. Infectious complications

A. Infection [1,2,5,6,8,10–13]

1. Definition

   a) Most frequently occurring complication of BMT, which exists when the body or part of the body is invaded by a pathogenic agent that mutiples (colonizes) and produces detrimental or injurious effects to the body.

   b) An opportunistic infection is one that is usually the consequence of defective functioning of the normal immune system. Such an infection is caused by microorganisms that lack virulent infection-producing properties, unless a defect or group of defects is present in the host's immune system. [3]

   c) The timing of post-transplant bacterial, fungal, viral, and protozoal infection varies (see Figure 5.1 on p. 125).

2. Etiology [2,3]

   a) Myelosuppression induced by pretransplant conditioning regimen and other marrow-suppressive medications

   b) Conditioning results in an absence of WBCs including granulocytes, monocytes/ macrophages, and lymphocytes. (Infections resulting from phagocyte disorders: *Staphylococcus aureus, Pseudomonas, Escherichia coli.*)

   c) Immunosuppression induced by the pretransplant preparative regimen, prophylaxis, or treatment for acute or chronic GVHD and the disease process of GVHD

(1) Abnormal T- and B-lymphocyte function, resulting in impaired cellular and humoral immune function. Infections that result from cellular defects include fungal (*Candida, Aspergillus*), protozoal *(Pneumocystis carinii, Toxoplasmosis),* and viral (herpes simplex virus [HSV]), varicella-zoster virus (VZV) and CMV. Infections that result from humoral defects include pyogenic organisms and *Streptococcus pneumonia.*

(2) Decreased serum immunoglobulin levels

3. Incidence

a) Occurrence of infection varies because of a number of host factors, which include underlying disease, host endogenous flora, and pretreatment infections.

b) Overall incidence rates:[11]

Causative organism	Overall incident rate
Herpes zoster	30% to 50%
Fungal infections	50%
Bacterial infection	
(Haemophilus, encapsulated bacteria)	50%
CMV infections	50%
Pneumocystis pneumonia	28%

c) Types of infection vary according to the different phases of the transplant process (Table 5.3).

Table 5.3 Infectious Complications and Occurrence in BMT Recipients

Organism	Common site

First Month Post-Transplant

Viral:

Herpes simplex virus (HSV)	Oral, esophageal, skin and gastrointestinal tract, genital
Respiratory syncytial virus (RSV)	Sinopulmonary
Epstein-Barr virus (EBV)	Oral, esophageal, skin and gastrointestinal tract

Bacterial:

Gram positives (S. epidermidis, S. auerus, Streptococci)	Skin, blood, sinopulmonary
Gram negatives (E. Coli, P. aeruginosa, Klebsiella)	Gastrointestinal, blood, oral, perirectal

Fungal:

Candida species (C. albican, glabratta krusei)	Oral, esophageal, skin
Aspergillus (fumagata, flavum)	Sinopulmonary

1–4 Months Post-Transplant

Viral:

Cytomegalovirus (CMV)	Pulmonary, hepatic, gastrointestinal
Enteric viruses (rotavirus, coxsackie, adenovirus)	Pulmonary, urinary, gastrointestinal, hepatic
RSV	Sinopulmonary
Parainfluenza	Pulmonary

Bacterial:

Gram positives	Sinopulmonary and skin

Fungal:

Candida species	Oral, hepatosplenic, integument
Aspergillus species	Sinopulmonary, CNS
Mucormycosis	Sinopulmonary
Coccidio mycosis	Sinopulmonary
Cryptococcus neoformas	Pulmonary, CNS

Table 5.3 *(continued)*

Organism	Common site
Protozoa:	
Pneumocystis carnii	Pulmonary
Toxoplasma gondii	Pulmonary, CNS

4–12 Months Post-Transplant

Viral:

CMV, echoviruses, RSV, varicella zoster (VZV)	Integument, pulmonary, hepatic

Bacterial:

Gram positives	
(S. peneumoniae, H. influenza	Sinopulmonary and blood
Pneumococci)	Sinopulmonary

Fungal:

Aspergillus	Sinopulmonary
Coccididio mycosis	Sinopulmonary

Protozoa:

Pneumocystis carinii	Pulmonary
Toxoplasma gondii	Pulmonary, CNS

Greater than 12 Months Post-Transplant

Viral:

VZV	Integument

Bacterial:

Gram positives	
(Streptococci, H. Flu,	Sinopulmonary and blood
encapsulated bacteria)	

Reprinted with permission from Ezzone and Camp-Sorrell, 1994.

4. Risk factors/etiology
   a) Hematologic/lymphoid malignancy
   b) Hematologic/lymphoid malignancy in relapse
   c) Excessive previous treatment
   d) Prolonged neutropenia and immune deficiency
   e) Allogeneic transplant recipient

     f)   GVHD and immunosuppressive therapy to prevent or treat acute or chronic GVHD

     g)   Altered mucosal barriers

     h)   Previous microorganism colonization prior to conditioning

     i)   Prolonged use of antimicrobials

     j)   Older age

     k)   Total body irradiation (TBI) in conditioning regimen

5. Clinical features/signs and symptoms (Table 5.4)

6. Management of fever in the neutropenic BMT patient

     a)   Thorough physical exam twice daily to identify potential sites of infection; culture potential sites if possible

     b)   With onset of fever (> 38°C), panculture: Obtain blood cultures from all CVL sites, peripheral blood culture (optional), throat, urine, and stool cultures for bacteria and fungus, and CMV buffy coat (optional).

     c)   Obtain chest x-ray with onset of fever.

     d)   Initiate broad-spectrum gram negative and gram positive antibiotic coverage based on transplant center's experience and pathogen history (2–3 drug combination usually indicated).

     e)   Modify antibacterials based on culture sensitivities.

     f)   Daily blood cultures with fever (rotate lumen cultured, or culture most frequently manipulated lumen from central venous line)

     g)   If defervescence results from broad-spectrum antibacterials, panculture with new fever spikes.

     h)   If fever continues despite broad-spectrum antibacterials, fungal infection should be presumed and systemic antifungal therapy initiated in the form of amphotericin B (minimum of 0.5 mg/kg/d).

Table 5.4 Clinical Features and Common Signs and Symptoms of Infection in BMT Patients

System	Signs & symptoms	Causes
General	Fatigue, weight loss Fever, chills, malaise, night sweats	All opportunistic infections *Mycobacterium avium* complex (MAC), hepatitis, CMV, tuberculosis (TB)
Abdominal	Hepatomegaly	Hepatitis, CMV, MAC, toxoplasmosis
	Splenomegaly	CMV, MAC
Anorectal	Anal pain/drainage	Herpes simple virus (HSV), CMV, fissures/fistulas (pseudomonas, Klebsiella)
Cardiopulmonary	Persistent dry cough, dyspnea, chest tightness, rales	*Pneumocystis carinii* pneumonia, bacterial infection, CMV, toxoplasmosis, cryptococcosis. *Aspergillus,* TB, MAC, respiratory syncytial virus, adenovirus, parainfluenza
Dermatologic	Skin discoloration, rash, vesicles, scaling, eruptions, necrotic ulceration	Varicella-zoster virus (VZV), HSV, fungus, *Pseudomonas*
Gastrointestinal	Diarrhea, anorexia, nausea, vomiting, esophagitis	Protozoal, bacterial, *Clostridium difficile,* CMV, HSV, rotavirus, coxsackievirus, Norwalk virus
Genitourinary	Rashes, lesions, ulcers, dysuria, hematuria	HSV, adenovirus, bacteria, BK virus (human polyoma)
Hematologic	Pancytopenia	Viral infections (CMV)
Neurologic	Headache, weakness, seizures, motor/sensory deficits	Cryptococcosis, toxoplasmosis, HSV, VZV, *Aspergillus*
Oral	White lesions/patches, ulcers, pain dysphagia, pharyngitis, esophagitis	Candidiasis, HSV, CMV, gram-negative bacteria

    i)   If fever continues despite broad-spectrum antibacterial and antifungal coverage, a diligent search for possible fever source is warranted (viral cultures, stool for electron microscopy, frequent chest x-ray, culture and/or biopsy suspected lesions, meticulous evaluation of pain).

j) Empiric coverage for highly suspected organisms

B. Bacterial enterocolitis
1. Definition: an enteric bacterial infection usually contracted from a food source that causes frequent, loose, or watery stools
2. Risk factors
   a) Neutropenia
   b) Ingesting food (especially eggs, dairy products, poultry) that is not well cleaned, is undercooked, or is poorly stored
3. Clinical features
   a) Early symptoms include vomiting and fever.
   b) Diffuse liquid diarrhea, which may be bloody
   c) Painful abdominal cramps
   d) Dehydration
4. Differential diagnosis
   a) Bacterial enteritis (*Yersinia, Salmonella, Shigella,* enterotoxic *E. coli, Clostridium difficile, Campylobacter jejuni, Klebsiella*)
   b) Viral enteritis (e.g., CMV, rotavirus, Norwalk virus, adenovirus)
   c) Gut GVHD
   d) Toxicity from conditioning therapy
5. Diagnostic studies
   a) Stool culture (should always send for ova and parasites and *C. difficile* toxin with any diarrheal illness).
   b) Fecal leukocytes: Presence of white cells suggests bacterial infection, although neutropenic BMT patients are unable to mount white cell response.
   c) Stool from viral culture and electron microscopy to rule out viral infection
   d) Serum electrolytes at least daily with high gastrointestinal losses, more frequently if losses are excessive

e) Stool electrolyte and osmotic gap:

Stool osmotic gap formula
= 290 - 2 X ([Na] X [K])

Secretory diarrheas tend to have elevated stool [Na] and a resultant lower osmotic gap (< 100 mOsm/L). In viral illness and conditioning-related toxicity, the stool tends to have decreased [Na] and increased stool osmotic gap (> 100 mOsm/L).[8]

f) Gastrointestinal endoscopy with culture and biopsy (rule out GVHD, and further evaluate infection)

6. Management
   a) Treat dehydration with IV/PO fluids and correct electrolyte abnormalities.
   b) Bowel rest for 24 to 48 hours, then BRAT (bananas, rice, applesauce, toast) diet if tolerated
   c) Continue total parenteral nutrition if already established.
   d) For culture-positive bacterial enterocolitis, administer co-trimoxazole (8 mg/kg divided qid for 21 days) **or** ciprofloxacin:
      (1) Children: 20 to 30 mg/kg/24 h divided q12h for 10 to 14 days
      (2) Adults: 250 to 500 mg PO q12h for 10 to 14 days

C. Bacterial pneumonia
   1. Causative organisms
      a) First month post-BMT: gram-positive organisms *(Staphylococcus epidermidis, Streptococcus)*, gram-negative organisms *(Pseudomonas aeruginosa, Klebsiella)*, and atypical organisms *(Legionella, Chlamydia, Mycobacterium, Mycoplasma)*
      b) One to four months post-BMT: gram-positive organisms

    c) Four to 12 months post-BMT: gram-positive organisms *(S. pneumoniae* [pneumococcal pneumonia], *Haemophilus influenzae)*

2. Risk factors
   a) Debilitation
   b) Chronic GVHD (pneumococcal pneumonia)
   c) Increased age at time of transplant

3. Clinical features
   a) Dry or productive cough
   b) Dyspnea/shortness of breath
   c) Infiltrates on chest x-ray; isolated area of consolidation

4. Differential diagnosis
   a) Viral pneumonia
   b) Fungal pneumonia
   c) Radiation pneumonitis/cytotoxic lung injury
   d) *P. carinii* pneumonia
   e) Bronchiolitis obliterans organizing pneumonia

5. Diagnostic studies
   a) Arterial blood gas to evaluate degree of hypoxemia
   b) Isolation of causative organism through culture of sputum (low yield)
   c) Bronchoalveolar lavage, transbronchial biopsy, computed tomography (CT)–guided needle or open lung biopsy samples for culture and pathology

6. Management of bacterial pneumonia[5]
   a) Drug choices are based on causative organism and sensitivities.
   b) Empiric treatment includes broad-spectrum gram-positive and gram-negative coverage (third-generation cephalosporin/aminoglycoside [see chapter 7])
      (1) Children: ceftriaxone or cefotaxime plus gentamicin or tobramycin

(2) Adults *(Mycoplasma, S. pneumoniae, Legionella,* and *H. influenzae)*: azithromycin, clarithromycin, erythromycin, or doxycycline (rifampin may be added for documented *Legionella)*

(3) Adults *(Klebsiella pneumoniae, Enterobacter, Chlamydia, S. aureus)*: erythromycin plus imipenem or ceftriaxone or cefotaxime

(4) Aspiration suspected, with severe mucositis *(S. pneumoniae, Bacteroides,* or other oral flora): clindamycin or metronidazole

(5) Pneumococcal pneumonia: penicillin G or third-generation cephalosporin IV q4h for 7 days

D. Bacteremia/bacterial sepsis [1–3,5,11,12,14]

1. Causative organisms

    a) First month post-BMT: gram-positive organisms *(S. epidermidis, Streptococcus)* and gram-negative organisms *(P. aeruginosa, K. pneumoniae)*

    b) One to four months post-BMT: gram positive organisms

    c) Four to 12 months post-BMT: gram-positive organisms *(Streptococcus, H. influenzae)*

2. Clinical features

    a) Gram-negative bacteremia causes massive vasodilation, resulting in deficient circulating blood volume, cardiac output, and tissue perfusion. Cellular hypoxia and acidosis result.

    b) Complications may include vascular collapse, adult respiratory distress syndrome (ARDS), renal failure, congestive heart failure, arrhythmias, DIC, and viral and fungal infections.

c) Signs and symptoms include
   (1) Warm shock: fever; widening pulse pressure; change in level of consciousness and behavior; flushing; warm, dry skin; tachycardia; tachypnea; decreased PO_2; urine output normal to slightly increased
   (2) Cool shock: cool skin, peripheral edema, tachycardia, hypotension, tachypnea, pulmonary congestion, progressive hypoxemia, oliguria, thirst
   (3) Cold shock: cold, clammy skin; tachycardia; thready pulse; severe hypotension; high central venous pressure; high pulmonary wedge pressure; respiratory failure; profound hypoxemia; metabolic acidosis; severe oliguria or anuria

3. Diagnostic studies
   a) Blood cultures: isolation of causative organism. All patients should have blood cultures done with the onset of fever whether neutropenic or not.
   b) Arterial blood gases: respiratory alkalosis related to hyperventilation, metabolic acidosis related to accumulation of organic acids
   c) Lactic acid
   d) BUN/creatinine: elevated related to renal hypoperfusion
   e) Electrolytes: variable abnormalities
   f) Chest x-ray: Rule out capillary leak or ARDS.

4. Management
   a) With above symptomatology, initiate empiric antibiotic therapy immediately after cultures are obtained (empiric choice is broad-spectrum coverage for gram-negative and gram-positive organisms and should be based on transplant center's pathogen history).
   b) Modify antibacterials based on culture sensitivities.

      c) Ensure hemodynamic stability: crystalloid/colloid to maintain blood pressure and perfusion of vital organs.

      d) Swan-Ganz thermodilutional catheter as needed to monitor and manage fluid status

      e) Vasopressors to maintain blood pressure if crystalloid/colloid ineffective

      f) Treat hypoxemia: oxygen support/mechanical ventilation if needed.

E. *Clostridium difficile*[5,8,14]

1. Definition: *C. difficile* causes a pseudomembranous enterocolitis infection secondary to broad-spectrum antimicrobial use or chemotherapy, which alters the normal balance of gut flora.

2. Risk factors
   a) Prior history of *C. difficile* colitis
   b) Recent chemotherapy
   c) Prolonged use of antibiotic therapy

3. Clinical features
   a) Fever
   b) Explosive, liquid diarrhea (may be bloody)
   c) Foul-smelling stool or flatulence
   d) Crampy abdominal pain

4. Differential diagnosis
   a) Viral enteritis (e.g., CMV, rotavirus, adenovirus)
   b) *Salmonella/Shigella* enteritis
   c) Giardiasis
   d) Chemotherapy/radiation (total body irradiation)-induced diarrhea
   e) Gut GVHD

5. Diagnostic studies
   a) Stool sample for *C. difficile* toxin (also send bacterial, fungal, and viral studies to rule out). Should be read at 24 and 48 hours. If negative and diarrhea persists, repeat due to possible sampling error (false-negative result).

      b) Repeat *C. difficile* stool sample after 10 to 14 days of therapy to ensure toxin has cleared.

      c) Electrolytes at least daily due to gastrointestinal losses

  6. Management

      a) Metronidazole

          (1) Children: 7.5 mg/kg q6h PO (preferred) or 15 mg/kg IV loading dose, then 7.5 mg/kg q6h for 10 to 14 days

          (2) Adults: 500 mg PO (preferred)/IV q6h for 10 to 14 days

      b) Alternative: oral vancomycin (no gastrointestinal absorption)

          (1) Children: 40 mg/kg PO tid or qid for 10 to 14 days

          (2) Adults: 125 mg PO qid for 10 to 14 days

      c) IV fluid replacement of stool losses

      d) Replace electrolytes based on laboratory values.

F. *Mycobacterium avium-intracellulare*

  1. Definition: infection caused by *M. avium* complex, which can be organ specific, but typically is disseminated.

  2. Clinical features:

      a) Diarrhea

      b) Abdominal pain

      c) Hepatomegaly/splenomegaly

      d) Persistent high fever

      e) Weight loss

      f) Enlarged lymph nodes may or may not be present.

  3. Differential diagnosis

      a) GVHD

      b) Epstein-Barr virus (EBV) lymphoma

      c) Hepatosplenic candidiasis

4. Diagnostic studies
   a) *M. avium-intracellulare* culture (requires special medium), including blood, stool, and bone marrow
   b) Lymph node and liver biopsy (if highly suspect)
5. Management: Treat if culture is positive for acid-fast bacteria.
   a) Clarithromycin, 500 mg to 1 g bid, plus clofazimine, 50 to 100 mg qd
   b) If no improvement, add one to two additional drugs:
      (1) Amikacin, 15 mg/kg/d IV bid
      (2) Ethambutol, 25 mg/kg/d qd for first 2 months
      (3) Rifampin, 10 to 15 mg/kg/d qd
   c) These drugs have considerable side effects, and toxicities should be monitored.
   d) Blood cultures for *M. avium intracellulare* should be negative if treatment is effective.

G. *Mycobacterium tuberculosis* [5,8,14]
   1. Definition
      a) Bacterial infection spread through droplet nuclei coughed up by persons with untreated tuberculosis (TB) of the lungs or larynx
      b) Most patients are asymptomatic but can develop clinical disease at any time, especially if rendered immunoincompetent.
      c) The lungs are the most common site for clinical TB; however, extrapulmonic disease is not uncommon in immunosuppressed BMT patients.
      d) Extrapulmonary sites include lymphatic TB, miliary disease (disseminated TB), meningitis, and bone or joints.
      e) Multidrug-resistant TB is becoming more common in recent years.
   2. Risk factors
      a) Close exposure to person with TB
      b) Asymptomatic colonization with TB pretransplant

    c) Allogeneic transplant recipient

    d) Chronic GVHD

3. Clinical features

    a) Productive, prolonged cough

    b) Fever, chills, night sweats

    c) Loss of appetite, weight loss

    d) Hemoptysis

    e) Arthralgias/myalgias

    f) Lymphadenopathy (+/- in BMT patients due to lymphopenia)

4. Differential diagnosis:

    a) *M. avium-intracellulare* infection

    b) Other bacterial, fungal, or viral infection/pneumonitis

    c) Relapsed Hodgkin's or non-Hodgkin's lymphoma

5. Diagnostic studies

    a) Pretransplant: purified protein derivative (PPD) tuberculin skin test with control (*Candida,* mumps, tetanus toxoid) due to possible anergy: positive if TB skin test is greater than 5-mm area of reaction

    b) Chest x-ray: area of lobar consolidation

    c) Sputum smear and culture

    d) Bronchoalveolar lavage, transbronchial biopsy, CT-guided needle or open lung biopsy samples for acid-fast bacteria, culture, immunofluorescent antibody and pathology

    e) Lumbar puncture with samples for acid-fast bacteria and culture to rule out meningeal involvement

6. Management

    a) PPD should be performed on all patients pre-BMT; if positive but no active disease, give prophylaxis optimally for three months pretransplant.

    b) Treat BMT patients prophylactically for significant exposures.

    c) Table 5.5 outlines current prophylaxis and treatment of TB.[8,14]

Table 5.5 Prophylaxis and Treatment of TB

Disease status	Drug regimen	Comments
PPD > 5 mm, asymptomatic		Delay BMT; attempt to give at least 3 mo pre-BMT if possible.
Isoniazid susceptible	Isoniazid for 9 mo	
Isoniazid resistant	Rifampin for 9 mo	
Positive bronchoalveolar lavage with pulmonary infiltrate and hilar lymphadenopathy	Standard—6 mo isoniazid, rifampin & pyrazinamide for 2 mo, then isoniazid & rifampin for 4 mo	If drug resistance possible, add streptomycin or ethambutol to initial therapy until susceptibility is known.
or	**or**	
Extrapulmonary other than meningitis, disseminated (miliary), or bone/joint	Isoniazid, rifampin, & pyrazinamide qd for 2 mo, then isoniazid & rifampin 2 times/wk for 4 mo	For hilar LAD: 6 mo of isoniazid & rifampin has been shown to be sufficient if drug resistance unlikely.
	Alternative—9 mo (low incidence of drug resistance) Isoniazid and rifampin daily for 9 mo	
	or	
	Isoniazid & rifampin daily for 1 mo, then isoniazid and rifampin 2 times/wk for 8 mo	
Meningitis, disseminated (miliary), or bone/joint	Isoniazid, rifampin, pyrazinamide, & streptomycin qd for 2 mo, then isoniazid & rifampin qd for 10 mo	Give streptomycin in initial therapy until drug susceptibility known. If resistance to streptomycin possible, may use capreomycin or kanamycin instead of streptomycin.*
	or	
	Isoniazid, rifampin, pyrazinamide, & streptomycin qd for 2 mo, then isoniazid & rifampin 2 times/wk for 10 mo	

* Capreomycin, kanamycin, ethionamide, para-aminosalicyclic, and cycloserine are difficult to manage and should only be prescribed and monitored by a health-care provider experienced in their use.

Data from Johnson, 1993; Red Book, 1991.

d) Table 5.6 outlines dosages and side effects of TB therapies.

Table 5.6 Dosages and Side Effects of Current TB Therapies

Drug	Form	Dosage	Maximum dose	Side effects
Isoniazid	Tablet: 100, 300 mg Syrup: 50 mg/5 mL Vial: 1 g	5–10 mg/kg/d PO, IM	300 mg	Transaminitis, peripheral neuropathy, hepatitis hypersensitivity
Rifampin	Capsule: 150, 300 mg Vial: 600 mg	10–20 mg/kg/d PO/IV	600 mg	Orange discoloration of secretions & urine, nausea, vomiting, hepatitis, febrile reaction, purpura (rare)
Pyrazinamide	Tablet: 500 mg	15–30 mg/kg/d PO	2 g	Hepatotoxicity, hyperuricemia
Streptomycin	Vial: 1 g, 4 g IM	20–40 mg/kg/d	1 g	Ototoxicity, nephrotoxicity
Ethambutol	Tablet: 100, 400 mg PO	15–25 mg/kg/d	2.5 g	Optic neuritis, skin rash

* Capreomycin, kanamycin, ethionamide, para-aminosalicyclic, and cycloserine are difficult to manage and should only be prescribed and monitored by a health-care provider experienced in their use.

Data from Johnson, 1993; Red Book, 1991.

e) Cases of TB are reportable to the state Boards of Health.

f) Consult the Infectious Disease service when managing a patient with TB.

g) Isolation: Patients highly suspect for TB should be in a private, negative-pressure room. Health-care providers should wear high-efficiency masks.

H. Oral (thrush)/esophageal candidiasis [8,12,14,15]

1. Definition: oral/esophageal fungal infection caused by *Candida albicans*
2. Risk factors
   a) Immunocompromised patients with defective T-lymphocyte function (early post-transplant and in patients on corticosteroids for GVHD)
   b) Also common in patients receiving antibiotics
3. Clinical presentations
   a) Pseudomembranous candidiasis is characterized by the presence of creamy white or yellowish plaques that can be located anywhere on the mucosa. They can be removed by scraping, revealing a bleeding mucosal surface.
   b) Erythematous or atrophic candidiasis is characterized by redness of the mucosa; the tongue will present with depapillation. Common locations include the hard and soft palate and the dorsum of the tongue.
   c) Angular cheilitis is characterized as a fissuring or cracking of the angles of the mouth (commissures). It is frequently associated with crusting, bleeding, white plaques.
   d) Hyperplastic candidiasis is characterized by white plaques that cannot be scraped off. Common locations include lateral borders of the tongue and buccal mucosa.
   e) Symptoms, in general, will vary and may include bad taste in the mouth, absence of taste, burning, pain when swallowing, and epigastric discomfort. Some individuals may be completely asymptomatic.
4. Differential diagnosis
   a) HSV infection (oral or esophageal)
   b) Conditioning-related mucosal breakdown/tissue damage

5. Diagnostic studies
    a) Made by clinical examination and/or culture
    b) Scrape the lesion (ensure platelets > 20,000); use KOH preparation to look for fungal mycelia, or culture base of lesion for fungus.
    c) Viral culture to rule out HSV
    d) Upper gastrointestinal endoscopy with cultures and brushings to evaluate esophageal complaints and need for systemic antifungals
6. Management [5,8,16]
    a) May treat presumptively based on clinical findings.
    b) Good control of oral candidiasis has been achieved by using a combination of topical antifungals, mouth rinses, and good oral hygiene.
    c) Topical antifungals include[*]:
        (1) Clotrimazole (Mycelex), 10-mg troches, dissolved in saliva up to 4 to 5 times a day for 1 to 2 weeks (adults and children). Takes 10 minutes to dissolve. No food or drink for 20 minutes (may affect compliance).
        (2) Nystatin suspension, 100,000 U/mL
            Adults: 5 to 10 mL qid or 1.3 million U/d divided qid
            Children: 4 to 6 mL qid
        (3) Nystatin tablets, 500,000 U/tablet
            Adults: 1 tablet PO qid
            Children: 1/2 tablet PO qid
        (4) Nystatin troches/pastilles, 200,000 U/dose (adults and children): 400,000 to 600,000 U qid

[*] With topical therapies, patients may experience poor tolerance due to bad taste and nausea (may require IV systemic therapy).

    d) Chlorhexidine 0.12% (Peridex), oral rinse, bid to qid, is used in conjunction with antifungals. It should be used after the initial episode is under control and can be used for maintenance in combination with good oral hygiene. Dosage:

(1) < 0.5 m^2: 5 mL/dose
(2) 0.5 to 1.0 m^2: 10 mL/dose
(3) 1.0 to 1.5 m^2: 15 mL/dose
(4) > 1.5 m^2: 15 mL/dose

e) Significant esophageal disease (or if patient is neutropenic with oral involvement only) may require systemic antifungal therapy.

(1) Fluconazole (Diflucan) is a systemic antifungal with fungicidal activity against *C. albicans*. Its use has resulted in an increase in infection rates of *Torulopsis glabrata* and *Candida krusei*. It is the drug of choice for treatment and prophylaxis. Dosage: greater than 50-kg patient: 200 to 400 mg/d qd IV/PO; 20- to 40-kg patient: 200 mg/d qd IV/PO; less than 20-kg patient: 3 to 8 mg/kg/d qd IV/PO.

(2) Amphotericin B (Fungizone) is a systemic antifungal with fungicidal activity against all species of *Candida*. It is effective against invasive fungus such as that seen with invasive esophageal candidiasis. Dosage: 0.5 to 1.5 mg/kg/d over 2 to 4 hours IV.

(3) Liposomal-encapsulate amphotericin B (Abelcet) may be used in patients with poor renal function. Generally used in the setting of documented fungal infections requiring long-term antifungal therapy. Dosage: 5 mg/kg/d over 2 to 4 hours.

f) Miscellaneous measures

(1) If patient is switched from topical to systemic antifungals for some other clinical reason, topicals may be discontinued while the patient is on systemic therapy.

(2) Encourage frequent oral hygiene q4h with saline or bicarbonate rinses prior to chlorhexidine 0.12% (Peridex) oral rinse and topical antifungals.

(3) Patient should use toothettes with frequent mouth care to encourage debridement.

(4) Foods with high sugar content should be avoided.

(5) Transfuse with platelets and PRBCs as needed for oral or esophageal bleeding.

I. Vaginal candidiasis [8,12,14,15]

1. Definition: Vaginal fungal infection is usually caused by *C. albicans*, but other species of *Candida* can be present.

2. Risk factors
   a) Immunocompromised patients with defective T-lymphocyte function (early post-transplant and in patients on corticosteroids for GVHD)
   b) Also common in patients receiving antibiotics
   c) Women with previous history of vaginal yeast infections pretransplant

3. Clinical features
   a) Intense itching and burning sensation in vaginal area
   b) Reddening of vagina and labia
   c) Thick white discharge with yeast-like odor (discharge may be thinner or clear if patient is neutropenic).

4. Differential diagnosis
   a) HSV infection (type I or II)
   b) Conditioning-related mucosal breakdown/ tissue damage
   c) Bacterial vaginosis

5. Diagnostic studies
   a) Diagnosis is made by clinical examination, KOH preparation, and/or fungal culture.

b) Swab vagina, and use KOH preparation to look for fungal mycelia or culture discharge.

c) Viral culture to rule out HSV

6. Management

a) Patients who have history of frequent candidal vaginitis infections pretransplant should receive prophylaxis during acute phase of BMT.

b) Treat with vaginal inserts: tablets, cream. Topical antifungals include Gynelotrimin/Mycelex/Lotrimin (clotrimazole), Terazol (terconazole), Mycostatin (nystatin), Femstat (butoconazole), and Monistat (miconazole nitrate). The recommended dosage is to use 1 insert per day for 7 days (minimum, or qd while neutropenic). Use at bedtime allows medication to remain in the vagina longer. BMT patients may require prolonged use if symptoms recur (especially while on steroids). Patients should avoid intercourse while on treatment.

c) Fluconazole (Diflucan) can be used for suppressive therapy during period of aplasia or while patient is on steroids or for short-term treatment. It is a systemic antifungal with fungicidal activity against *C. albicans*. Its use has resulted in an increase in infection rates of *T. glabrata* and *C. krusei*. If systemic treatment is used, there is no need for vagina insert. Treat PO (if tolerated) for 10 days. Dosage:

(1) > 50-kg patient: 200 to 400 mg/d qd IV/PO

(2) 20 to 40-kg patient: 200 mg/d qd IV/PO

(3) < 20-kg patient: 3 to 8 mg/kg/d qd IV/PO

J. Hepatosplenic candidiasis[5,14-16]

1. Definition: invasive fungal infection involving the liver and spleen by *Candida* species (e.g., *C. albicans*, *C. tropicalis*, *C. krusei*)

2. Risk factors
   a) Hematologic malignancy
   b) Extensive chemotherapy treatment pretransplant
   c) History of previous *Candida* central venous access device (CVAD) infection or fungemia
   d) Prolonged immunosuppression (delayed engraftment/on corticosteroids for GVHD)
3. Clinical features
   a) Unexplained fever
   b) Hyperbilirubinemia
   c) Elevated liver transaminases
   d) Upper quadrant pain
   e) Hepatosplenomegaly
4. Differential diagnosis
   a) Veno-occlusive disease of the liver
   b) GVHD of the liver
   c) CMV or other viral hepatitis
5. Diagnostic studies
   a) Liver function studies
   b) Abdominal CT to image high-attenuated invasive fungal lesions. Makes presumptive diagnosis in patients at too high risk for liver biopsy.
   c) Liver biopsy for pathology and culture; provides definitive diagnosis and documents response to treatment.
6. Management
   a) Requires long-term systemic antifungal therapy. May require more than six months of therapy.
   b) Systemic antifungal of choice is amphotericin B (Fungizone), which has fungicidal activity against all species of *Candida*. The dosage is 0.5 to 1.5 mg/kg/d over 2 to 4 hours IV. Therapy usually begins daily; once stable, may switch to every other day or 3 times a week.
   c) Due to the long-term nature of this therapy, liposomal-encapsulate amphotericin B (Abelcet)

is often preferred to spare renal function. It provides identical antifungal activity as that of Fungizone. The dosage is 5 mg/kg/d over 2 to 4 hours. Therapy usually begins daily; once stable, may switch to every other day or 3 times a week.

d) Patients who fail to respond to amphotericin B or who suffer severe toxicity may respond to fluconazole, which provides good fungicidal activity against most species of *Candida*. Dosage: 200 to 400 mg qd for 6 to 12 months.

e) Liver imaging and biopsy are used to determine length of required antifungal therapy. It is unknown when and how often these studies should be performed.

K. Fungal septicemia[5]

1. Definition: Fungal blood infection caused by *Candida* species (*C. albicans, C. tropicalis, C. krusei, C. guilliermondii, C. parapsilosis, C. pseudotropicalis, C. lusitaniae, C. rugosa*) or *T. glabrata*. Is commonly secondary to a colonized CVAD. Is often fatal.

2. Risk factors
   a) Neutropenia
   b) Hematologic malignancy
   c) Extensive chemotherapy treatment pretransplant
   d) History of previous *Candida* CVAD infection or fungemia pretransplant
   e) Colonization of other site(s) with *Candida* species
   f) Prolonged immunosuppression (delayed engraftment/on corticosteroids for GVHD)

3. Clinical features
   a) High fever and chills
   b) Myalgias/arthalgias
   c) Hemodynamic instability
   d) Symptoms of warm, cool, and cold shock (see p. 147)

4. Differential diagnosis: bacterial (gram-negative septicemia)
5. Diagnostic studies
   a) Blood cultures for bacteria and fungus: Isolation of causative organism. All patients should have blood cultures done with the onset of fever whether neutropenic or not.
   b) Culture of exit site drainage (if present) for bacteria and fungus
   c) Arterial blood gases: respiratory alkalosis related to hyperventilation, metabolic acidosis related to accumulation of organic acids
   d) Lactic acid
   e) BUN/creatinine: elevated related to renal hypoperfusion
   f) Electrolytes: variable abnormalities
   g) Chest x-ray: Rule out capillary leak or ARDS.
6. Management
   a) Remove CVAD as soon as feasible, and provide alternative access.
   b) Crystalloid, colloid, and vasopressors to maintain hemodynamic stability
   c) Systemic antifungal of choice is amphotericin B (Fungizone), which has fungicidal activity against all species of *Candida*. The dosage is 0.5 to 1.5 mg/kg/d over 2 to 4 hours IV. Therapy usually begins daily; once stable, may switch to every other day or 3 times a week to total dose of approximately 0.5 to 1.0 g with complete resolution of fungemia.
   d) Due to the long-term nature of this therapy, liposomal-encapsulate amphotericin B (Abelcet) is often preferred to spare renal function. It provides identical antifungal activity as that of

Fungizone. The dosage is 5 mg/kg/d over 2 to 4 hours. Therapy usually begins daily; once stable, may switch to every other day or 3 times a week.

   e) Fluconazole may be used if *Candida* species is known to be fluconazole sensitive. It provides good fungicidal activity against some species of *Candida*. Dosage: 200 to 400 mg qd for 6 to 12 months.

L. Aspergillosis[15,17]

1. Definition: Opportunistic infection that primarily invades the lung and other organs such as the brain and pericardium. Is responsible for approximately 10% of all interstitial pneumonia. The most common species are Aspergillus fumigatus and Aspergillus flavus. Is almost always fatal.

2. Risk factors
   a) Allogeneic transplant recipient
   b) Pulmonary colonization pretransplant (usually not known)
   c) Prolonged neutropenia
   d) High-dose corticosteroids

3. Clinical features
   a) Are often subtle: persistent fever, mild productive cough, pleuritic-type chest pain.
   b) Chest x-ray: rapidly progressing nodular infiltrate, often cavitating lesions that cross lung fissures
   c) As disease progresses, fever worsens, rales develop, pulmonary infiltrates appear, and if brain metastasis is present, there are neurological changes.

4. Differential diagnosis*
   a) Bacterial pneumonia, especially cavitary TB, atypical bacterial or *Legionella* pneumonia
   b) Other fungi: *Cryptococcus neoformans*, *Candida* species

c) Protozoa: *P. carinii, Toxoplasma gondii*

d) Viral: CMV, HSV, VZV, RSV, parainfluenza

* Unable to establish definitive diagnosis without bronchoalveolar lavage/tissue. Time sequence post transplant and x-ray picture are important when establishing a differential diagnosis.

5. Diagnostic studies
   a) Chest x-ray: classic pattern of rapidly progressing nodular infiltrate, often cavitating lesions that cross lung fissures
   b) Identification of organism in sputum (rare), bronchoalveolar lavage or open lung biopsy. Specimens should be sent for pathology, bacterial and fungal cultures, viral culture, immunofluorescent antibody, or rapid shell, silver stain to rule out *P. carinii,* acid-fast bacilli, *Mycoplasma,* and *Legionella.*

6. Management
   a) Surgical resection of fungating lesion if possible (isolated "fungal balls" may sometimes be effectively resected).
   b) Support oxygenation (via O₂ or mechanical ventilation)
   c) Aggressive systemic antifungal therapy is required even if fungal lesion is resectable.
   d) Systemic antifungal of choice is amphotericin B (Fungizone), which has fungicidal activity against species of *Aspergillus*. The dosage is 1.0 to 1.5 mg/kg/d over 2 to 4 hours IV. Therapy is daily; once stable, may switch to every other day or 3 times a week to total dose of approximately 2.0 to 2.5 g. May use less if response is good.
   e) Due to the long-term nature of this therapy, liposomal-encapsulate amphotericin B (Abelcet) may be preferred to spare renal function. It provides identical antifungal activity as that

of Fungizone. The dosage is 5mg/kg/d over 2 to 4 hours. Therapy usually begins daily; once stable, may switch to every other day or 3 times a week to total dose of approximately 10 to 15 g. May use less if response is good.

f) Itraconazole has fungicidal activity against species of Aspergillus and may be more effective than amphotericin B. It is difficult to use in critically ill patients, since its only form is oral. The dosage in adults is 200 to 400 mg PO. The dosage in children is unknown. It should be taken with a carbonated beverage for maximum absorption.

g) Use of 5 FC, rifampin, tetracycline in combination with amphotericin B has questionable efficacy.

M. *Pneumocystis carinii* pneumonia (PCP)[5,12,18]

1. Definition: Common opportunistic organism infecting the lung. Is thought to infect most humans in early childhood and then remains dormant. Becomes active in immunodeficient persons; most commonly 30+ days post-BMT. Infection is rare in patients compliant with prophylaxis.

2. Risk factors
   a) Allogeneic transplant recipient
   b) Immunocompromised patients with defective T-lymphocyte function (early post-transplant and in patients on corticosteroids for GVHD)
   c) Pretransplant history of PCP
   d) Lack of proper PCP prophylaxis pre- and post-transplant

3. Clinical features
   a) Dry, nonproductive cough
   b) Shortness of breath, tachypnea
   c) Hypoxemia, restrictive defect
   d) Less specific symptoms such as fever, malaise, weight loss

e) Chest x-ray reveals diffuse interstitial alveolar pneumonia that is bilateral and symmetrical

4. Differential diagnosis [*]
   a) Bacterial pneumonia, especially atypical bacterial or *Legionella* pneumonia
   b) Other fungi: *C. neoformans, Candida* species, aspergillosis
   c) Protozoa: *T. gondii*
   d) Viral: CMV, HSV, VZV, respiratory syncytial virus (RSV), parainfluenza

[*] Unable to establish definitive diagnosis without bronchoalveolar lavage or tissue. Time sequence post-transplant and x-ray picture are important when establishing a differential diagnosis.

5. Diagnostic studies
   a) Chest x-ray reveals diffuse interstitial alveolar pneumonia that is bilateral, symmetric, and rapidly progressing.
   b) Arterial blood gases/O_2 saturation reveal decreased PO_2 and saturation.
   c) Induced sputum/bronchoalveolar lavage, or open lung biopsy for silver staining. Specimens should also be sent for pathology, bacterial, and fungal cultures, viral culture, immunofluorescent antibody, or rapid shell, acid-fast bacilli, *Mycoplasma,* and *Legionella.*
   d) Gallium scan: not necessarily required if definitive diagnosis obtained with bronchoalveolar lavage

6. Management [5]
   a) Support oxygenation (via O_2 or mechanical ventilation).
   b) For acutely ill patients (PO_2 < 70 mm Hg), give prednisone, 40 mg PO bid for 5 days.

c) Drug of choice is co-trimoxazole (Bactrim, Septra). The dosage is 20 mg (trimethoprim)/kg/d IV divided q6–8 hours for 21 days. Allergy to sulfa can cause rash and fever. If severe, drug should be discontinued (may lead to Stevens-Johnson syndrome). Is also myelosuppressive.

d) If unable to tolerate co-trimoxazole due to myelosuppression or already low blood counts, use dapsone plus trimethoprim. The dosage is dapsone, 100 mg/d PO, plus trimethoprim, 5 mg/kg PO q6h for 21 days (if able to tolerate PO). Can cause hemolysis of red blood cells in the absence of glucose-6-phosphate-dehydrogenase (G6PD); order test for G6PD before starting. Patients with history of sulfa reaction (rash, fever), may also react to dapsone.

e) Alternative to co-trimoxazole or dapsone plus trimethoprim is pentamidine, 4 mg/kg/d IV for 21 days or 600 mg in 6 mL of sterile water qd for 21 days by aerosol nebulizer. If aerosolized pentamidine is used, rule out pulmonary TB with two to three acid-fast bacteria smears.

f) Following 21 days of treatment, patient should be switched to prophylaxis (see chapter 3).

g) Corticosteroids are often added to the above regimens in documented cases of PCP.[19] If used, it should be started within 72 hours of initiating anti-PCP therapy. Dosage (prednisone):
   (1) 40 mg bid days 1 to 5
   (2) 40 mg qd days 6 to 10
   (3) 20 mg qd days 11 to 21

N. *Toxoplasma gondii* infection[5,14,18]

1. Definition: Infection caused by protozoan parasite, *T. gondii*. Most frequently occurring CNS infection in BMT patients; can also cause pneumonia. Approximately 30% of U.S. population are infected with *T. gondii* during life; may be reactivated when the immune system is damaged.

2. Risk factors
   a) Allogeneic transplant recipient
   b) Previous colonization with *T. gondii.*

3. Clinical features
   a) CNS toxoplasmosis: mild to severe headache, fever, CNS impairment (neurological problems, changes in mental status, seizures), possible destruction of retina, coma.
   b) *Toxoplasma* pneumonia: fever, cough/shortness of breath, rales, bilateral pulmonary infiltrates on chest x-ray

4. Differential diagnosis
   a) CNS toxoplasmosis: other CNS infection (*C. neoformans,* aspergillosis, *Candida* species, *Listeria pneumoniae, S. pneumoniae, E. coli,* alpha streptococcus, HSV, VZV), cyclosporine-induced neurotoxicity, metabolic encephalopathy, malignant CNS disease, CNS bleed or vascular event
   b) *Toxoplasma* pneumonia*: other pneumonia, atypical bacteria, *Legionella, C. neoformans, Candida* species, aspergillosis, PCP, CMV, HSV, VZV, RSV, parainfluenza

* Unable to establish definitive diagnosis without bronchoalveolar lavage/tissue. Time sequence post-transplant and x-ray picture are important when establishing a differential diagnosis.

5. Diagnostic studies
   a) *T. gondii* IgM antibody
   b) CT scan/magnetic resonance imaging (MRI) for ring-enhancing lesions
   c) Brain biopsy is indicated if *T. gondii* antibody is negative, single lesion, or progressive symptoms, or no improvement after 14 days of treatment.
   d) Lumbar puncture: cerebrospinal fluid (CSF) for profile, cytology, culture, IFA, electron microscopy
   e) Bronchoalveolar lavage/open lung biopsy: Specimens should also be sent for pathology, bacterial and fungal cultures, viral culture, immunofluorescent antibody, or rapid shell, silver stain, acid-fast bacteria, *Mycoplasma,* and *Legionella.*

6. Management
   a) Pyrimethamine (Daraprim), 100 mg PO day 1, then 50 to 75 mg daily for 4 to 5 weeks; plus sulfadiazine, 4 to 8 g PO/IV; plus folinic acid, 10 mg PO for 3 to 6 weeks. Side effects include decreased white blood cells, red blood cells, and platelets; crystals in urine; fever; rash; abdominal pain; headaches; and abnormal liver function tests.
   b) Pyrimethamine (Daraprim), 100 mg PO day 1, then 50 to 75 mg daily for 4 to 5 weeks; plus clindamycin, 900 mg IV q6h for 3 weeks. Side effects include diarrhea, inflammation of large intestine *(C. difficile),* rash, abnormal liver function tests, abdominal pain.

O. Cytomegalovirus (CMV) infection[12-14,20-23]
   1. Definition: Virus in the herpes family. CMV infection can occur in the gastrointestinal tract, lungs, liver, brain, retina, and other organs; occurs most commonly in the lung of allogeneic BMT recipients greater

than 30 days post-transplant. Infection occurs one of three ways:

a) Reactivation of latent CMV
b) An acquired viral pathogen from an infected marrow donor
c) An acquired viral pathogen through a blood transfusion

2. Risk factors
   a) Allogeneic BMT recipient who is seropositive for CMV or has a donor that is seropositive
   b) Recipient of a blood product that is seropositive for CMV that was not leuko-reduced or leukopoor filtered.
   c) Inadequate CMV prophylaxis for seropositive patients
   d) Acute GVHD

3. Clinical features
   a) CMV pneumonitis: fever, shortness of breath, hypoxia; "fluffy," usually bilateral interstitial infiltrates on chest x-ray; diminished breath sounds bilaterally on auscultation
   b) Liver: elevated liver transaminases and bilirubin, ascites, hepatomegaly
   c) Retina: blurred vision, floaters, loss of peripheral vision in one or both eyes, loss of vision in isolated fields
   d) Gastrointestinal: diarrhea, loss of gastrointestinal mucosa, esophagitis
   e) CNS: CNS impairment (non-focal neurologic findings, seizures, changes in mental status), headache, coma

4. Differential diagnosis
   a) Pulmonary*: bacterial pneumonia (especially atypical bacterial or *Legionella* pneumonia), *C. neoformans*, *Candida* species, aspergillosis,

coccidioidomycosis, PCP, *T. gondii,* HSV, VZV, RSV, parainfluenza.

* Unable to establish definitive diagnosis without bronchoalveolar lavage/tissue. Time sequence post-transplant and x-ray picture are important when establishing a differential diagnosis.

  b) Liver: viral hepatitis (VZV, hepatitis B, hepatitis C), TB or *M. avium-intracellulare* infection, hepatic GVHD, drug toxicity
  c) Retina: aspergillosis or other fungal pathogen
  d) Gastrointestinal: bacterial enteritis (*Yersinia, Salmonella, Shigella,* enterotoxic *E. coli, C. difficile, C. jejuni, Klebsiella*), viral enteritis (rotavirus, Norwalk virus, adenovirus), gut GVHD, toxicity from conditioning therapy
  e) CNS: other CNS infection (*C. neoformans,* aspergillosis, *Candida* species, *L. pneumoniae, S. pneumoniae, E. coli,* alpha streptococcus, HSV, VZV), cyclosporine-induced neurotoxicity, metabolic encephalopathy, malignant CNS disease, CNS bleed or vascular event

5. Diagnostic studies
  a) CMV IgM antibody titer
  b) CMV buffy coat
  c) Urine culture for CMV excretion
  d) Pulmonary: Bronchoalveolar lavage/open lung biopsy to identify "inclusion bodies" and polymerase chain reaction to identify CMV virus. Specimens should also be sent for pathology, bacterial and fungal cultures, viral culture, immunofluorescent antibody, or rapid shell, silver stain, acid-fast bacteria, *Mycoplasma,* and *Legionella.*
  e) Gastrointestinal: stool for CMV antigen and culture. Stool should always be sent for ova and parasites and *C. difficile* toxin with any diarrheal

illness. Stool for viral culture and electron microscopy to identify other viral pathogens.

    f) Ophthalmologic diagnosis; use of "Amsler grid."

    g) CNS: lumbar puncture—CSF for profile, cytology culture, IFA, electron microscopy

6. Management: Treatment of CMV is often empiric.

    a) Ganciclovir (Cytovene) inhibits viral replication. The dosage is 5 mg/kg/12 h IV for 2 weeks, then 5 times a week until day +120. May cause low blood counts/marrow suppression (may necessitate modification or change in therapy).

    b) Foscarnet (Foscavir): Elevation of serum creatinine is seen in 50% of patients treated (may necessitate change or modification in therapy).

      (1) Dosage: 40 to 60 mg/kg/8 h IV

      (2) Induction: 60 mg/kg IV over 2 hours q8h for 14 days

      (3) Maintenance: 90 to 120 mg/kg daily until day +120

    c) Intravenous immune globulin is often used in combination with ganciclovir or foscarnet in the treatment of CMV disease. Dosage: 400 to 600 mg/kg/day qd or every other day for 10 doses.

P. Herpes simplex virus (HSV) infection[12,13,24]

1. Definition: a vesicular eruption of skin or mucous membranes caused by infection with HSV 1 or 2

    a) Most cases are secondary to viral reactivation.

    b) Usually occurs early post-transplant, but may occur once patient is off prophylaxis.

    c) Acyclovir-resistant strains of HSV are emerging.

    d) Can also be caused from primary infection.

    e) HSV encephalitis is also seen in immunocompromised patients.

2. Risk factors

    a) Seropositive for HSV

    b) Prior history of repeated HSV infection

c) GVHD on steroids

d) Inability to tolerate adequate HSV prophylaxis

3. Clinical features

   a) Lesions are painful vesicles, usually several millimeters in diameter, on an erythematous base. Intraoral lesions appear as erythematous ulcerations.

   b) Lesions most frequently occur intraorally or extralabially; in the vagina, on the penis, and around the anal opening; and on buttocks and thighs. Occasionally other body parts are affected.

   c) Type 1 usually affects skin and mucous membranes above the umbilicus.

   d) Type 1 can also manifest as acute keratoconjunctivitis with intense swelling of the eyelid with no exudate. Herpetic vesicles may be found near the affected eye.

   d) Type 2 usually affects skin and mucous membranes below the umbilicus.

   e) After primary infection, the virus remains latent in the dorsal root ganglia of nerve cells that are in the area of the original lesions.

   f) Lesions are infectious until fully crusted or until intraoral lesions have resolved.

4. Differential diagnosis of oral lesions

   a) Gram-negative bacteria: *Klebsiella, Proteus, E. coli, Enterobacter, Pseudomonas.* Such lesions are usually gray in appearance.

   b) *Pseudomonas* ulcers: gray in appearance with blue-black eschar surrounded by an erythematous halo

   c) *C. albicans*: Lesions are curdy, white patches or clumps that cause bleeding and red, raw appearance when removed, or pseudomembranous coating (fungus and epithelial cells) that wipes

off; or erythema that is patchy and diffuse or
white and exudative.
5. Differential diagnosis of genital lesions
   a) Genital warts
   b) *Lymphogranuloma venereum*: Appear as 2- to
      3-mm painless vesicle or nonindurated ulcer.
   c) *Molluscum contagiosum* virus: Appear as 1- to
      5-mm, smooth, rounded, firm, shiny flesh-colored,
      pearly-white papules on anogenital area and
      trunk.
   d) Conditioning-related perianal skin breakdown
6. Diagnostic studies
   a) Direct visualization of classic herpetic
      lesion/vesicle
   b) HSV IgM antibodies (IgG antibody will document
      past history of disease.)
   c) Microscopic examination (from swab of lesion
      base): identification of multinucleated giant cells
      with intranuclear inclusion
   d) Tissue culture: Erupt vesicle, and swab base
      of lesion. Culture is the only true test of active
      disease; a positive result is usually available in
      one to two days.
7. Management
   a) Acyclovir (Zovirax) is gold standard of therapy:
      (1) Adult: 200 mg PO 5 times a day (if able to
          tolerate PO) or 250 mg/m^2 IV q8h
      (2) Children: 250 mg/m^2 IV q8h
      (3) For frequent recurrences: 200 to 800 mg bid
          for suppression
      (4) Acyclovir ointment may be used alone for iso-
          lated, small lesions (should not be used for
          lesions that occur within the first 40 days
          post-transplant).
   b) Foscarnet may be used in acyclovir-resistant
      disease. Elevation of serum creatinine is seen in

50% of patients treated (may necessitate change or modification in therapy).

    (1) Dosage: 40 to 60 mg/kg/8 h IV

    (2) Induction: 60 mg/kg IV over 2 hours q8h for 14 days

    (3) Maintenance: 90 to 120 mg/kg until day +120.

c) Patients should wear gloves when applying topical medication.

d) Keep the affected areas as clean as possible.

e) Meticulous oral care: Use precautions when handling oral secretions.

f) Avoid touching lesions and then other parts of body; wash hands after touching lesions.

g) Medicate for pain; use topical analgesic if appropriate.

Q. Herpes zoster infection [12,13,24]

1. Definition: reactivation of varicella-zoster virus (VZV)

    a) May be localized to a single dermatome (shingles) or disseminated.

    b) Usually occurs four to five months post-transplant.

    c) May also be associated with visceral involvement (pulmonary and hepatic most common).

    d) VZV encephalitis is also seen in immunocompromised patients with disseminated disease.

2. Risk factors

    a) Seropositive for VZV

    b) Diagnosis of Hodgkin's disease

    c) Prior history of repeated VZV infection

    d) GVHD on steroids

3. Clinical features

    a) Appear as patches of raised, erythematous papules that evolve into vesicles.

    b) Lesions follow paths of large dermatomes (shingles) or may be disseminated.

    c) Commonly occur on legs, buttocks, head, arms, and back.
    d) For exposed patients, vesicles may occur 1 to 7 days after exposure.
    e) Shingles may present as a prodrome of pain along the affected nerve and fever.
    f) CNS infection: headache, altered mental status (is often fatal)
    g) Hepatic infection: hyperbilirubinemia, transaminitis
    h) Pulmonary infection: interstitial pneumonitis

4. Differential diagnosis
    a) Early in the disease course, rash may be mistaken for drug rash, acute GVHD, or fungal or viral skin rash.
    b) Vesicles are diagnostic of classic VZV infection.
    c) Visceral disease is rarely seen without cutaneous manifestations.

5. Diagnostic studies
    a) Visual examination of vesicles; further studies usually not required for definitive diagnosis
    b) Tanck test
    c) Viral culture
    d) Ophthalmalogic examination if trigeminal dermatome affected
    e) Liver function tests and chest x-ray with onset of disease
    f) Lumbar puncture: Send CSF for viral culture, immunofluorescent antibody.

6. Management
    a) Acyclovir, 500 mg/m^2 IV q8h. For infection in first 100 days post-BMT, if patient is on immunosuppression for GVHD, or if visceral disease is expected
    b) May use oral acyclovir 800 mg 5 times a day for 1 week, if isolated to a single dermatome.

    c) If progresses to more than one dermatome on oral therapy, change to intravenous acyclovir.

    d) For varicella exposure[8]: If patient is actively receiving intravenous immune globulin (IVIG), observe for outbreak and isolate for two weeks. Other exposed post-BMT patients should receive varicella immune globulin (VZIG). VZIG should be administered within 96 hours of exposure and provides three weeks of protection. VZIG dosage:

      (1) Less than or equal to 10 kg: 125 U IM

      (2) 10.1 to 20 kg: 250 U IM

      (3) 20.1 to 30 kg: 375 U IM

      (4) 30.1 to 40 kg: 500 U IM

      (5) Greater than 40 kg: 625 U IM (not > 2.5 mL /injection site)

    e) Keep lesions as clean and dry as possible.

    f) Affected areas may itch; try to avoid scratching.

    g) Wear loose cotton clothing to minimize irritation.

    h) Do not touch lesions and then other body orifices to avoid auto-inoculation.

R. Human herpes virus type 6 (HHV-6) infection[25,26]

    1. Definition: newly recognized (1986) herpesvirus pathogen capable of causing infection in immunocompromised patients

      a) Healthy people are primarily infected with a benign febrile illness (roseola infantum).

      b) After primary infection, similar to other herpesviruses, HHV-6 can persist in the host in a latent form that has been detected in circulating monocytes and the epithelia of the bronchial and salivary glands.

      c) Reactivation can lead to interstitial pneumonitis, hepatitis, encephalitis, and bone marrow failure.

    2. Risk factors

      a) Allogeneic BMT recipient with past HHV-6 exposure

b) Acute GVHD on steroids

c) Others unknown

3. Clinical features

   a) HHV-6 interstitial pneumonitis: fever, shortness of breath, hypoxia; "fluffy," usually bilateral interstitial infiltrates on chest x-ray; diminished breath sounds bilaterally on auscultation

   b) HHV-6 hepatitis: elevated liver transaminases and bilirubin, ascites, hepatomegaly

   c) HHV-6 encephalitis: headache, altered mental status

   d) HHV-6 marrow failure: pancytopenia in a patient with previous signs of engraftment

4. Differential diagnosis

   a) Pulmonary*: bacterial pneumonia (especially atypical bacterial or *Legionella* pneumonia), *C. neoformans, Candida* species, aspergillosis, coccidioidomycosis, PCP, *T. gondii,* HSV, VZV, RSV, parainfluenza

* Unable to establish definitive diagnosis without bronchoalveolar lavage/tissue. Time sequence post-transplant and x-ray picture are important when establishing a differential diagnosis.

   b) Liver: viral hepatitis (VZV, hepatitis B, hepatitis C), TB or *M. avium-intracellulare* infection, hepatic GVHD, and drug toxicity

   c) CNS: other CNS infection (*C. neoformans,* aspergillosis, *Candida* species, *L. pneumoniae, S. pneumoniae, E. coli,* alpha streptococcus, HSV, VZV), cyclosporine-induced neurotoxicity, metabolic encephalopathy, malignant CNS disease, CNS bleed or vascular event

   d) Marrow failure: primary graft failure, CMV or other viral infection, GVHD, drug-induced myelosuppression

5. Diagnostic studies

a) HHV-6 Igm serology
b) Identification relies either on restriction endonu-
clease analysis or DNA sequencing (done on lung
tissue, liver tissue, CSF, or bone marrow).
c) Several laboratories are attempting to develop
an HHV-6 rapid shell culture.

6. Management
a) Unclear whether current antivirals (acyclovir,
ganciclovir, foscarnet) are effective in treating
HHV-6 disease but are often used in cases of
documented or suspected disease.
b) Intravenous immune globulin may be used alone
or in combination with acyclovir, ganciclovir,
or foscarnet in the treatment of HHV-6 disease.
Dosage: 400 to 600 mg/kg/d qd or every other
day for 10 doses.

S. Parainfluenza virus[27,28]
1. Definition: an uncommon (2.2%) RNA virus that
infects the upper and lower respiratory tract and
may lead to serious/fatal interstitial pneumonia in
immunocompromised patients
2. Risk factors
a) Isolation of RSV from the upper respiratory tract
places the immunocompromised BMT patient at
risk for lower tract disease.
b) Prolonged use of steroids
c) None other known
3. Clinical features
a) Presents as typical viral respiratory infection.
b) Two clinically distinct groups can be identified
on the basis of the presence or absence of lower
respiratory tract involvement.
c) Upper tract symptoms include fever, cough,
coryza, and otitis media. Sinus films may reveal
opacification. Chest x-ray is clear.
d) Lower tract symptoms include fever, cough,

coryza, wheezing, and shortness of breath. Sinus films may reveal opacification. Chest x-ray reveals diffuse interstitial pulmonary infiltrates. Arterial blood gases show hypoxemia.

4. Differential diagnosis*
   a) Bacterial pneumonia, especially atypical bacterial or *Legionella* pneumonia
   b) Fungi: *C. neoformans, Candida* species, aspergillosis, coccidioidomycosis
   c) Protozoa: PCP, *T. gondii*
   d) Viral: HSV, VZV, RSV

* Unable to establish definitive diagnosis without bronchoalveolar lavage/tissue. Time sequence post-transplant varies with parainfluenza. X-ray picture is that of other viral pneumonias.

5. Diagnostic studies
   a) Sinus films and chest x-ray
   b) Parainfluenza culture (nasopharyngeal, throat, or bronchoalveolar lavage sample) with onset of upper or lower tract symptoms. Is often underdiagnosed due to poor culturing techniques in the past.
   c) Pulmonary: Bronchoalveolar lavage/open lung biopsy for culture. Specimens should also be sent for pathology, bacterial and fungal cultures, viral culture, immunofluorescent antibody, or rapid shell, silver stain, acid-fast bacteria, *Mycoplasma,* and *Legionella.*

6. Management
   a) Aerosolized ribavirin has been used with some success if used early in the disease. Administer by aerosol 12 to 18 hours daily for 3 to 7 days. Dilute 6-g vial in 300 mL preservative-free sterile water to a final concentration of 20 mg/mL. Must be administered with Viratek Small Particle Generator

(SPAG-2).
- b) Intravenous immune globulin may be used, although efficacy is unknown.
- c) Treat hypoxemia: oxygen support/mechanical ventilation if needed.

T. Respiratory syncytial virus (RSV) infection[28-30]

1. Definition: viral infection affecting the upper and lower respiratory tracts common in healthy children. Increasing prevalence in BMT and other immunocompromised patients

2. Risk factors
   - a) Allogeneic BMT recipients
   - b) Children less than 12 to 18 months of age
   - c) Pretransplant immunosuppression
   - d) GVHD on steroids
   - e) Chronic lung disease pretransplant

3. Clinical features
   - a) Presents as typical viral respiratory infection.
   - b) Early presentation of upper tract symptoms: fever, nonproductive cough, coryza, otitis media
   - c) Symptoms progress to wheezes, shortness of breath, dyspnea, and hypoxia.
   - d) Chest x-ray reveals bilateral interstitial infiltrates.
   - e) Some patients will demonstrate opacity on sinus films.

4. Differential diagnosis*
   - a) Bacterial pneumonia, especially atypical bacterial or *Legionella* pneumonia
   - b) Fungi: *C. neoformans, Candida* species, aspergillosis, coccidioidomycosis
   - c) Protozoa: PCP, *T. gondii*
   - d) Viral: HSV, VZV, parainfluenza

* Unable to establish definitive diagnosis without bronchoalveolar lavage/tissue. Time sequence post-transplant varies with RSV. X-ray picture is that of other viral pneu-

monias.

5. Diagnostic studies
   a) Chest x-ray and sinus films
   b) Antigen test available in most institutions
   c) Obtain specimens from bronchoalveolar lavage, sputum, throat, sinus aspirate, or lung biopsy for immunofluorescence or enzyme-linked immunosorbent assay for RSV.
   d) RSV culture of above stated tissue
   e) Pulmonary: Bronchoalveolar lavage/open lung biopsy for culture. Specimens should also be sent for pathology, bacterial and fungal cultures, viral culture, immunofluorescent antibody, or rapid shell, silver stain, acid-fast bacteria, *Mycoplasma,* and *Legionella.*
   f) Frequent O_2 saturation measurements to document effectiveness of ribavirin

6. Management
   a) Aerosolized ribavirin has been used with some success in BMT patients if used early in the disease. Administer by aerosol 12 to 18 hours daily until RSV is cleared (per antigen, culture, or antibody testing). Dilute 6-g vial in 300-mL preservative-free sterile water to a final concentration of 20 mg/mL. Must be administered with Viratek Small Particle Generator (SPAG-2).
   b) Intravenous immune globulin has been shown to decrease viral shedding and improve O_2 saturation. It is often used in combination with ribavirin. Dosage: 400 to 600 mg/kg/d qd every other day for 10 doses.
   c) RSV immune globulin: not yet commercially available. Animal studies promising
   d) Treat hypoxemia: oxygen support/mechanical ventilation if needed.

U. Adenovirus infection[2,6,13,17,31]

1. Definition: Viral infection seen in immunocompromised patients, most commonly associated with hemorrhagic cystitis in BMT patients. Has also been associated with interstitial pneumonitis, viral enteritis, and viral hepatitis.

2. Risk factors
   a) Prolonged immunosuppression
   b) Previous bladder injury
   c) Allogeneic BMT recipient

3. Clinical features
   a) Hemorrhagic cystitis, which may begin as microscopic hematuria and progress to frank bladder hemorrhage
   b) Interstitial pneumonitis: fever, cough, shortness of breathing, dyspnea. Chest x-ray reveals bilateral interstitial infiltrates.
   c) Gastroenteritis: diarrhea, abdominal cramping
   d) Liver/hepatitis: transaminitis

4. Differential diagnosis*
   a) Hemorrhagic cystitis: cyclophosphamide-induced or BK (human polyoma) viruria
   b) Interstitial pneumonitis: bacterial pneumonia (especially atypical bacterial or *Legionella* pneumonia), *C. neoformans, Candida* species, aspergillosis, coccidioidomycosis, PCP, *T. gondii,* HSV, VZV, RSV, parainfluenza
   c) Gastroenteritis: GVHD, bacterial, enteritis, *C. difficile* colitis, CMV, rotavirus, or coxsackievirus viral enteritis
   d) Liver/hepatitis: GVHD, drug-induced liver toxicity or hepatitis, CMV, HSV, VZV, EBV hepatitis, hemolysis

* Unable to establish definitive diagnosis without bronchoalveolar lavage/tissue. Time sequence post-transplant and x-ray picture are important when establishing a differential diagnosis.

5. Diagnostic studies
   a) Adenovirus antigen or culture of urine, lung tissue (bronchoalveolar lavage specimen), stool culture, gastrointestinal mucosal biopsy, or culture of liver biopsy specimen
   b) Pulmonary: Bronchoalveolar lavage/open lung biopsy for culture/antigen detection. Specimens should also be sent for pathology, bacterial and fungal cultures, viral culture, immunofluorescent antibody, or rapid shell, silver stain, acid-fast bacteria, *Mycoplasma,* and *Legionella.*
   c) Stool samples or gastrointestinal biopsies should also be sent to rule out GVHD (biopsy), bacterial, *C. difficile,* CMV, HSV, rotavirus, coxsackievirus, or other viral pathogens (viral studies by immunofluorescent antibody, antigen detection, culture, or rapid shell).
   d) Follow liver function studies closely (at least qd with acute elevations).
   e) Liver biopsy may be required with worsening liver function studies and should be sent for pathology (to rule out GVHD), fungal and viral studies.
6. Management
   a) No antiviral therapy available for adenovirus
   b) Intravenous immune globulin has been used.
   c) For acute hemorrhagic cystitis, consult urology service. Continuous bladder irrigation, silver nitrate, alum, or prostaglandin instillations may be required to stop bladder bleeding.

V. Viral enteritis[2,5,13,31]

1. Definition: viral infection of the gastrointestinal tract
   a) Usual pathogens include CMV, HSV, adenovirus, rotavirus, Norwalk virus, and coxsackievirus.
   b) Commonly occurs more than 30 days post-transplant.
   c) Viral enteritis may trigger flare of acute GVHD, or viral superinfection can occur in the face of gut GVHD.

2. Risk factors
   a) Allogeneic BMT recipient
   b) Very young patients
   c) Pretransplant immunodeficiency
   d) GVHD on steroids

3. Clinical features
   a) Profuse, liquid diarrhea
   b) Abdominal pain/cramping
   c) Fever
   d) Epigastric pain/dysphagia (CMV esophagitis)
   e) Dehydration
   f) Abdominal distension/ileus in severe cases

4. Differential diagnosis
   a) Bacterial enteritis or *C. difficile*
   b) Parasitic infection: *Giardia lambia, Cryptosporidium,* or *Strongyloides*
   c) Conditioning-related toxicity
   d) Acute GVHD

5. Diagnostic studies
   a) Stool viral studies: culture, rapid shell, antigen detection, immunofluorescent antibody
   b) Stool for bacteria culture, ova and parasites, *C. difficile* toxin to rule out other infectious causes.
   c) Endoscopic examination with cultures and biopsy if GVHD suspected

6. Management
   a) Identify and treat underlying cause. Treat CMV
      with ganciclovir or foscarnet with or without
      intravenous immune globulin. Treat HSV with
      acyclovir (if sensitive) or foscarnet. Intravenous
      immune globulin may be used with other viral
      pathogens. Has also been used PO, but efficacy
      of this route of administration is unknown.
   b) Correct fluid, electrolyte, and acid-base
      abnormalities.
   c) Provide symptomatic relief. Antidiarrheal agents
      such as diphenoxylate hydrochloride with atropine
      sulfate (Lomotil) are not recommended in the face
      of enteric pathogens. The recommended dosage
      for Octreotide acetate (Sandostatin) is 1 to 10
      µg/kg/24 h.
   d) Protect skin in the perirectal area from breakdown.
      Moisture barriers or ointments should be used
      preventively (Desitin, Carrington Moisture
      Barrier Cream, 1:1 zinc oxide, and A & D
      ointment mixture).

III. Graft Versus Host Disease (GVHD)[32–45]

A. Acute GVHD
   1. Definition
      a) A common complication of allogeneic BMT in
         which an immunologic response occurs in the
         marrow recipient whereby immunologically
         competent T cells from the donor marrow attack
         the seemingly "foreign" host, resulting in varying
         degrees of severity
      b) Damage occurs to three target organs: the skin,
         gastrointestinal tract, and liver.
      c) Acute GVHD is defined as occurring within the
         first 100 days post-transplant.

2. Etiology: From an immunologic standpoint, GVHD is initiated when:
   a) Genetically determined histocompatibility differences exist between the bone marrow recipient and the bone marrow donor.
   b) Immunocompetent cells in the donor's marrow that can recognize the foreign histocompatibility antigens of the host and can therefore mount an immunologic reaction against them are present
   c) The bone marrow recipient is unable to react against and reject the donor marrow.
   d) It is thought that the underlying mechanism of GVHD is alloaggression resulting from histocompatibility differences. It is unclear, however, what the exact immunologic events are that cause the disease or bring about associated phenomena such as autoimmunity, immunodeficiency, and immune dysfunction.
3. Risk factors
   a) Matched unrelated donor transplant
   b) HLA-mismatched donor transplant
   c) Sex-matched transplant, with a female-to-male graft having increased incidence, especially with female donors who are multiparous or have had a previous transfusion(s)
   d) Increasing age of recipient or donor
   e) Transfusion of nonirradiated blood products and increased number of post-transplant transfusions
   f) Disease status at time of transplant (in relapse)
   g) Viral or enteric infections (prior herpesvirus infection)
   h) Microorganism colonization
   i) Low pretransplant performance status or Karnofsky score

4. Clinical features: See Table 5.7 for clinical staging and grading of acute GVHD. (Symptoms usually arise near the time of marrow engraftment, but can occur anytime within the first 100 days post-transplant.)

   a) Skin manifestations first appear as macular/papular rash or erythema, which may be described as pruritic and "sunburn"-like. It commonly first appears on palms, soles, and ears; as the rash intensifies, involvement spreads to the trunk, face, and extremities and becomes more confluent. In severe forms, bullous lesions and epidermal necrolysis may develop. Isolated skin involvement is not uncommon.

   b) Liver manifestations: Acute GVHD usually presents with abnormal liver function studies; no specific abnormal findings are diagnostic. Elevation in conjugated bilirubin is most common. Elevated liver transaminases are also common. Hepatomegaly and right upper quadrant tenderness are present in more severe cases. Isolated liver involvement is rare.

   c) Gut manifestations: Lower gastrointestinal GVHD first manifests as watery diarrhea, which may be voluminous and is usually forest-green in appearance. Nausea, vomiting, and severe abdominal cramping are seen as the disease progresses. Isolated gut involvement is rare. This is the most difficult form of GVHD to treat.

5. Differential diagnosis

   a) Skin manifestations: drug rash, Stevens-Johnson syndrome, infection (cutaneous candidiasis, early VZV), erythema multiforme

   b) Liver manifestations: CsA toxicity, other drug toxicity, viral hepatitis (hepatitis A, B, or C), other infection (CMV, HSV, VZV, EBV), hemolytic-uremic syndrome, veno-occlusive disease

Table 5.7 Clinical Staging and Grading of Acute GVHD

Staging by Organ

Organ	Stage	Parameters
		Rash
Skin	I	< 25% BSA
	II	25–50% BSA
	III	Generalized erythroderma
	IV	Bullae & desquamation
		Total bilirubin (mg/dL)
Liver	I	2.0–3.5
	II	3.5–8.0
	III	8.0–15.0
	IV	> 15.0
		Volume of diarrhea (mL/24 h)
Gut	I	Adults: 500–1000 mL/d Children: 10–15 mL/kg/d
	II	Adults: 1000–1500 mL/d Children: 15–20 mL/kg/d
	III	Adults: 1500–2000 mL/d Children: 20–30 mL/kg/d
	IV	Adults: > 2000 mL/d Children: > 30 mL/kg/d

Overall Clinical Grade

Grade	Description
0	Stage I clinical skin GVHD (with grade 2 histology)
I	Stage II clinical skin GVHD (with ≥ grade 2 histology)
II	Stage II–III clinical skin GVHD (with ≥ grade 2 histology) and stage II–IV clinical liver and/or gut GVHD. Only one system stage III or greater.
IV	Stage II–IV clinical skin GVHD (with > grade 2 histology) and stage II–III clinical liver and/or gut GVHD. Two or more systems stage III or greater.

c) Gastrointestinal manifestations: conditioning-related toxicity, enteric pathogens (bacteria, *C. difficile*, parasites, viruses), medication side effects

6. Diagnostic studies
   a) Skin biopsy: Histology reveals lymphocytic infiltration with epidermal necrolysis.
   b) Liver function tests: Follow daily with acute elevations.
   c) Liver biopsy: Not commonly done due to high risk of intracapsular hemorrhage. If histologic diagnosis is desired, skin or gut biopsies are preferred.
   d) Endoscopic rectal or upper gastrointestinal biopsy reveals lymphocytic infiltration with inflammation and destruction of mucosal and submucosal glands.

7. Management
   a) Steroids form the "backbone" of GVHD therapy. Therapy is usually initiated when the patient is clinical grade 2 or greater. Therapy starts with methy-prednisolone, 0.5 to 3.0 mg/kg IV divided q8–12h. Some centers may increase up to 10 mg/kg divided tid if patient is unresponsive after 2 to 3 days of "standard" doses. Short-course megadose steroids (500 mg to 1 g/d) may be used for 2 to 3 days for hyperacute GVHD. Standardly, once control is achieved, steroids are tapered every 4 days to 2 weeks.
   b) Patients who fail steroid therapy have a very poor prognosis but may go on to alternative immunosuppressive therapy: antithymocyte globulin, 10 to 20 mg/kg/d for 5 to 7 days. Intradermal skin test should be administered prior to dose. Ensure emergency anaphylaxis kit is available (epinephrine, diphenhydramine,

hydrocortisone) at bedside. Premedication with steroids, diphenhydramine, and acetaminophen is required. Patients who do not experience an acute reaction may still develop serum sickness. ATG will "rescue" a small number of steroid-resistant patients.

c) CsA, 1.5 mg/kg IV q12h, should remain in the therapeutic range while treating acute GVHD. CsA is highly utilized as a prophylactic agent but does not play a large role in the treatment of acute GVHD (see chapter 3 for more information on CsA prophylaxis).

d) Other agents that have been used to treat GVHD (with little success) include anti–T-cell immunotoxins, antilymphocyte globulin, and OKT 3.

e) Follow-up: Patients with acute GVHD run a high risk of developing chronic GVHD. Immunodeficiency is often severe secondary to the disease itself and its treatment. Patients will require additional intravenous immune globulin, prophylactic antimicrobials (see chapter 3), and careful monitoring for opportunistic infections.

B. Chronic GVHD[33, 35, 38, 39, 46–48]

1. Definition

a) A chronic, systemic, multiorgan syndrome that bears some clinical resemblance to the collagen-vascular diseases.[46]

b) The initiating event is an immune attack by donor T cells on host cells, which differ by histocompatibility antigens.

c) Histologic features include epithelial cell damage, a mononuclear cell inflammatory infiltrate, fibrosis, and in the lymphoid system, hypocellularity and atrophy.

2. Etiology: Several mechanisms have been described that contribute to the pathogenesis of chronic GVHD.
   a) Initiation by donor T cells
   b) Persistence of circulating alloreactive T cells
   c) Development of autoreactive T cells
   d) Development of counterbalancing regulatory cells
   e) Development of circulating autoantibodies
3. Risk factors
   a) History of acute GVHD
   b) Increased age (> 20 years)
   c) T cell–depleted marrow recipient
   d) Recipient of alloimmune female donor (pregnancy or blood transfusion recipient)
   e) Recipient or donor CMV-positive (controversial)
4. Clinical features:
   a) Occurs more than 100 days post-transplant.
   b) May occur as part of a continuous spectrum, with acute GVHD merging into chronic GVHD.
   c) May also occur after a period when no GVHD has been present.
   d) May also be de novo (no history of acute GVHD).
   e) No specific grading criteria has been established, although the Karnofsky performance score is a practical method for assessing the severity of chronic GVHD.
   f) Multiple systems are affected.[46]
   g) Skin: Hypo- or hyperpigmentation, patchy erythema accompanied by scaling, and erythematous or violaceous papules often covered by lichen planus with striae. Later, dermal and subcutaneous fibrosis may cause thickening and hardening of the skin, resembling localized or generalized scleroderma with hair loss in the affected areas. Skin fibrosis may result in joint contractures, skin ulceration, poor wound

healing, and poor vascular access. Sun exposure may worsen skin manifestations.

h) Mouth: Earliest changes include white striae on the mucosa of the cheeks, lips, or palate that resemble lichen planus. Erythema progresses to painful ulcerations. Destruction of the minor salivary glands results in decreased salivary flow and dry mouth.

i) Eyes: Keratoconjunctivitis sicca results in painful, dry eyes and complaints of "grittiness." Sterile conjunctivitis, uveitis, and cicatricial lagophthalmos have also be described.

j) Sinuses: frequent sinusitis related to sicca syndrome and predisposition for gram-positive sinusitis, especially pneumococcus

k) Gastrointestinal tract: Dysphagia due to esophageal web, epithelial desquamation seen on endoscopy, and retrosternal pain due to acid reflux. Lower gastrointestinal symptoms are less common than in acute GVHD but include diarrhea and abdominal pain. Malabsorption and submucosal fibrosis are seen in advanced cases.

l) Liver: Increased bilirubin and elevation in alkaline phosphatase, often out of proportion to changes in transaminases and bilirubin. Liver biopsy reveals focal portal inflammation and bile duct obliteration, which may progress to sclerosis.

m) Pulmonary: Large airway disease is occasionally noted with cough and bronchorrhea. Small airway disease is more common and is characterized by obliterative bronchiolitis. Symptoms include progressive dyspnea, wheezing, pneumothorax, and a restrictive defect on pulmonary function tests. Obliterative bronchiolitis is associated with a history of *P. aeruginosa* chest infection and low serum IgG. Other rare pulmonary findings include lymphoid interstitial pneumonitis and pulmonary fibrosis.

n) Vagina: Inflammation, stricture formation, and stenosis have been described with web formation.

o) Muscle: Occasional cases of polymyositis have been reported. Symptoms include severe proximal muscle weakness. Muscle biopsy reveals necrotic muscle fibers, interstitial inflammation, and IgG deposits in immune fluorescent staining.

p) Nervous system: Nerve entrapment associated with subcutaneous fibrosis, incapacitating peripheral neuropathy, and myasthenia gravis. CNS involvement with focal lymphohistiocytic aggregates has been reported.

q) Urologic system: renal involvement (nephrotic syndrome) and bladder involvement (severe cystitis)

r) Hematopoietic system: Eosinophilia and thrombocytopenia, platelet-bound autoantibodies, autoimmune hemolytic anemia, and reduced hematopoietic progenitor cells are seen upon examination of the bone marrow. The bone marrow may become hypoplastic. Marrow fibrosis with transfusion-dependent anemia, a leukoerythroblastic picture, and thrombocytopenia may also occur with chronic GVHD.

s) Lymphoid system: severe lymphoid hypocellularity and atrophy and functional asplenia (predisposition to pneumococcal infections)

t) Growth, development, and endocrine: decreased growth rates, which normalize when chronic GVHD is controlled; delayed puberty, if patient received total body irradiation; and autoimmune hyperthyroidism

u) Infection: Bacterial, fungal, and viral infections are the most frequent cause of death with chronic GVHD. Encapsulated gram-positive cocci are the most common bacterial pathogen. VZV infection occurs in about 80% of patients with chronic GVHD. Late interstitial pneumonitis is caused by a variety of organisms (risk of PCP if not on prophylaxis).

5. Diagnostic studies: Specific tissue diagnoses are dependent on clinical findings and systems affected.
   a) Skin biopsy examined by light microscopy
   b) Oral or lip biopsy
   c) Eyes: Patients with chronic GVHD should have Schirmer's testing three times yearly.
   d) Chest x-ray and sinus films per clinical symptoms
   e) Upper endoscopy to evaluate for esophageal web, biopsies (rectal/colonic)
   f) Liver biopsy
   g) Bronchoalveolar lavage or open lung biopsy to diagnose pulmonary interstitial pneumonitis, lymphoid interstitial pneumonitis, pulmonary fibrosis
   h) Muscle biopsy and electromyogram
   i) Urinalysis, renal function studies, renal ultrasound
   j) CBC, differential, antiplatelet antibodies, Coombs' test (direct and indirect), haptoglobin
   k) Bone marrow aspirate and biopsy to evaluate hypoplasia, fibrosis
   l) Radioisotopic scan of the spleen to evaluate for atrophy
   m) Endocrine: growth charts, growth hormone levels, gonadal function studies, thyroid function studies
   n) Infection work-up based on clinical findings with focus on pneumococcus, HSV, VZV

6. Immunosuppression therapy
   a) Long-term administration of CsA post-BMT has been found to decrease the incidence of chronic GVHD; therefore, a slow taper (5%/wk) is recommended starting about seven weeks post-BMT.
   b) For GVHD flare, resume CsA at 12.5 mg/kg/d (if renal function can tolerate).
   c) If symptoms do not improve on CsA alone, start prednisolone at 2 to 3 mg/kg/d for 2 weeks followed by rapid taper to 1 mg/kg on alternate days for approximately 9 months.
   d) Azathioprine (Imuran), 1 mg/kg/d, may be added as a steroid-sparing agent in severe cases.
   e) Thalidomide appears effective in some steroid-resistant patients with lichenoid and sclerodermatous cutaneous chronic GVHD, as well as oral, ocular, and hepatic GVHD not responsive to steroids or CsA. Thalidomide is generally given at a dose to achieve a plasma level of 5 µg/mL.
   f) FK-506 has demonstrated efficacy in rescuing patients who have failed steroids.[49] The dosage is 0.15 mg/kg bid PO or 0.15 mg/kg/d IV. The dose may be adjusted upward until a clinical response is seen or to maintain a blood level of 1 to 2 ng/mL. The dose should be lowered if renal dysfunction is encountered.
7. Additional therapy for chronic GVHD
   a) Psoralen ultraviolet A phototherapy has been effective for cutaneous and oral chronic GVHD.
   b) Photopheresis: Extracorporeal ultraviolet A phototherapy using psoralen as a light-sensitizing agent has been used experimentally as prophylaxis for patients at high risk for chronic GVHD.
   c) Physical/occupational therapy to maximize functional capacity
   d) Ursodiol for hepatic involvement

8. Infection prophylaxis
    a) PCP prophylaxis
        (1) Co-trimoxazole (Bactrim, Septra) dosage:
            Adults: 1 double-strength tablet qd or bid
            PO 3 times a week
            Children: 5 to 10 mg/kg (trimethoprim)/d or
            150 mg/m^2 qd or bid PO 3 times a week
        (2) Dapsone (Avlosulfon) provides effective
            PCP prophylaxis in BMT patients who cannot
            take co-trimoxazole due to myelosuppression
            (platelet count < 100,000 µL &/or absolute
            neutrophil count < 1000/ßL).[3] Patients who are
            hypersensitive to co-trimoxazole will also be
            hypersensitive to dapsone. Dosage:
            Adults: 100 mg PO qd or 3 times a week
            Children: 1 mg/kg PO qd or 3 times a week
            Should not be used in patients with
            G6PD deficiency.
        (3) Pentamidine (Pentam 300) can be used for
            patients who cannot tolerate co-trimoxazole
            or dapsone due to hypersensitivity, hemolysis,
            or myelosuppression. Dosage:
            Adults: 4 mg/kg/dose IV q2wk or 300 mg
            inhaled q2wk
            Children: 4 mg/kg/dose IV q2wk
            (inhaled doses difficult to administer in
            younger children)
    b) Penicillin is recommended to decrease risk of
       pneumococcal infection. Dosage:
        (1) Adults: penicillin, ampicillin, or amoxicillin,
            250 mg PO bid
        (2) Children (< 40 kg): 20 to 40 mg/kg PO bid
    c) Monthly intravenous immune globuline to
       maintain IgG above 500 mg/dL. Dosage: 150 to
       500 mg/kg/dose IV once a month.
    d) All fevers in this population should be
       evaluated formally.

9. Experimental therapies for chronic GVHD
   a) Cytokines: Studies have shown a decreased incidence of GVHD in patients who received Granulocyte-monocyte colony-stimulating factor.
   b) Oxpentifylline (and similar compounds) decreases transcription of messenger RNA for tumor necrosis factor and appears to reduce the number of transplant-related complications, including acute GHVD.
   c) Cytokine antagonists: Cloned soluble receptors for a number of interleukins and cytokines have shown promise in several animal models of T cell immunity and are currently being explored in animal models of GVHD.

IV. Pulmonary Complications[50-59]

A. Pulmonary interstitial pneumonitis
   1. Definition: An inflammatory process involving the intra-alveolar lining of the lungs.
   2. Pathogenesis (see Figure 5.4)[59]
      a) Immunosuppression
      b) Lung damage from high-dose chemotherapy and radiation therapy. The following conditioning agents are commonly associated with interstitial pneumonitis damage:[59] Bleomycin, busulfan, carmustine, cyclophosphamide, mitomycin, total body irradiation, mantal radiation, melphalan, methotrexate, procarbazine, vincristine.
      c) Opportunistic microorganisms. The following microorganisms are frequently associated with interstitial pneumonitis:[59] adenovirus *Aspergillus, Candida,* coccidioidomycosis, *Crytococcus,* cytomegalovirus, HSV, histoplasmosis, *Klebsiella, Mycoplasma,* pneumococcus, *P. carnii, Pseudomonas,* RSV, *Toxoplasma,* VZV, *Legionella.*

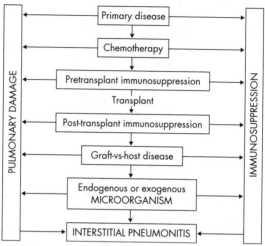

Figure 5.4 outlines possible pathways for the pathogenesis of interstitial pneumonitis. (Reprinted with permission from Wikle, 1991.)

     d) Often the cause is idiopathic.

     e) The cause may be polymicrobial.

  3. Risk factors

     a) Allogeneic transplant recipient

     b) Immunosuppressive agents (steroids, CsA, methotrexate)

     c) High-dose cytoxan in conditioning regimen

     d) GVHD (acute and chronic)

     e) Blood product transfusions (transmission of CMV)

     f) High-dose rate of radiation therapy

     g) High total lung dose of radiation therapy

     h) Single-fraction radiation therapy

     i) Total body irradiation

     j) Increased age at time of transplant

     k) CMV seropositivity at time of BMT

4. Clinical features
   a) Overall clinical symptoms include fever, dry cough, dyspnea, shortness of breath, tachypnea, low PO_2 and oxygen saturation, and interstitial infiltrates on chest x-ray.
   b) Bacterial interstitial pneumonitis occurs in the first six months post-transplant. Risk factors include neutropenia, B-cell immunodeficiency, and chronic GVHD. Chest x-ray often reveals consolidation of the alveolar sacs. *Legionella* pneumonia may start as a unilateral process that rapidly progresses to a bilateral interstitial pneumonitis.
   c) Viral interstitial pneumonitis occurs six to eight weeks post-transplant. CMV is the most common causative organism. Risk factors include CMV seropositivity and prolonged immunosuppression for GVHD. Chest x-ray reveals bilateral "fluffy" interstitial infiltrates.
   d) Fungal interstitial pneumonitis can be divided into three categories: opportunistic organisms that invade the lung (*Aspergillus, Cryptococcus*), opportunistic organisms that reach the lung from another site (*Aspergillus, Candida*), and systemic mycoses that lie dormant for years and reactivate during immunosuppression (coccidioido mycosis, mucormycosis, histoplasmosis). The presenting clinical symptoms are fever and often pleuritic-type chest pain. Chest x-ray often reveals a nodular, rapidly progressing infiltrate.
   e) Parasitic interstitial pneumonitis is most commonly caused by *Pneumocystis*. It presents with dry cough, tachypnea, and rapidly progressing hypoxemia. Chest x-ray may lag behind clinical symptoms but then reveals bilateral, symmetric lower-lobe infiltrates. Gallium scan is sometimes used to evaluate infiltrates.

f) Drug-induced interstitial pneumonitis presents in two clinical syndromes: subacute, with fever, cough, and dyspnea occurring weeks to several month post-transplant; and chronic, associated with exertional dyspnea, tachypnea, and a restrictive defect, often seen months post-transplant in patients who have received a number of pulmonary toxins.

(1) Bleomycin toxicity is seen in patients who receive more than 150 U but can occur at lower doses if patient receives radiation, alkylating agents, or high tensions of oxygen. It causes fibrosis. Chest x-ray reveals bilateral infiltrates. Chest x-ray findings and physical examination may be preceded by abnormal pulmonary function tests.

(2) Carmustine toxicity usually occurs six months after receiving the drug and results in interstitial fibrosis, alveolar septal thickening, and protein-filled alveoli. Chest x-ray findings are reticulonodular in nature.

(3) Methotrexate pulmonary toxicity is independent of the dose the patient receives. Pulmonary function tests show a restrictive defect with low DLCO. Hypersensitivity to methotrexate is the most common pulmonary toxicity. It does not respond to leucovorin but is reversible when the drug is stopped.

(4) Cyclophosphamide (and occasionally busulfan) can cause intra-alveolar inflammation and edema leading to fibrosis. Chest x-ray reveals complete "whiting out" of both lung fields.

(5) Melphalan rarely causes pulmonary toxicity, but may occasionally cause damage to the alveolar epithelium, which can progress to fibrosis.

(6) Cytarabine (ArA-C) can increase pulmonary vascular permeability leading to noncardiogenic pulmonary edema and capillary leakage.

g) Radiation-induced pulmonary damage is the major cause of BMT-related pulmonary damage. The degree of damage is related to the amount of radiation to the lung, dose delivery rate, and fractionation of doses. Symptoms usually occur six to eight weeks following radiation and include progressive dyspnea, high spiking fevers, dry cough, and chest pain. It may progress to pulmonary fibrosis with chronic cyanosis, nail clubbing, orthopnea, and cor pulmonale. Chest x-ray appears as "ground glass."

5. Diagnostic studies are aimed at identification of cause.
   a) Chest x-ray (two views if possible): Some centers screen for interstitial pneumonitis with weekly films for first 100 days post–allogeneic BMT.
   b) Pulmonary function tests, oxygen saturation, arterial blood gases
   c) Sputum examination (low yield): Gram's stain and culture
   d) Transbronchial biopsy/bronchoalveolar lavage: Specimens should be sent for Gram's stain, culture for aerobic and anaerobic bacteria, mycobacteria, fungi, viruses, *Mycoplasma*, *Legionella*, and CMV culture and polymerase chain reaction.
   e) Open lung biopsy: Send specimens for above studies.
   f) High-resolution CT scan of the chest with contrast not only allows detailed imaging of the extent and location of the affected area but also may indicate the possible nature of the lesion. May also facilitate needle-guided biopsy.

6. Management
   a) Treatment is often presumptive and includes antibacterial, antifungal, antiparasitic, and antiviral therapy pending bronchoalveolar lavage/biopsy/culture results.

b) Treatment is focused on appropriate antimicrobial therapy for causative organisms (see section II).

c) Drug-induced or radiation pneumonitis: Most agents respond to high-dose corticosteroid therapy.

d) Maintenance of adequate oxygenation frequently requires mechanical/positive pressure ventilation.

B. Pulmonary edema

1. Definition: Usually appears early post-BMT and is most often related to the pretransplant conditioning regimen. The syndrome is presumed to be due primarily to leaky pulmonary vasculature. May also be due to left-sided heart failure.

2. Risk factors
   a) High-dose cytarabine in preparative regimen
   b) High-dose cyclophosphamide in preparative regimen
   c) Previous chest irradiation
   d) TBI in preparative regimen
   e) Underlying cardiac disease

3. Differential diagnosis
   a) Interstitial pneumonitis
   b) Cardiac failure
   c) Radiation pneumonitis
   d) Intra-alveolar hemorrhage

4. Clinical features
   a) Tachypnea and orthopnea
   b) Rales and diminished breath sounds
   c) Lethargy, restlessness
   d) Weight gain
   e) Chest x-ray displays decreased interstitial markings, "fluffy" infiltrates, and possible cardiac enlargement (if cardiac in origin). Kerley's B lines may also be present.

5. Diagnostic studies
   a) Chest x-ray is diagnostic if infiltrates improve with fluid restriction and diuretics.
   b) Oxygen saturation
   c) Arterial blood gases if hypoxemia is severe

d) Transbronchial biopsy/bronchoalveolar lavage if no improvement with fluid restriction and diuretics to rule out other pathology
e) Echocardiogram to evaluate cardiac status
6. Management
   a) Aggressive diuresis: May require routine dosing. Loop diuretics first: Thiazide diuretic may be added 30 minutes prior to loop diuretic.
      (1) Adults: Start with furosemide, 20 mg IV; double dose if not effective; may give up to 500 mg/day.
      (2) Children: 1 mg/kg/dose q6–12h; may increase by 1 mg/kg/dose.
   b) Measure weight twice a day; strict intake and output.
   c) Fluid restriction: Concentrate IV fluids, medications, and oral fluids as much as possible.
   d) For true congestive heart failure: fluid restriction, diuretics, nitroglycerine, and dobutamine
   e) Maintain adequate oxygenation; severe cases may require mechanical ventilation.

C. Bronchiolitis obliterans organizing pneumonia
   1. Definition: Various immunologic, toxic, or inflammatory insults to the lung may lead to the characteristic lesion associated with bronchiolitis obliterans organizing pneumonia. These lesions consist of exudates with plugs of granulation and connective tissue in the distal airways extending into the alveoli. A small amount of interstitial inflammation and fibrosis is also present. Usually occurs two to four months post-transplant.
   2. Risk factors
      a) Chronic GVHD
      b) Matched unrelated donor transplant
      c) Haploidentical donor transplant
      d) FK-506 for GVHD prophylaxis
   3. Differential diagnosis
      a) Infectious interstitial pneumonitis
      b) Drug-induced or radiation pneumonitis

4. Clinical features
   a) Present with progressive dyspnea preceded by a flu-like illness.
   b) Pulmonary funciton tests show a restrictive defect.
   c) Chest x-ray or CT scan reveals patchy, predominately peripheral infiltrates distinguishable from bronchopneumonia.
5. Diagnostic studies
   a) Chest x-ray
   b) CT scan of the chest with contrast
   c) Pulmonary function tests
   d) Bronchoalveolar lavage/transbronchial biopsy/open lung biopsy: Specimens should be sent for histopathology, Gram's stain, culture for aerobic and anaerobic bacteria, mycobacteria, fungi, viruses, *Mycoplasma*, *Legionella*, CMV culture/polymerase chain reaction (PCR).
6. Management
   a) High-dose corticosteroids
   b) Additional antimicrobial therapy based on broncho-alveolar lavage/transbronchial biopsy/open lung biopsy, since concomitant infection is common.

D. Diffuse alveolar hemorrhage
   1. Definition: Bleeding into the intra-alveolar space most likely secondary to pulmonary injury from the conditioning regimen. Occurs within two to three weeks post–transplant. This process is different from a pulmonary hemorrhage caused by trauma, thrombocytopenia, or infections such as aspergillosis. Mortality is about 80%.
   2. Risk factors
      a) Autologous BMT/stem cell recipient
      b) Severe mucositis (frequent association)
      c) Renal insufficiency (frequent association)
      d) Leukocyte recovery (frequent association)
   3. Differential diagnosis

a) Infectious interstitial pneumonitis
b) Drug-induced or radiation pneumonitis
c) Pulmonary edema

4. Clinical characteristics
a) Rapidly progressive dyspnea, cough, hypoxemia (no hemoptysis)
b) Chest x-ray reveals diffuse consolidation.
c) Bronchoalveolar lavage fluid is extremely bloody.

5. Diagnostic studies
a) Chest x-ray (frequent due to rapidly progressive nature)
b) Oxygen saturation and arterial blood gases
c) Bronchoalveolar lavage/transbronchial biopsy/open lung biopsy: Specimens should be sent for histopathology, Gram's stain, culture for aerobic and anaerobic bacteria, mycobacteria, fungi, viruses, *Mycoplasma*, *Legionella*, CMV culture/polymerase chain reaction (PCR).

6. Management
a) High-dose corticosteroids
b) Maintain adequate oxygenation; often requires mechanical ventilation.

E. Miscellaneous pulmonary complications (rare)
1. Occult pulmonary hemorrhage
a) May evolve as a primary or secondary event in thrombocytopenic patients.
b) May result from trauma or secondary to an underlying infection such as aspergillosis.
c) Treated with platelet and red cell transfusion support.

2. Malignant infiltration
a) May be secondary to the infusion of autologous bone marrow or PBSCs contaminated with malignant cells.
b) Leukemic infiltration can also be associated with pulmonary compromise associated with fever.

3. Pulmonary embolism secondary to the infusion of fat

or bone spicules from poorly filtered bone marrow

4. Leukoagglutinin reaction

   a) Causes a febrile pneumonitis syndrome that stems from the interaction in the blood between preformed antibodies and antigens.

   b) Symptoms occur within the first 24 hours following a blood product transfusion and include the abrupt onset of fever, rigors, tachypnea, nonproductive cough, and respiratory distress.

   c) Such reactions are most commonly associated with the transfusion of granulocytes.

   d) This reaction can be avoided by using transfusions that are washed, packed, or frozen if possible.

5. Pulmonary VOD

   a) An unusual response to high-dose chemotherapy and TBI

   b) Some relationship between hepatic VOD and pulmonary complications has been described, although not well defined.

V. Cardiac complications[60-70]

A. Figures 5.5, 5.6, and 5.7 review normal cardiac physiology.

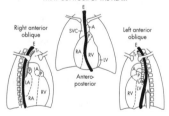

Figure 5.5 Outlines the normal chest x-ray contours of the heart. (Reprinted with permission from Johnson, 1993.)

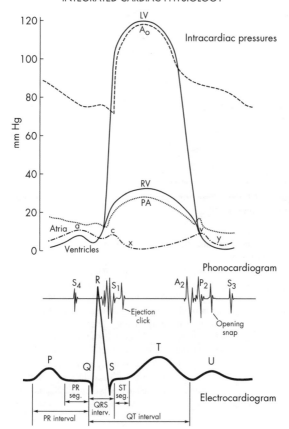

Figure 5.6 Depicts the normal cardiac cycle. (Reprinted with permission from Johnson, 1993.)

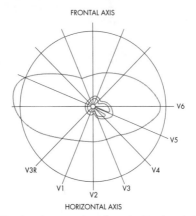

Figure 5.7 Depicts the normal cardiac axis. (Reprinted with permission from Johnson, 1993.)

B. Cardiac complications of BMT are rare. They include the following:
1. Chemotherapy-induced cardiac damage
   a) Patients with previous anthracycline history (doxorubicin doses > 450 mg/m^2, daunorubicin) are at particular risk for cardiomyopathy. Heart damage caused by anthracyclines is from a loss of myocardial fibrils, mitochrondrial changes, and cellular necrosis. Damage is irreversible. Anthracycline cardiomyopathy usually occurs very early post-transplant, since the conditioning regimen adds to the already present cardiac insult.

b) Cyclophosphamide at high doses (120 to 200 mg/kg pretransplant) can cause myocardial necrosis, thickening of the left ventricular wall, serosanguineous pericardial effusion, and a fibrinous pericarditis. Such damage may worsen if the patient has received other cardiotoxic drugs or total body irradiation. Damage is usually irreversible.

2. Radiation-induced cardiac damage is rare with fractionated and low-dose-rate total body/total lymphoid irradiation; however, there is a synergistic effect between chemotherapy and radiation. Patients with a history of prior chest irradiation are at highest risk for cardiac damage. Either they should have their chest shielded or TBI should not be used in the pretransplant conditioning regimen. Radiation-induced cardiac damage has been associated with the development of pericardial effusions and constrictive pericarditis. Radiation may also have a synergistic effect with the hyperlipidemia seen with high-dose steroids.

3. Cardiac infections are rare, but can affect the pericardium, endocardium, and myocardium, *Candida, Aspergillus, Pseudomonas, Clostridium, Streptococcus, Toxoplasma,* coxsackievirus, and adenovirus have all been implicated in cardiac infections.

   a) Bacterial infections of the heart usually seed from the gut or oral cavity. Acute infective endocarditis is related to the presence of bacteremia. Bacteremia (especially *S. auerus*) predisposes the patient to valvular disease. Valvular vegetations may break off and become emboli. Bacterial infections of the heart are not always associated with central venous line infection.

   b) Deep-seated fungal infections produce multiple fungal emboli that may infect the heart (rare).

Death from myocardial infarction secondary to *Aspergillus* embolization has been reported. *Aspergillus* is most often associated with pericarditis and endocarditis secondary to extrapulmonary spread.

   c) Viral infections of the heart are not well documented. The most common viral infections are adenovirus and coxsackievirus. Viruses generally attack the myocardium and often go undetected.

  4. GVHD and cardiac damage

   a) There have been a small number of reports of an acute inflammatory endocarditis associated with the onset of severe, acute GVHD.

   b) Concentric intimal sclerosis of the major coronary arteries and lymphocytic infiltration of the myocardium have been noted in chronic GVHD.

C. Risk factors for the development of cardiac complications post-BMT

  1. History of anthracyclines pretransplant

  2. History of irradiation to the chest

  3. Diagnosis of thalassemia major or Hurler's syndrome

  4. Total conditioning dose of cyclophosphamide of more than 150 mg/kg

  5. Cyclophosphamide as pretransplant conditioning, especially if patient has had high-dose cytarabine or 6-thioguanine

  6. Sepsis (bacteremia or line infection)

  7. History of mitral valve disease

  8. Baseline cardiac ejection fraction of less than 50%

D. Clinical characteristics

  1. Anthracycline cardiac toxicity

   a) Chronic weight gain

   b) Peripheral edema

   c) Tachycardia

    d) Pulmonary edema

    e) Dyspnea with exertion

    f) Orthopnea

    g) Rales/rhonchi

    h) S^4 may be present.

    i) Echocardiogram reveals markedly diminished left ventricular ejection fraction.

2. Cyclophosphamide-induced cardiac toxicity

    a) Signs of refractory congestive heart failure one to 10 days following high-dose infusion

    b) Pulmonary edema

    c) Cardiomegaly on chest x-ray (see Figure 5.5 on p. 206 for normal x-ray contours of the heart).

    d) Poor peripheral perfusion

    e) Systemic edema

    f) S^4 may be present (see Figure 5.6 on p. 207 for the normal cardiac cycle).

    g) Electrocardiogram reveals decreased voltage (see Figure 5.7 on p. 208 for the normal cardiac axis).

    h) Symptoms may progress to hemorrhagic myocarditis, cardiac tamponade, and death.

3. Radiation-induced cardiac damage

    a) Dyspnea with exertion

    b) Chest pain (pericarditis)

    c) Pericardial friction rub

    d) Distant heart sounds (restrictive pericarditis)

4. Bacterial infections of the heart

    a) Fever, chills, cough, malaise, headache

    b) History of bacteremia or line infection

    c) New murmur, pericardial friction rub, symptoms of congestive heart failure

    d) ECG may show conduction or rhythm disturbance.

    e) Echocardiogram may reveal valvular vegetations.

    f) May present with symptoms of embolus if vegetations embolize.

5. Fungal infections of the heart
   a) Resemble those features of bacterial endocarditis.
   b) Most cases have some radiologic or clinical sign or symptom of respiratory infection or pleuritis (substernal chest pain).
   c) Complaints include substernal chest pain that is refractory to pain medication.
   d) ECG may reveal ischemic changes.
   e) Echocardiogram may show echotic fungal lesions in the endocardium.
   f) May also have elevated cardiac iosenzymes.
   g) Most patients will likely develop congestive heart failure and/or cardiac arrest and die.
6. Viral infections of the heart
   a) Features resemble those of bacterial endocarditis/myocarditis.
   b) Symptoms are associated with decreased myocardial contractility, decreased cardiac output, and secondary pulmonary edema.
7. GVHD cardiac damage
   a) Usually associated with severe or hyperacute GVHD.
   b) Features resemble those of bacterial endocarditis/myocarditis and coronary artery disease.
   c) Symptoms are associated with decreased myocardial contractility, decreased cardiac output and secondary pulmonary edema, and intimal sclerosis of the coronary arteries.

E. Diagnostic studies
   1. ECG
   2. Echocardiogram: Rule out vegetations, intracardiac infection, diminished ventricular function.
   3. Cardiac isoenzymes: determine myocardial damage.
   4. Chest x-ray: view cardiac size, pulmonary edema.
   5. Cardiac biopsy: Determine extent of drug-induced myocardial damage, cardiac infection.

F. Management
1. Chemotherapy- or radiation-induced cardiac damage
   a) Astute fluid management and restriction
   b) Diuretics
   c) Digitalis or afterload reduction
   d) Pericardiocentesis in patients with pericardial effusions or tamponade
2. Bacterial infections of the heart
   a) Removal of central line if considered source of bacterial seeding
   b) Long-term gram-positive bacterial coverage (e.g., vancomycin)
   c) Astute fluid management
3. Fungal infections of the heart
   a) Removal of central line if considered source of fungal seeding
   b) Long-term antifungal therapy with Amphotericin B
   c) Astute fluid management
   d) Digitalis if indicated
   e) Diuretics
   f) Nitroglycerin and narcotics for pain relief
4. Viral infections
   a) Little can be offered in the way of antiviral therapy since most viruses go undetected. If a virus is detected, ganciclovir may be used if the virus was caused by CMV; ribavirin may be used for adenovirus or coxsackie virus
   b) High-dose IVIG
   c) Astute fluid management
   d) Digitalis if indicated
   e) Diuretics
5. GVHD-induced cardiac damage
   a) Usual management of acute and chronic GVHD
   b) Lipid-lowering agents
   c) Astute fluid management

d) Digitalis if indicated

e) Diuretics if indicated

f) Nitroglycerin if indicated

VI. Gastrointestinal complications

A. Most BMT patients develop some type of gastrointestinal complication following their transplant. The main complications are summarized in Table 5.8.

Table 5.8 Common Gastrointestinal Complications in Bone Marrow Transplantation

Organ	< 21 days	> 21 days
Mouth	Mucositis Infection: *Candida*, herpes simplex	Infection: *Candida*, herpes simplex GVHD: acute & chronic Xerostomia
Esophagus	Mucositis Reflux: esophagitis	Infection: *Candida*, herpes simplex Reflux: peptic GVHD (acute & chronic)
Stomach	Malory-Weiss tear Gastritis	Infection: CMV Peptic ulceration
Duodenum	Duodenitis	Infectious CMV duodenitis Peptic ulceration GVHD: acute & chronic
Small intestine	Colitis Neutropenic colitis	Infectious CMV colitis Pseudomembranous colitis GVHD: acute

B. Diarrhea

1. Definition: mucosal damage resulting in inflammation leading to significant passage of frequent, loose, or watery stool or hemorrhage

2. Etiology

a) Acute (self-limiting, < 14 days), infectious: *C. jejuni, C. difficile, E. coli, Klebsiella, rotavirus, Shigella*

b) Chronic
   (1) Infectious: *E. coli, Shigella, Salmonella, Giardia, Candida*
   (2) Inflammatory: pseudomembranous colitis secondary to antibiotic therapy caused by *C. difficile*, GVHD of gut
   (3) Medications: chemotherapy, nonabsorbable antibiotics, metoclopramide, oral magnesium, antacids
   (4) Hospital diets
3. Clinical features
   a) Acute diarrhea: developing after four days
   b) Chronic diarrhea: lasting at least two weeks, or frequent recurrences after the initial presentation
   c) Abdominal cramping and pain
   d) Exudative diarrhea presents as mucous, watery, or hemorrhagic diarrhea. This type is accompanied by frequent stools.[71]
   e) Malabsorption or secretory diarrhea presents as large-volume (> 1000 mL/d), foul-smelling, light-colored stools that persist in the absence of oral intake.[71]
   f) Osmotic diarrhea is characterized by hypermotility and frequent stools.[71, 72]
   g) Bacterial or viral infections: abdominal pain, vomiting with abrupt onset
4. Laboratory studies[73]
   a) Endoscopy evaluation with biopsy to distinguish a definitive diagnosis. Platelet count should be 50,000/L, and coagulation parameter should be within normal limits.
   b) Stool for occult blood (Hemoccult): Blood present in the stool may indicate bacterial infection or inflammation

c) Stool for electrolytes: Secretory diarrhea usually has an elevated stool sodium. Malabsorption or viral illness usually has a decreased sodium and increased stool osmotic gap (> 100 mOsm/L).

d) Stool for fecal leukocytes: Leukocytes are indicative of bacterial infections.

e) Stool for ova and parasites and stool culture for enteric pathogens

5. Management

a) Treatment is dependent on the cause.

b) Management should focus on correction of fluid and electrolyte abnormalities and on preventing or correcting resultant malnutrition and nutrient deficiencies.

c) Diarrhea interferes with the absorption of oral CsA and may require use of the parenteral route.

d) Try to determine the type of diarrhea. Osmotic diarrhea is caused by the accumulation of poorly absorbed solutes in the intestine. It will usually diminish with fasting or resting the gut. Secretory diarrhea is caused by the abnormal secretion of water and electrolytes in the intestine. This type of diarrhea persists despite fasting. Secretory diarrhea may be caused by bacterial enterotoxins or secretory hormones (i.e., gastrin, bile acids, and fatty acids).

e) Administer the appropriate antimicrobial therapy: vancomycin or metronidazole for *C. difficile*, acyclovir for HSV, and foscarnet or ganciclovir for CMV.

f) Dietary modification to eliminate bowel stimulants or irritants will restore normal bowel function.

g) If infectious causes have not been identified, pharmacologic agents to relieve symptoms and restore normal bowel function include absorbents (i.e., aluminum hydroxide), absorbents (i.e., kaolin), anticholinergics (i.e., belladonna, atropine sulfate), opiate derivatives (i.e., codeine, paregoric), and antisecretory agents (i.e., clonidine).

h) If skin is intact, apply methylated spirits or witch hazel (Tucks Premoistened Pads).Wash anal area after each bowel movement using mild or no soap, dry thoroughly, and apply powder. Try to keep skin dry; if unable, protect with zinc oxide ointment. Vesicle or bulla formation is suggestive of fungal infections; treat with clotrimazole 1% solution.

C. Nausea and vomiting

1. Definition: an impending feeling of vomiting and/or the forceful expulsion of gastric contents
2. Etiology
   a) Chemotherapy
   b) Radiation therapy
   c) Medications: amphotericin, co-trimoxazole, CsA, nystatin
   d) GVHD: upper gastrointestinal tract and liver
   e) Hepatic disease: viral hepatitis
   f) Viral or fungal infections: involving the esophagus, stomach, intestine
3. Clinical features
   a) Nausea and vomiting develop seven to 21 days post-transplant due to the conditioning regimen.
   b) Intractable retching
   c) Persistent vomiting after 14 days may be due to acute GVHD or intestinal infection.
   d) Hiccuping
4. Laboratory studies: serum chemistries to document dehydration, acid-base, electrolyte status
5. Differential diagnosis
   a) Bowel obstruction
   b) Electrolyte imbalance
   c) Induced by support drugs (e.g., narcotics)

6. Management
   a) Identify the causative agent.
   b) Provide supportive measures when the diagnosis is unclear.
   c) Ensure electrolyte replacement to prevent metabolic alkalosis.
   d) Refer to chapter 2.
   e) Review the patient's drug profile to determine agents that may be emetic.
   f) Consider the use of nonpharmacologic interventions such as relaxation approaches (e.g., rhythmic breathing, hypnosis, massage, muscle relaxation techniques, music, visual imagery).
   g) Employ dietary interventions to minimize irritation to the gastrointestinal tract: Clear liquids only should be taken until 12 hours have passed without vomiting. Liquids should be small quantities (i.e., 15 mL every 10 min). If vomiting does not occur, double the amount. Gradually increase the amount until 8 ounces has been taken every hour. Advance to full liquids and bland food after an 8-hour period without vomiting (i.e., saltine crackers, bland soups, rice, mashed potatoes, bananas, rice, applesauce, toast).

D. Mucositis
   1. Definition: Painful desquamation of the oral and pharyngeal epithelium causing alteration to the oropharyngeal mucosa. Mucositis occurs in 36% to 89% of patients after transplant conditioning regimens.[74-76]
   2. Etiology: The character and severity vary according to specific agents contained in the conditioning regimen, type of transplant, infecting organism and the occurrence of GVHD.[75,77]

a) Conditioning regimen containing high dose busulfan, etoposide, melphalan, thiotepa, or TBI
b) GVHD prophylactic regimen (e.g., Methotrexate)
c) Viral infection: HSV
d) Fungal infection: *Candida*

3. Clinical features: Mucositis develops within one to two weeks after the administration of the conditioning regimen, usually peaking between seven and 11 days.[78] The presentation of this condition coincides with the neutropenic period.
   a) Erythema leading to mouth ulceration and sloughing of the oral mucosa
   b) Isolated ulcerations with or without pseudomembranous plaques
   c) Dry mucous membrane
   d) Nonpurulent, shiny erythematous erosions usually consistent with bacterial infections
   e) White or yellow plaques are usually consistent.
   f) Xerostomia
   g) Dysphagia
   h) Pain
   i) Anorexia with or without weight loss
   j) Sensitivity to acidic foods

4. Laboratory studies
   a) Culture for *C. albicans*
   b) Culture for herpesvirus

5. Management
   a) Prophylactic acyclovir, 200 mg tid PO or 2 50 mg tid IV
   b) Frequent oral care
   c) Avoidance of foods that are acidic
   d) Frequently rinsing of the mouth (i.e., baking soda, dilute hydrogen peroxide solution)

     e) Narcotic analgesia for pain control, which may require parenteral morphine sulfate or fentanyl patch

     f) Use of viscous lidocaine by swish and swallow or the combination of BAX solution (equal parts of diphenhydramine elixir [Benadryl], an antacid, and viscous lidocaine [Xylocaine])

E. GVHD of the gut

  1. Definition: diarrhea along with fluid, protein, and mineral depletion and malabsorption, leading to severe nutritional depletion

  2. Etiology: histoincompatible difference between the patient and the donor, mounting an immune response against the antigens, having an effect on the gastrointestinal mucosa

  3. Risk factors: GHVD usually occurs in conjunction with skin or liver involvement.

  4. Clinical features

     a) Mouth/esophagus: dysphagia, odynophagia, esophageal ulcerations, anorexia, weight loss

     b) Small intestine: diarrhea (i.e., watery and can be large volume [up to 15 L/d]), abdominal cramps, nausea, vomiting, hemorrhage and frank bleeding from ulceration

  5. Differential diagnosis

     a) Neutropenic colitis

     b) Infectious colitis

     c) CMV enteritis

  6. Laboratory studies

     a) Endoscopy with biopsy will demonstrate crypt cell necrosis.

     b) Barium swallow of the esophagus and small bowel follow-through

     c) Electrolytes to determine degree of hypoproteinemia and hypoalbuminemia

d) Abdominal x-ray will demonstrate luminal irregularities indicating mucosal edema.

7. Management

a) Determine the diagnosis by endoscopic tissue biopsy examination.

b) NPO due to diarrhea and fluid along with protein and mineral depletion. Total parenteral nutrition is usually required along with rehydration.

c) Medications should be given parenterally because of rapid intestinal transit leading to impaired absorption.

d) Immunosuppressive therapy (CsA) should be given IV, usually at a dose of 1.5–3 mg/kg/24 h. Corticosteroids may be required, depending on the severity of the disease. The starting dose of methylprednisolone is 0.5–3 mg/kg/d. A third type of immunosuppressive therapy, antithymocyte globulin, may be required.

e) If acute paralytic ileus develops, decompress with nasogastric intubation and suction.

f) Intestinal distention may develop if excessive opiates have been used.

g) Continue to assess for the development of gram-negative septicemia, which presents frequently with gut GVHD.

h) GVHD diet, consisting of a bland diet with advancing food selections, must be instituted once symptoms of diminish.

i) Prokinetic agents (i.e., cisapride) can assist in esophageal clearing.

j) H$_2$ receptor antagonists (i.e., Ranitidine or famotidine) or acid pump inhibitors (i.e., omeprazole) will reduce acid secretion.

F. Infectious complications of the GI tract
    1. Definition: direct bacterial invasion of the
       gastrointestinal tract with local release of an
       a) Enterotoxin
       b) Neutropenic colitis
       c) Infectious colitis
    2. Etiology
       a) Bacterial infections: *C. difficile*
       b) Fungal infections: *Candida, Cryptosporidium*
       c) Viral infections: CMV, HSV type 1
    3. Clinical features
       a) Pain localized at the right iliac fossa (typhilitis)
       b) Diarrhea
    4. Differential diagnosis
       a) Gastritis
       b) Duodenitis or erosion
       c) GVHD
       d) Antibiotic-associated diarrhea
    5. Laboratory studies
       a) Chest x-ray or abdominal film revealing
          peritoneum
       b) Endoscopy or colonoscopy: biopsy results
          by immunoperoxidase staining can provide a
          result in six hours;[79] biopsy for polymerase chain
          reaction analysis.
       c) Stool for occult blood (Hemoccult): Blood
          present in the stool may indicate bacterial
          infection or inflammation.
       d) Stool for electrolytes: Secretory diarrhea usually
          has an elevated stool sodium. Malabsorption or
          viral illness usually has a decreased sodium and
          increased stool osmotic gap (> 100 mOsm/L).
       e) Stool for fecal leukocytes: Leukocytes are
          indicative of bacterial infections.
       f) Stool for ova and parasites and stool culture for
          enteric pathogens

6. Management
   a) Broad-spectrum antibiotic therapy including aminoglycosides and metronidazole
   b) Growth factors (e.g., granulocyte or granulocyte-macrophage colony-stimulating factor) to enhance neutrophil recovery
   c) Surgical debridement may be required in extreme cases.
   d) If endoscopy findings reveal yellow plaques of mucosal edema, this is consistent with *C. difficile* infection. Empiric treatment with vancomycin or metronidazole is recommended.

VII. Renal and hepatic complications

A. Drug-induced renal complications (nephrotoxicity)
   1. Definition: toxic effect of drug(s) on the kidney resulting in acute tubular necrosis, acute tubulointerstitial disease, chronic tubulointerstitial disease, or glomerulonephritis
   2. Etiology: Exposure to CsA, aminoglycosides, sulfonamides, vancomycin, cephalosporins, cisplatin, contrast media, methotrexate, allopurinol, cyclophosphamide, IV acyclovir, IV ganciclovir, foscarnet, pentamidine, and so on
   3. Risk factors
      a) Cumulative effect of chemotherapy or antibiotic therapy
      b) Increasing age
      c) History of diabetes mellitus
      d) Underlying renal dysfunction
      e) Volume depletion/dehydration
   4. Clinical features
      a) Oliguria (may initially demonstrate mild polyuria)
      b) Edema
      c) Hypertension

5. Differential diagnosis
   a) Sepsis (especially CMV or disseminated fungal)
   b) Renal hypoperfusion
   c) Renal impairment secondary to VOD
   d) Hemolytic-uremic syndrome
6. Laboratory studies
   a) BUN (elevated)
   b) Serum creatinine (elevated)
   c) Urinary protein may be positive.
   d) Renal biopsy
7. Management
   a) Discontinue any drug with potential for nephrotoxicity, if possible.
   b) Reduce the dose of any essential medication with potential for nephrotoxicity.
   c) Monitor peak and trough drug levels; modify dose appropriately.
   d) Increase fluid intake.
   e) If severe, patient may require dialysis.

B. Acute renal failure
   1. Definition: sudden deterioration of renal function
   2. Etiology
      a) Prerenal: decreased renal blood flow, decreased cardiac output, hypotension, hypovolemia, renovascular thrombosis/obstruction, sepsis
      b) Intrarenal: exposure to nephrotoxic drugs, prolonged ischemia, malignant hypertension, tumor lysis syndrome/hyperuricemia
      c) Postrenal: bilateral ureteral obstruction, bladder obstruction, hemorrhagic cystitis, obstruction by tumor
   3. Risk factors
      a) Prior history of hypertension, diabetes mellitus, or vascular disease
      b) Exposure to nephrotoxic drugs
      c) Volume depletion/dehydration

      d) Sepsis
      e) Exposure to cyclophosphamide (hemorrhagic cystitis)
  4. Clinical features
      a) May demonstrate oliguria
      b) Edema (central > peripheral)
  5. Differential diagnosis
      a) Drug toxicity
      b) Hemolytic-uremic syndrome
  6. Laboratory studies
      a) BUN (elevated)
      b) Serum creatinine (mild failure > 2.0 mg/dL; severe > 5.0 mg/dL)
      c) BUN/creatinine ratio (intrarenal = 10:1; pre- or postrenal = 15:1)
      d) Renal sonogram to rule out obstruction
  7. Management
      a) Determine cause and correct.
      b) Discontinue any nephrotoxic drug, if possible.
      c) Reduce cumulative doses of all medications.
      d) Monitor fluids and electrolytes; replace appropriately.
      e) Daily weight
      f) Intake and output
      g) Renal-dose dopamine may be used to improve renal perfusion.
      h) If severe, patient may require dialysis.

C. Hemolytic-uremic syndrome
  1. Definition: syndrome of hemolytic anemia, renal insufficiency, and thrombocytopenia that occurs at least 30 days after BMT[80]
  2. Etiology: Appears to involve damage to the endothelium, causing activation of platelets with subsequent thrombocytopenia and microangiopathic hemolysis.
  3. Risk factors

a) Intensive pretransplant conditioning regimens (especially TBI)
b) HLA nonidentical transplant
c) Use of cyclosporine
d) CMV infection
e) GVHD

4. Clinical features
   a) Fatigue, pallor
   b) Bruising, bleeding, petechiae
   c) Fever
   d) CNS complaints
   e) Renal failure

5. Differential diagnosis
   a) Drug effect
   b) DIC
   c) Sepsis
   d) Acute renal failure

6. Laboratory studies
   a) Lactate dehydrogenase (elevated)
   b) Decreased platelet count
   c) Low hemoglobin/hematocrit
   d) Schistocytes and fragmented cells on review of blood smear
   e) Serum creatinine (elevated)

7. Management
   a) Plasma exchange via pheresis
   b) Corticosteroid therapy
   c) Discontinue use of cyclosporine
   d) RBC and platelet support as needed

8. Follow-up: close follow-up of blood counts, lactate dehydrogenase (LHD), and serum creatinine

D. Veno-occlusive disease of the liver

1. Definition: Most common cause of serious hepatic dysfunction within the first 20 days post-transplant. Involves obliteration of terminal hepatic venules and small lobular veins, resulting in acute liver congestion.

Varies in severity.

2. Etiology: Hepatotoxity of chemotherapy and/or radiotherapy used for conditioning therapy. Effect may be cumulative with standard chemotherapy used to treat the patient prior to transplant.

3. Risk factors
   a) Underlying liver disease or dysfunction, especially hepatitis
   b) Heavily pretreated patients (high dose or prolonged treatment)
   c) CMV-positive serology
   d) Age greater than 15 years
   e) Conditioning therapy containing high-dose busulfan
   f) HLA-mismatched related donor
   g) Matched unrelated donor
   h) Any hematologic malignancy other than acute lymphoblastic leukemia
   i) Pretransplant acyclovir therapy
   j) Persistent fever during the conditioning regimen

4. Clinical features
   a) Weight gain secondary to sodium and water retention
   b) Jaundice
   c) Abdominal discomfort (especially right upper quadrant)
   d) Hepatomegaly
   e) Ascites
   f) Peripheral edema
   g) Thrombocytopenia
   h) Encephalopathy
   i) Multiorgan failure

5. Differential diagnosis
   a) Infection (bacterial, viral, or fungal)
   b) Acute GVHD
   c) Drug toxicity (hepatotoxicity)

        d) Pancreatitis

        e) Peritonitis

        f) Pericarditis/congestive heart failure

   6. Laboratory studies

        a) Serum bilirubin (elevated > 2.0 mg/dL)

        b) Aspartate transamine (elevated)

        c) Alkaline phosphatase (elevated)

        d) Protein C (decreased)

        e) Factor VII (decreased)

   7. Management

        a) Mild cases may resolve spontaneously.

        b) Treatment is primarily supportive; early detection is essential.

        c) Maintain fluid and electrolyte balance (intake and output, daily weight).

        d) Restrict sodium intake.

        e) Discontinue or reduce the dose of any hepatotoxic or nephrotoxic drug.

        f) Spironolactone diuresis may be utilized.

        g) Hypertransfusion of RBCs or salt-poor albumin may be used to maintain renal perfusion.

        h) Vitamin K may be used to correct associated coagulopathy.

        i) Abdominal paracentesis may be required.

        j) Platelet support as necessary

        k) Pentoxyfilline, tissue plasminogen activator, and heparin are of questionable use.

E. Acute GVHD of the liver

   1. Definition: common cause of liver dysfunction in allogeneic transplant patients before day 100

   2. Etiology: immunologic response of immunocompetent donor T lymphocytes against recipient tissues, especially the skin, gastrointestinal tract, and liver

3. Risk factors
   a) Allogeneic transplants with a higher degree of antigenic disparity
   b) Known history of acute GVHD of skin or gastrointestinal tract
4. Clinical features
   a) Mild hepatomegaly
   b) Right upper quadrant tenderness
   c) Jaundice
   d) Skin and/or gastrointestinal manifestations of GVHD
5. Differential diagnosis
   a) VOD
   b) Drug toxicity (hepatotoxicity)
   c) Infection (bacterial, viral, or fungal)
6. Laboratory studies
   a) Serum bilirubin (elevated)
   b) Alkaline phosphatase (elevated)
   c) Serum transaminase levels (elevated)
   d) Liver biopsy one to two weeks after onset may reveal cholestasis.
7. Management: Increase immunosuppressive therapy (e.g., cyclosporine, steroid, antithymocyte globulin).
8. Follow-up
   a) Many patients will develop chronic GVHD.
   b) Continue to monitor laboratory parameters closely.
   c) Patient may continue to require higher doses of immunosuppressant drugs for longer period of time.

F. Chronic GVHD of the liver
   1. Definition: A common cause of liver dysfunction in transplant patients after day 100; may appear years later.
   2. Etiology: Complex immunopathology results in immunodeficiency and an autoimmune response. May occur following acute GVHD or de novo.

3. Risk factors
   a) Previous acute GVHD of liver
   b) Older age at transplant
4. Clinical features
   a) Chronic liver disease
   b) Anorexia
   c) Weight loss
   d) Jaundice (fluctuating)
   e) Other manifestations of chronic GVHD
      (e.g., skin, eye)
5. Differential diagnosis
   a) Chronic viral infection (hepatitis, CMV)
   b) Infiltrative liver disease
   c) Hepatotoxic drug reaction
   d) Cholestasis/biliary obstruction
6. Laboratory studies
   a) Alkaline phosphatase (elevated up to five to 10
      times normal)
   b) Aspartate transaminase (elevated up to three to six
      times normal)
   c) Serum bilirubin (elevated)
   d) Liver biopsy: small bile duct injury and
      marked cholestasis
7. Management: immunosuppressive therapy
8. Follow-up: Alkaline phosphatase may remain
   persistently elevated.

G. Hepatobiliary infections
   1. Definition: Viral, bacterial, or fungal infection
      of the liver
   2. Etiology:
      a) Cytopenia, immunosuppression, and low serum
         immunoglobulin levels post-transplant
      b) Viral infections are most common (hepatitis B
         or C, CMV, HSV, EBV, VZV, or adenovirus).

3. Risk factors
   a) Acute and chronic GVHD suppress T- and B-cell function.
   b) Antibiotic therapy may allow fungal overgrowth.
4. Clinical features
   a) Abdominal discomfort (especially right upper quadrant)
   b) Fever
   c) Hepatomegaly
5. Differential diagnosis
   a) VOD
   b) GVHD
   c) Drug toxicity (hepatotoxicity)
6. Laboratory studies
   a) Hepatitis screen
   b) Viral titers (CMV, EBV, HSV, VZV)
   c) Blood cultures
   d) Liver function tests (elevated)
   e) Ultrasound or CT may reveal fungal lesions or abscess.
   f) Liver biopsy may assess lesions or determine viral agent.
7. Management
   a) Appropriate antimicrobial therapy
   b) Avoid hepatotoxic medications.
8. Follow-up
   a) In the post-transplant setting, hepatitis C can rapidly evolve to cirrhosis.
   b) Interferon-α therapy should be considered.

VIII. Neurologic complications

A. Neurologic complications occur in more than 50% of BMT recipients. Complications arise from the following:
   1. Underlying disease leading to neurologic infection, hemorrhage, or degeneration
   2. The initial therapy causing increased risk factors

3. The transplant conditioning regimen
4. Post-transplant immunosuppressive therapy
5. Post-transplant therapy causing organ toxicity
   and failure[81]

B. Seizures

1. Definition: A paroxysmal event representing
   abnormal electrical activity in cerebral neurons.
   Partial or generalized seizures occur in more than
   10% of BMT recipients.[81]

2. Etiology
   a) Drug-related chemotherapy: busulfan, cytoarabine
      (high-dose), cyclophosphamide, L-asparaginase,
      methotrexate
   b) Support medications: CsA, corticosteroids
   c) Disease: relapse or primary disease, new
      CNS malignancy
   d) Infection: focal infection, infarct
   e) Metabolic: hypocalcemia, hypoglycemia,
      hyperglycemia, hypomagnesemia,
      hyponatremia, hypoxia

3. Clinical features
   a) Partial (focal) seizures with no change in level
      of consciousness: motor symptoms that start
      with one muscle group and spread to the muscle
      groups, sensory symptoms (e.g., paresthesias,
      visual changes), autonomic symptoms (e.g.,
      tachycardia, loss of bowel and bladder function)
   b) Partial seizures can lead to impairment in level
      of consciousness.
   c) Generalized seizures (also known as petit mal
      seizures): characterized by sudden onset of motor
      activity, accompanied with a blank stare
   d) Myoclonic seizures: sudden shock-type
      contraction of large muscles
   e) Clonic seizures: repetitive involuntary contraction
      of muscles

f) Tonic seizures: sustained involuntary contraction of muscle

g) Tonic-clonic or grand mal seizures: may be preceded by an aura, tonic involuntary contraction of muscles, loss of consciousness, loss of bladder or bowel function, postictal period

4. Laboratory studies

a) Serum electrolytes, serum glucose, BUN, creatinine

b) Serum CsA level

c) CBC with differential

5. Management

a) Initial management of generalized seizures lasting one to two minutes in duration is supportive care since most seizures are self-limiting. Maintain a clear airway by turning patients on their side, do not try to pry open airway, and protect the patient from head injury.

b) Recurring or prolonged seizures are best treated with intravenous benzodiazepine (diazepam, 1 to 2 mg, or clonazepam, 1 to 2 mg). Benzodiazepines are not likely to cause bone marrow suppression.

c) If phenytoin, carbamazepine, or phenobarbital is used for maintenance therapy, it will reduce cyclosporine levels. Increase cyclosporine doses and carefully monitor the patient to maintain the appropriate immunosuppression.

d) When titrating doses to achieve adequate blood concentrations, use therapeutic range in combination with clinical symptoms to determine appropriate dosage.

e) Gradually taper drug therapy instead of an abrupt withdrawal.

C. CNS infection

1. Definition: Infections in the CNS occur in 7% to 14% of BMT patients, with up to 77% of the infected patients immunocompromised and death as the end result. The primary cause of death is delay in diagnosis as a result of suppression of symptoms.[82, 83]

2. Etiology (see Table 5.9)

   a) During the first month after transplant, the most common types of CNS infections are bacterial.

Table 5.9 Causes of CNS Infections

Causative agent	Organism
Viruses	Adenovirus
	Cytomegalovirus
	Herpes simplex virus
	Papovaviruses
	Varicella-zoster virus
Bacteria	*Pseudomonas*
	Haemophilus influenzae
	Staphylococci
	Streptococci
Fungi	*Aspergillus*
	Mucoraceae
	Histoplasma
	Candida
	Cryptococcus neoformans
Protozoa	*Toxoplasma*
	Strongyloides stercoralis

   b) Bacterial infections are caused primarily by intravenous lines, paranasal sinuses, or ulceration in the gastrointestinal tract.

   c) The second period of infection occurs one month to one year after transplant. The types of infection that are most prevalent during this period are fungal, parasitic, and viral.

   d) *Aspergillus* accounts for 30% to 50% of CNS infections.[83]

e) *C. albicans* infects approximately 12% of BMT recipients, most often in the first 35 days after transplant.[83, 84]

f) *Cryptococcus* is rarely encountered in the BMT patient.

g) *T. gondii* is seen in the BMT patient early post-transplant.[82]

h) HSV reactivates and is shed in the oral secretions of 80% of seropositive patients during the first several weeks after BMT.[85]

i) HVZ has the highest incidence of presentation in the fourth or fifth month after BMT.[86]

j) Infections are caused by hematogenous spread from the lungs, the gastrointestinal tract, or an infected central venous catheter.

3. Clinical features
   a) Focal neurologic signs
   b) Fever
   c) Headache
   d) Confusion
   e) Paresthesias
   f) Tremors
   g) Facial nerve palsy
   h) Hearing loss associated with cranial nerve infection

4. Differential diagnosis: drug-related toxicity or a CNS bleed

5. Laboratory studies
   a) Head CT scan, preferably with contrast, is indicated in patients with focal neurologic deficits or diminished level of consciousness.
   b) CSF culture specimens should be obtained once a mass has been excluded. CSF examination should include: cell count with differential and Gram's stain, protein, and glucose. The CSF protein is usually elevated (> 100 mg/dL), and the glucose is decreased (< 45 mg/dL).

    c) Bacterial cultures for blood, nasal, and catheter should be obtained simultaneously.

    d) Viral cultures

    e) Stereotactic biopsy if a brain abscess is suspected

6. Management

    a) Management of bacterial or fungal infections requires antibiotic therapy according to conventional guidelines based on sensitivity results. High-dose antibiotic therapy should be administered.

    b) If antifungal infection is required, aggressive therapy is warranted; however, significant neurologic toxicity may occur.

    c) Antifungal therapy may cause an increase in cyclosporine levels

    d) CMV: Ganciclovir therapy, 5 mg/kg q12h for 14 days with dosage adjustment in cases of renal failure. Repeat cultures in five to seven days to evaluate for resistance to ganciclovir.

    e) HSV and VZV: HSV infection appears to be uncommon. VZV infection occurs in 28% of autologous transplant patients and 50% of allogeneic patients who survive beyond six months.[87] HSV and VZV are treated with high-dose acyclovir, 10 to 15 mg/kg 5 times daily for seven to ten days.

    f) *S. aureus* infection produces high mortality and may be a result of staphylococcal bacteremia. Initially, oxacillin, 2 g IV, should be given. First-generation cephalosporins should not be used because they do not penetrate the CSF. In penicillin-resistant or allergic patients, vancomycin, 1 g IV q12h is the drug of choice.

D. Drug-related neurotoxicity
1. Definition
   a) The neurotoxicity of specific drugs affecting BMT patients has been well described after oral, intravenous, and intrathecal drug administration, with both acute and chronic presentations.
   b) BMT patients are exposed to a variety of chemotherapeutic agents with varying potential for neurologic toxicity.
2. Etiology: drugs that have been associated with neurotoxicity, including chemotherapeutic agents as a part of the conditioning regimen and immunosuppressive support drugs
   a) Busulfan
   b) Cytarabine
   c) Carmustine
   d) Methotrexate (oral, intravenous, and intrathecal), with toxicity appearing to be dose-related
   e) Antibiotics and antivirals
   f) CsA
3. Busulfan: Generalized seizures have been associated with 10% of the patients receiving high-dose busulfan therapy (4 mg/kg/day for 4 days). Since busulfan crosses the blood-brain barrier, it has the ability to increase the CSF concentration of the drug, leading to a direct neurotoxic effect.[88, 89]
   a) Clinical features: ataxia, confusion, diplopia, seizures (usually not focal)
   b) Management: Prophylactic anticonvulsant therapy, with a therapeutic value being reached for two days prior to the initiation of the busulfan in the conditioning regimen. An oral phenytoin loading dose of 18 mg/kg is adequate, followed by daily maintenance doses of 5 mg/kg.

4. Cytarabine: Diffuse sensorimotor neuropathy and acute demyelinating neuropathy can occur; however, there are several contributing factors leading to CNS damage from the primary treatment, conditioning regimen, and metabolic and immunosuppressive therapy.

   a) Clinical features: Symptoms generally evolve within 24 hours from the last dose and may be irreversible. Symptoms will appear when cumulative doses of 24 to 36 g have been administered. Symptoms include dysarthria, confusion, nystagmus, cognitive loss, tremor, lack of coordination, and somnolence.

   b) Management: Therapy should be immediately discontinued with the presentation of symptoms. Recovery may be slow and may not be complete.

5. Carmustine: High-dose carmustine (300 to 600 mg/m^2) is used in conditioning regimens for Hodgkin's disease.

   a) Clinical feature: seizures[90]

   b) Management: Prophylactic anticonvulsant therapy, with a therapeutic value being reached for two days prior to the initiation of the busulfan in the conditioning regimen. An oral phenytoin loading dose of 18 mg/kg is adequate, followed by daily maintenance doses of 5 mg/kg.

6. Methotrexate: The primary neurotoxicity of methotrexate is well described in the literature. The toxicity is associated with focal mineralizing microangiopathic and neuroaxonal dystrophy.

   a) Clinical features: Aphasia, hemiparesis, and mental status changes present typically five to seven days after a second or subsequent course of methotrexate therapy without toxic serum levels.

   b) Laboratory studies: Electroencephalogram shows focal abnormalities. CT scans are usually unrevealing.

c) Management: Further treatment is permitted after symptoms have resolved.

7. CsA: Neurologic complications associated with CsA are common and are usually reversible after temporary discontinuation of CsA. There is evidence that TBI and etoposide increase the risk of CsA toxicity.[91–93]

a) Clinical features: Earliest signs are disorientation, confusion, impairment of concentration, and memory deficits. Other clinical features include ataxia, blurred vision to the degree of cortical blindness, headaches, tremor, and seizures. As encephalopathy deepens, agitation occurs.

b) Laboratory studies: CT scan will demonstrate hypodense white areas of enhancement, indicating leukoencephalopathy. MRI identifies diffuse or patchy plaques. Electroencephalogram demonstrates diffuse slow-wave dysrhythmia.

c) Management: CsA should be withheld for several days and then restarted at a reduced dose. In the event of seizure activity, anticonvulsant therapy should be initiated; however, the use of phenytoin enhances the metabolism of corticosteroids. Headache may be relieved with propranolol. Magnesium replacement may reverse seizure-related symptoms.

E. Encephalopathies

1. Definition:

a) Encephalopathy in the transplant patient is usually metabolic and associated with gram-negative sepsis or due to the use of sedative and hypnotic drugs.

b) Hypoxic encephalopathy usually carries the risk of permanent neurologic dysfunction, occurring from interstitial pneumonia or from the hypoxemia-associated form of RBC lysis in patients with the hemolytic-uremic syndrome.

   c) Hepatic encephalopathy may occur from GVHD-related liver involvement or from hepatic failure associated with VOD.

   d) Renal failure resulting in uremic encephalopathy has been identified with nephrotoxic drugs (e.g., CsA, cisplatin).

   e) Electrolyte and acid-base imbalance occurs in the transplant patient and is often associated with encephalopathy.[82]

  2. Etiology: The causes of metabolic encephalopathy have multiple interacting pathologies.

   a) Electrolyte and acid-base imbalance (e.g., calcium, magnesium, or phosphate depletion)

   b) Hypoglycemia or hyperglycemia

   c) Hypoxia

   d) Hepatic failure

   e) Metabolic

   f) Renal failure

  3. Clinical features

   a) Delirium

   b) Depression of the sensorium, which manifests as lethargy or stupor leading to coma

   c) Extensor and flexor posturing to noxious stimuli

   d) Focal neurologic findings

   e) Hemiplegia

F. Immune-medicated peripheral nerve disorders

  1. Definition: Immune-mediated neurologic complications of BMT affect the peripheral nervous system. These conditions include myasthenia gravis, polymyositis, and inflammatory demyelinating polyneuropathy.

  2. Myasthenia gravis: An immune mediated disorder of the neuromuscular junction, in which autoantibodies to the acetylcholine receptor produce a clinical syndrome of muscle weakness.

      a) Clinical features: extraocular muscle weakness leading to ptosis, facial muscle weakness, proximal limb muscle weakness

      b) Diagnosis is based on the distribution of muscle weakness and the clinical symptoms of fatigability over the time of presentation of the signs and symptoms.

      c) Treatment: prednisone therapy, therapeutic plasmapheresis, intravenous immune globulin infusion therapy, cautious use of drugs that affect neuromuscular transmission (e.g., antibiotics, cardiac antiarrhythmic agents, parenteral magnesium)

3. Polymyositis: A disorder seen in allogeneic BMT and a well-established complication of chronic GVHD.[94] The majority of BMT patients developing myositis have undergone allogeneic BMT for aplastic anemia. The time to onset has been between four months and four years, with most patients experiencing acute GVHD.

      a) Clinical features: dysphagia, proximal muscle weakness, muscle tenderness, cardiac muscle weakness

      b) Diagnostic study: Nerve biopsy is nonspecific.

      c) Treatment: corticosteroids

G. Hiccups

1. Definition: Hiccups are symptomatic of a brain stem and spinal focal lesion; however, they can occur as a benign drug-related presentation following sedative withdrawal or prolonged use of steroid therapy or as gastric distention, esophageal irritation, or phrenic nerve irritation.

2. Treatment

      a) Reduction in gastric distention: peppermint water (relaxes esophageal sphincter) or antiflatulents (simethicone)

b) Central suppression of the hiccup reflex: prochlorperazine, 5 mg tid PO or 25 mg IV, or chlorpromazine

c) Induction of hypercapnia by breath holding or rebreathing into a paper bag

d) Benzodiazepines with metoclopramide, 10 to 20 mg PO q4h, often ameliorates intractable hiccups

e) Clonazepam, 0.5 mg tid, increased to 1 mg if needed. This agent can be helpful if the hiccups have a central origin.

f) A small number of patients have intractable hiccups.

References

1. Ford R, Ballard B. Acute complication after bone marrow transplantation. *Semin Oncol Nurs.* 1988;4:15–24.

2. Ezzone S, Camp-Sorrell D, eds. *Manual for Bone Marrow Transplant Nursing: Recommendations for Practice and Education.* Pittsburgh: Oncology Nursing Press, Inc; 1994.

3. Caudell KA, Whedon MB. Hematopoietic complications. In: Whedon MB, ed. *Bone Marrow Transplantation: Principles, Practice and Nursing Insights.* Boston: Jones and Bartlett; 1991:135–159.

4. Deeg HJ, Klingemann HG, Phillips GL, eds. *A Guide to Bone Marrow Transplantation: When Should Marrow Transplantation Be Considered?* New York: Springer-Verlag; 1988.

5. Sanford JP, Gilbert DN, Gerberding JL, et al., eds. *The Sanford Guide to Antimicrobial Therapy.* 24th ed. Dallas: Antimicrobial Therapy, Inc; 1996.

6. Treleaven J and Wiernik P, eds. *Bone Marrow Transplantation.* London, England: Mosby-Wolfe; 1995.

7. Fuller AK. Platelet transfusion therapy for thrombocytopenia. *Semin Oncol Nurs.* 1990;6:123–128.

8. Johnson K, ed. *The Harriet Lane Handbook.* 13th ed. St. Louis: Mosby; 1993.

9. Voogt PJ. Rejection of bone marrow graft by recipient-derived cytotoxic T-lymphocytes against minor histocompatibility antigens. *Lancet.* 1990;335:131–134.

10. Cunningham R. *Prevention of Infection in Patients Receiving Myelosuppressive Chemotherapy.* New York: Triclinica Communications; 1992.

11. Mangan K, Klump I, Rosenfeld T, et al. Bone marrow transplantation. In: Makowka L, ed. *The Handbook of Transplantation Management.* Austin, Tex: RG Landis; 1991:374–376.

12. Wingard J. Management of infectious complications of bone marrow transplantation. *Oncology.* 1990;4:69–72.

13. Meyers JD. Infection in marrow recipients. In: Mandell GL, Douglas RG, Bennett JE, eds. *Principles and Practice of Infectious Diseases*. New York: Wiley and Sons; 1985:1674–1676.

14. Committee on Infectious Diseases. *The Red Book*. Washington, DC: American Academy of Pediatrics; 1993.

15. Drutz DJ. Invasive fungal disease. *Convers Infect Control*. 1985;6:1–12.

16. Saag DA, Dismukes WE. Azoles antifungal agents: emphasis on new trizoles. *Antimicrob Agents Chemother*. 1988;32:1–8.

17. Wikle TJ. Pulmonary and cardiac complications of bone marrow transplantation. In: Whedon MB, ed. *Bone Marrow Transplantation: Principles, Practice, and Nursing Insights*. Boston: Jones and Bartlett; 1991:182–205.

18. Michel G, Thuret I, Scheiner C, et al. Lung toxoplasmosis after HLA mismatched bone marrow transplantation. *Bone Marrow Transplant*. 1990;14:445–457.

19. NIH-University of California Expert Panel for Corticosteroids as Adjunctive Therapy for Pneumocystis Pneumonia. Consensus statement on the use of corticosteroids as adjunctive therapy for pneumocystis pneumonia in the acquired immunodeficiency syndrome. *N Engl J Med*. 1990;323:1500–1504.

20. Bacigalupo A, van Lint E, and Tedone F. Early treatment of CMV infections in allogeneic bone marrow transplant recipients with foscarnet or ganciclovir. *Bone Marrow Transplant*. 1994;13:753–758.

21. Emanuel D, Cunningham I, and Jules-Elysee K. Cytomegalovirus pneumonia after bone marrow transplantation successfully treated with the combination of ganciclovir and high-dose intravenous immune globulin. *Ann Intern Med*. 1988;109:777–782.

22. Ho M. Observations from transplantation contributing to the understanding of pathogenesis of CMV infection. *Transplant Proc*. 1991;23:104–109.

23. Volker DL. Clinical characteristics of cytomegalovirus infection. *Nursing Acumen: A Guide to Viral Infection in the Hematology/Oncology Patient.* 1992;3:1–2.

24. Whedon, MB. Viral infection in the BMT patient. *Nursing Acumen: A Guide to Viral Infection in the Hematology/Oncology Patient.* 1991;3:1–3.

25. Cone R, Hackman RC, Huang ML, et al. Human herpes virus type 6. *N Engl J Med.* 1993;329:156–161.

26. Lusso P, Gallo RC. Human herpes virus 6 in AIDS. *Immunol Today.* 1995;16:67–71.

27. Wendt CH, Weisdorf DJ, Jordan MC. Parainfluenza virus respiratory infection after bone marrow transplantation. *N Engl J Med.* 1992;326:921–926.

28. Heilman CA. Respiratory syncytial virus and parainfluenza viruses. *J Infect Dis.* 1990;161:402–406.

29. Harrington RD. An outbreak of respiratory syncytial virus in a bone marrow transplant center. *J Infect Dis.* 1992;165:987–993.

30. Englund JA, Sullivan CJ, Jordan MC, et al. Respiratory syncytial virus infection in immunocompromised adults. *Ann Intern Med.* 1988;109:203–208.

31. Vanecek KS. Gastrointestinal complications of bone marrow transplantation. In: Whedon MB, ed. *Bone Marrow Transplantation: Principles, Practice, and Nursing Insights.* Boston: Jones and Bartlett; 1991.

32. Beatty PG. The use of unrelated donors for bone marrow transplantation. *Marrow Transplant Rev.* 1991;1:1–7.

33. Bortin MM, Atkinson K, van Bekkum BW, et al. Factors influencing the risk of acute and chronic graft versus host disease in humans: a preliminary report from the IBMTR. *Bone Marrow Transplant.* 1989;4(suppl 1):222–224.

34. Deeg HJ, Klingemann HG, Phillips GL, eds. *A Guide to Bone Marrow Transplantation: When Should Marrow Transplantation Be Considered?* New York: Springer-Verlag, 1988.

35. Ezzone SD, Camp-Sorrell D, eds. *Manual for Bone Marrow Transplant Nursing: Recommendations for Practice and Education.* Pittsburgh: Oncology Nursing Press, Inc; 1994.

36. Fay JW, Nash RA, Wingard JR, et al. FK-506-based immunosuppression for prevention of graft versus host disease after unrelated donor marrow transplantation. *Transplant Proc.* 1995;56:1374.

37. Ford R, Ballard B. Acute complication after bone marrow transplantation. *Semin Oncol Nurs.* 1988;4:15–24.

38. Holmes W. Cyclosporin immunosuppression: clinical practice issues. *Curr Issues Cancer Nurs Pract.* 1993;1:1–7.

39. Kanfer E. Graft versus host disease. In: Treleaven J, Wiernik P, eds. *Bone Marrow Transplantation.* London, England: Mosby-Wolfe; 1995:143–153.

40. Vanecek KS. Gastrointestinal complications of bone marrow transplantation. In: Whedon MB, ed. *Bone Marrow Transplantation: Principles, Practice, and Nursing Insights.* Boston: Jones and Bartlett; 1991.

41. Vogelsang GV. Acute graft versus host disease following marrow transplantation. *Marrow Transplant Rev.* 1993;2:49–53.

42. Treleaven J, Wiernik P, eds. *Bone Marrow Transplantation.* London, England: Mosby-Wolfe; 1995.

43. Gale RP, Bortin MM, van Bekkum BW, et al. Risk factors for acute graft versus host disease. *Br J Haematol.* 1987;67:397–406.

44. Ferrara J, Deeg HJ. Graft versus host disease. *N Engl J Med.* 1991;324:667–674.

45. Hagglund H, Bostrom L, Remberger M. Risk factors for acute graft versus host disease in 291 consecutive HLA identical bone marrow transplant recipients. *Bone Marrow Transplant.* 1995;16:747–754.

46. Atkinson K. Chronic graft versus host disease following marrow transplantation. *Marrow Transplant Rev.* 1992;2:1–7.

47. Caudell KA. Graft versus host disease. In: Whedon MB, ed. *Bone Marrow Transplantation: Principles, Practice, and Nursing Insights.* Boston: Jones and Bartlett; 1991.

48. Sullivan K. Commentary: Prevention and treatment of chronic graft versus host disease. *Marrow Transplantation Reviews: Issues in Hematology, Oncology, and Immunology.* 1992;2:8–9.

49. Tzakis AG, Abu-Elmagd K, Fung JJ, et al. F.K. 506 rescue in chronic graft versus host disease. *Transplant Proc.* 1991;23:3225–3227.

50. Bortin MM, Gale RD, Weiner R, et al. Factors associated with interstitial pneumonitis after bone marrow transplantation. *Lancet.* 1982;1:437–441.

51. Bortin MM. Pathogenesis of interstitial pneumonitis following allogeneic bone marrow transplantation for acute leukemia. In: Gale RP, ed. *Recent Advances in Bone Marrow Transplantation.* New York: Alan R. Liss, 1983:445–460.

52. Cardozo BL. Interstitial pneumonitis following bone marrow transplantation; pathogenesis and therapeutic considerations. *European Journal of Cancer and Clinical Oncology.* 1985;21:43–47.

53. Fort JA, Graham-Pole J. Pulmonary complication of bone marrow transplantation. In: Johnson FL, Pochedlym C, eds. *Bone Marrow Transplantation in Children.* New York: Raven Press, Ltd; 1989:397–406.

54. Granena A, Carreras E, Rozman C, et al. Interstitial pneumonitis after BMT: 15 years experience at a single institution. *Bone Marrow Transplant.* 1993;13:453–458.

55. Krowka MJ, Rosenow EC, Hoagland HC. Pulmonary complications of bone marrow transplantation. *Chest.* 1985;87 (no. 2):237–246.

56. Meyers JD, Flourney N, Wade JC, et al. Biology of interstitial pneumonia after marrow transplantation. In: Gale RP, ed. *Recent Advances in Bone Marrow Transplantation.* New York: Alan R. Liss, Inc.; 1983:406–421.

57. Quabeck K. The lung as a critical organ in marrow

transplantation. *Bone Marrow Transplant.* 1994;14:519–528.

58. Weiner RS, Bortin MM, Gale RP, et al. Interstitial pneumonitis after bone marrow transplantation: assessment of risk factors. *Ann Intern Medicine.* 1986;104(no. 2):168–175.

59. Wikle-Shapiro TJ. Cardiopulmonary complications of bone marrow transplantation. In: Whedon MB, Wujik, D, eds. *Bone Marrow Transplantation: Principles, Practice, and Nursing Insights.* Boston: Jones and Bartlett. In press.

60. Atkinson JB, Connor DH, Robinowitz M, et al. Cardiac fungal infections: review of autopsy findings in 60 patients. *Human Pathol.* 1984;15:935–942.

61. Buja LM, Ferrans VJ, Graw RG, et al. Cardiac pathologic findings in patients treated with bone marrow transplantation. *Human Pathol.* 1976;7:15–45.

62. Carlson K, Smedmyr B, Backlund L, et al. Subclinical disturbances in cardiac function at rest and in gas exchange during exercise are common findings after autologous bone marrow transplantation. *Bone Marrow Transplant.* 1994;14:949–954.

63. Cazin B, Gorin NC, Laporte JP, et al. Cardiac complications after bone marrow transplantation. *Cancer.* 1986;57:2061–2069.

64. Keung YK, Lau S, Elkayan U, et al. Cardiac arrhythmia after infusion of cryopreserved stem cells. *Bone Marrow Transplant.* 1994;14:363–367.

65. Kupari M, Volin L, Timonen T, et al. Cardiac involvement on bone marrow transplantation: electrocardiographic changes, arrhythmias, heart failure, and autopsy findings. *Bone Marrow Transplant.* 1990;5:91–98.

66. Lopez-Jimenez J, Cervero C, Munoz A, et al. Cardiovascular toxicities related to the infusion of cryopreserved graft: results of a controlled study. *Bone Marrow Transplant.* 1994;13:789–793.

67. Minow RA, Benjamin RS, Lee ET, et al. Adriamycin cardiomyopathy: risk factors. *Cancer.* 1977;39:1397–1402.

68. Pihkala UM, Saanen U, Lundstrom M, et al. Effects of bone marrow transplantation on myocardial function in children. *Bone Marrow Transplant.* 1994;13:149–155.

69. von Herbay A, Dorken B, Mall G, et al. Cardiac damage in autologous bone marrow transplant patients: an autopsy study. *Klinische Wochenschrift.* 1988;66:1175–1181.

70. Johnson K, ed. *The Harriet Lane Handbook.* 13th ed. St. Louis: Mosby; 1993.

71. Cascinu S. Drug therapy in diarrheal diseases in oncology/hematology patients. *Crit Rev Oncol/Hematol.* 1995;18:37–50.

72. Fruto LV. Current concepts: management of diarrhea in acute care. *JWOCN.* 1994;21:199–20.

73. Jones B, Kramer S, Saral R. Gastrointestinal inflammation after bone marrow transplantation: Graft versus host disease or opportunistic infection. *Am J Roentgenology.* 1988;277–281.

74. McGuire DB, Altomonte V, Peterson DE, et al. Patterns of mucositis and pain in patients receiving preparative chemotherapy and bone marrow transplantation. *Oncol Nurs Forum.* 1993; 20:10:1493–1502.

75. Zerbe MB, Parkerson SG, Ortlieb ML, et al. Relationships between oral mucositis and treatment variables in bone marrow transplant patients. *Cancer Nurs.* 1992;15:3 196–205.

76. Woo SB, Sonis ST, Monopoli MM, et al. A longitudinal study of oral ulcerative mucositis in bone marrow transplant recipients. *Cancer.* 1993;72:1612–1617.

77. Dorr RT, Von Hof DD. *Cancer Chemotherapy Handbook.* Norwalk: Appleton & Lange; 1994.

78. Bearman SI, Appelbaum FR, Buckner CD. Regimen-related toxicity in patients undergoing bone marrow transplantation. *Journal of Clinical Oncology.* 1988;6:1562–1568.

79. Einsele H, Ehninger G, Steidle M, et al. Polymerase chain reaction to evaluate antiviral therapy for cytomegalovirus disease. *Lancet*. 1991;338:1170–1172.

80. Juckett M, Perry EH, Daniels BS, Weisdorf DJ. Hemolytic uremic syndrome following bone marrow transplantation. *Bone Marrow Transplant*. 1991;7:405–409.

81. Garrick R. Neurological complications. In: Atkinson K, ed. *Clinical Bone Marrow Transplantation: A Reference Textbook*. Cambridge, England: Cambridge University Press; 1994:480–497.

82. Patchell RA, White CL, Clark AW, et al. Neurologic complications of bone marrow transplantation. *Neurology*. 1985;35:300–306.

83. Mohrmann RL, Mah V, Vinters HV. Neuropathologic findings after bone marrow transplantation: an autopsy study. *Hum Pathol*. 1990;21:630–639.

84. Verfaillie C, Weisdorf D, Haake R, et al. *Candida* infections in bone marrow transplant recipients. *Bone Marrow Transplant*. 1991;8:177–184.

85. Meyers JD. Infection in recipients of bone marrow transplants. *Curr Clin Top Infect Dis*. 1985;6:261–292.

86. Locksley RM, Flournoy N, Sullivan KM, Meyers JD. Infection with varicella zoster virus infection after marrow transplantation. *J Infect Dis*. 1985;152:1172–1181.

87. Schuchter LM, Wingard JR, Piantadosi S, et al. Herpes zoster infection after autologous bone marrow transplantation. *Blood*. 1989;74:1424–1427.

88. DeLa Camara R, Tomas JF, Fiquera A, et al. High dose busulfan and seizures. *Bone Marrow Transplant*. 1991;7:363–364.

89. Hassas M, Ehrsson H, Smedmyr B, et al. Cerebrospinal fluid and plasma concentrations of busulfan during high-dose therapy. *Bone Marrow Transplant*. 1989;4:113–114.

90. Jagannath S, Armitage JO, Dickie KA, et al. Prognostic factors for response and survival after high dose cyclophosphamide, carmustine, and etoposide with autologous bone marrow transplantation for relapsed Hodgkin's disease. *J Clin Oncol.* 1989;7:179–185.

91. Ghany AM, Tutschka PJ, McGhee RB, et al. Cyclosporin associated seizures in bone marrow transplantation recipients given busulfan and cyclophosphamide preparative therapy. *Transplantation.* 1991;52:310–315.

92. Kahan BD. Cyclosporine. *N Engl J Med.* 1989;321:1725–1738.

93. Reece DE, Frei-Lahr DA, Sherperd JS, et al. Neurologic complications in allogeneic bone marrow transplant patients receiving cyclosporin. *Bone Marrow Transplant.* 1991;8:393–401.

94. Schmidley JW, Galloway P. Polymyositis following autologous bone marrow transplantation in Hodgkin's disease. *Neurology.* 1990;40(6):1003–1004.

Bibliography

Andrykowski MA, Altmaier EM, Barnett RL, et al. Cognitive dysfunction in adult survivors of allogeneic marrow transplantation: relationship to dose of total body irradiation. *Bone Marrow Transplant.* 1990;6:269–279.

Ballard B. Renal and hepatic complications. In: Whedon MB, ed. *Bone Marrow Transplantation: Principles, Practice, and Nursing Insights.* Boston: Jones and Bartlett; 1991.

Bertheau P, Hadengue A, Cazals-Hatem D, et al. Chronic cholestasis in patients after allogeneic bone marrow transplantation. *Bone Marrow Transplant.* 1995;16:261–265.

Bicknell SL, McCallum O, Wright LF. Urinary tract disorders. In: Rakel RE, ed. *Textbook of Family Practice.* 6th ed. Philadelphia: W. B. Saunders Company; 1995.

Ferrara JL, Deeg HJ. Graft versus host disease. *N Engl J Med.* 1991;324:667–674.

Gluckman E. Veno-occlusive disease. In: Atkinson K, ed. *Clinical Bone Marrow Transplantation: A Reference Textbook*. Cambridge, England: Cambridge University Press; 1994.

Hwang TL, Yung WKA, Estey EH, Fields WS. Central nervous system toxicity with high dose Ara-C. *Neurology*. 1985;35:1475–1479.

Locasciulli A, Bacigalupo A, VanLint MT, et al. Hepatitis C virus and liver failure in patients undergoing allogeneic bone marrow transplantation. *Bone Marrow Transplant*. 1995;16:407–411.

Mouser JF, Hak LJ. Acute and chronic renal diseases. In: Herfindal ET, Gourley DR, eds. *Textbook of Therapeutics: Drug and Disease Management*. 6th ed. Baltimore: Williams & Wilkins; 1996.

Or R, Mehta J, Nagler A, Cracium I. Neutropenic enterocolitis associated with autologous bone marrow transplantation. *Bone Marrow Transplant*. 1992;9:833–835.

Rabinowe SN, Soiffer RJ, Tarbell NJ, et al. Hemolytic-uremic syndrome following bone marrow transplantation in adults for hematologic malignancies. *Blood*. 1991;77:1837–1844.

Reed EC, Wolford JL, Kopecky KJ. Ganciclovir for the treatment of cytomegalovirus gastroenteritis in bone marrow transplant patients: a randomized, placebo-controlled trial. *Ann Intern Med*. 1990;112:505–520.

Schiller GJ, Nimer SD, Gajewski JL. Abdominal presentation of varicella-zoster infection in recipients of allogeneic bone marrow transplantation. *Bone Marrow Transplant*. 1991;7:489–491.

Schubert MM, Williams BE, Lliod ME, et al. Clinical assessment scale for the rating of oral mucosal changes following bone marrow transplantation. *Cancer*. 1992;69:2469–2477.

Shuhart MC, McDonald GB. Gastrointestinal and hepatic complications. In: Foreman SJ, Blume KG, Thomas ED, eds. *Bone Marrow Transplantation*. Boston: Blackwell Scientific Publications; 1994.

Speicher CE. *The Right Test.* 2nd ed. Philadelphia: W. B. Saunders Company; 1993.

Van Bekkum DW. What is graft versus host disease: clinical significance and response to immunosuppressive therapy? *Blood.* 1990;76:110–111.

Vickers CR. Gastrointestinal complications. In: Atkinson K, ed. *Clinical Bone Marrow Transplantation: A Reference Textbook.* Cambridge, England: Cambridge University Press; 1994:435–443.

Vickers CR. Hepatic complications. In: Atkinson K, ed. *Clinical Bone Marrow Transplantation: A Reference Textbook.* Cambridge, England: Cambridge University Press; 1994:444–451.

Weisdorf SA, Snover DC, Haake R. Acute upper gastrointestinal graft versus host disease: clinical significance and response to immunosuppressive therapy. *Blood.* 1990;76:624–629.

Weisdorf SA, Roy J, Snover D. Inflammatory cells in graft versus host disease of the rectum: immunopathologic analysis. *Bone Marrow Transplant.* 1991;7:297–301.

CHAPTER 6

Diagnostic Test Interpretations

I. Hematology

A. Peripheral blood smear interpretation: Wright's stain technique

1. Place air-dried blood smears, film side up, on staining rack.
2. Cover blood smear with Wright's stain, and leave on for two to three minutes.
3. Rinse with equal amount of distilled water and until a greenish metallic sheen appears. Leave diluted stain on smear for two to four minutes.
4. Flood with water, and wash until stained smear is pinkish-red. Blot dry.

B. Reticulocyte count

1. Mix equal amounts of new methylene blue or brilliant cresyl blue with whole blood. After 10 to 20 minutes, prepare thin smears on a slide.
2. Count the number of reticulocytes per 1000 red cells. The reticulocytes contain reticulum or blue granules.
3. The amount should be reported as a percentage of red blood cells.

C. Anemia is defined by specific norms, and in the transplant patient, it is a result of inadequate production of red cells, excessive loss of red cells due to hemolysis or bleeding, or increased pooling and destruction of red cells due to an enlarged spleen. About seven to ten days after the ablative conditioning regimen, circulating nucleated red cells will be evident in buffy coat preparations. Circulating reticulocytes, however, will not be evident until about two to three weeks after marrow infusion. Return of normal erythropoiesis is generally first evident by the appearance of reticulocytes in the circulating blood.[1]

1. Etiology: Anemia due to dyserythropoiesis can be caused by
   a) Inadequate production of red cells due to insufficient marrow stem cells
   b) Chronic graft-versus-host disease (GVHD) involving the marrow
   c) Drugs (e.g., antimicrobial agents)
   d) Immune hemolytic anemia, ABO-mismatched transplants
   e) Lack of erythropoietin production, leading to insufficient stimulus of red cell production, common in the allogeneic bone marrow transplant (BMT) patient[2]
   f) Renal toxicity associated with cyclosporin A
   g) Red cell aplasia
   h) Sideroblastic anemia

2. Laboratory studies
   a) Complete blood count with differential and reticulocyte count
   b) Blood smear to examine morphology of cells
   c) Stool for occult blood
   d) Urinalysis for blood, bilirubin, glucose, protein
   e) Serum bilirubin, blood urea nitrogen, creatinine
   f) Bone marrow aspirate and biopsy examination

D. Thrombocytopenia: The megakaryocyte is the last cell to arrive in the myeloid engraftment process. Most patients are transfusion dependent for the first several weeks after transplant. Platelet counts are not normal until one to three months after transplant. Prolonged thrombocytopenia post-BMT is a complication, with two distinct types of thrombocytopenia described: transient benign thrombocytopenia and chronic persistent thrombocytopenia.[3]

1. Etiology
   a) Acute and chronic GVHD
   b) Alloimmune mechanism
   c) Autoimmune mechanism with a positive antiplatelet antibody test
   d) Purging agents
   e) Cryopreservation techniques
   f) Viral infections
2. Laboratory studies
   a) Transient benign thrombocytopenia: Platelet count remains normal, falls, and returns to normal.
   b) Chronic persistent thrombocytopenia: Platelet count is usually not achieved despite normal granulocyte and reticulocyte count.
   c) Platelet antibodies studies
   d) Megakaryocyte colony-stimulating activity: These levels peak after the administration of the conditioning regimen and for two weeks after the transplant, which corresponds to hematopoietic recovery.[4] Patients who fail to engraft do not show a spike.

II. Blood component replacement

A. Red blood cell transfusions

Volume of cells (mL) =
$$\frac{\text{Estimated blood volume X desired hematocrit change}}{\text{Hematocrit of packed red blood cells}}$$

1. The usual hematocrit of packed red blood cells is 65%. One unit of packed red blood cells will raise the hemoglobin 1 G/dL or the hematocrit 3%.
2. One unit can be transfused over two to four hours.

3. If the unit has not been leukocyte depleted, it should be administered with a leukocyte filter. Filtering will collect the remaining white cells in the product. Removing the white cells will minimize the potential for alloimmunization and in turn will prevent transfusion reactions.

B. Platelet transfusions

$$\text{Platelet increment/}\mu L = \frac{30{,}000 \times \text{number of units}}{\text{estimated blood volume (L)}}$$

1. Random-donor pooled concentrate products: pooled products from multiple donors
2. Single-donor products: products from a single donor obtained by apheresis. They are used in patients with antibodies from multiple transfusions to reduce the potential for alloimmunization.
3. HLA-matched products: products specifically matched to the patient's human leukocyte antigen (HLA) type
4. Post–platelet transfusion blood counts can be obtained as soon as 10 minutes after the completion of the transfusion.
5. One unit of platelets raises the platelet count 10,000/μL in the absence of platelet antibodies or factors that destroy platelets.
6. Platelet transfusions can be administered as rapidly as the patient can tolerate them.
7. Factors that contribute to poor responses to platelet transfusions
   a) Sepsis
   b) Fever
   c) Splenomegaly
   d) Disseminated intravascular coagulation (DIC)
   e) Drug-induced antibodies (e.g., vancomycin, quinidine, phenytoin, co-trimoxazole)

f) Bleeding

g) Platelet antibodies

C. Irradiated blood products

    1. Many blood products contain viable lymphocytes capable of being transfused to the recipient.

    2. Irradiation with the use of 1500 rads prior to transfusion can prevent GVHD in the immunocompromised transplant patient.

D. Cytomegalovirus (CMV)-negative blood products

    1. Desired in BMT patients who are CMV antibody negative to minimize transmission of CMV

    2. Patients who are CMV positive usually receive CMV untested products.

    3. CMV-negative products require a longer time to prepare and are more expensive than CMV untested products.

III. Blood chemistries, electrolytes, and minerals

A. Hyperglycemia is a frequent occurrence in patients in middle age or older age undergoing BMT. The type of hyperglycemia that generally occurs is type II maturity-onset diabetes; however, insulin therapy is usually required, but ketoacidosis is rare.

    1. Etiology

        a) Limitation of endogenous insulin production: pentamidine used for the treatment of pneumocystis pneumonitis. Damage is caused to the beta cells of the pancreas.

        b) Development of insulin resistance: Corticosteroids (cause an enhanced hepatic glucose output, which results in insulin resistance), infection, inflammation, emotional stress.

    2. Diagnostic studies

        a) Plasma glucose monitoring indications for further diagnostic testing: random plasma glucose monitoring greater than 160 mg/dL, fasting glucose greater than 115 mg/dL

b) Glucose measurements are necessary to document efficacy and to guide modification of therapy.

c) Plasma glucose measurement is appropriate for screening and diagnosis and the traditional therapeutic parameter. Avoid fingerprick or cutaneous puncture in the presence of thrombocytopenia. Monitoring should be achievable on the basis of two to three blood glucose measurements in a 24-hour period.

d) Capillary blood glucose measurement allows for rapid measurement of glucose in whole blood. This is a method of monitoring that is portable, convenient, and a cost-effective alternative to frequent plasma glucose determinations.

e) Reduction of insulin dose should be considered when corticosteroid dose reduction occurs or when treatment of an infection is effective.

B. Hypocalcemia can occur secondary to magnesium deficiency. Magnesium is necessary for both the release of parathyroid hormone and its peripheral action. Hypomagnesemia results in hypocalcemia that does not respond to calcium replacement.

1. Etiology

a) Magnesium deficiency occurs in the BMT patient as a result of cisplatin therapy, cyclosporin A therapy, diuretic therapy, and chronic diarrhea (e.g., post-conditioning therapy or secondary to GVHD).

b) Other causes of hypocalcemia include renal disease.

2. Diagnostic studies

a) Serum calcium

b) Serum magnesium

c) Serum phosphate

C. Hyperphosphatemia is a complication of treatment when the phosphorous level rises to 4.5 mg/dL. Rapid tumor lysis releases large amounts of uric acid, potassium, and phosphate. Elevated blood phosphate levels can persist for four to five days and can exceed 20 mg/dL. High phosphate levels should be lowered rapidly to avoid or reverse renal damage.

   1. Etiology: tumor lysis syndrome after conditioning therapy
   2. Diagnostic studies
      a) Serum phosphate (elevated)
      b) Serum calcium

D. Hypernatremia is usually caused by a loss of water from the body fluids. Any hypotonic fluid loss (i.e., diaphoresis, fever, hyperventilation, vomiting) will cause hypernatremia. Polyuria will usually be the presenting symptom; however, if the solute intake is low, urine output may not exceed 2 L/d.

   1. Etiology: Serum sodium elevations in the BMT patient are encountered due to decreased oral intake.
      a) Anorexia
      b) Mucositis
      c) Vomiting
   2. Diagnostic study: serum sodium (elevated)

E. Hyponatremia is also known as syndrome of inappropriate antidiuretic hormone. Antidiuretic hormone is normally released from the posterior pituitary gland in response to increased osmolality or decreased volume of plasma. The release of antidiuretic hormone is normally inhibited by decreased plasma osmolality and increased plasma volume. The hormone acts by increasing water resorption from the renal collecting tubules.

1. Etiology
    a) Renal losses: nephropathy, drugs (diuretics, amphotericin, chemotherapy [i.e., cyclophosphamide], narcotics)
    b) Extrarenal losses: gastrointestinal or skin
2. Diagnostic studies
    a) Renal losses: urine volume (increased), urine sodium (increased), specific gravity (decreased)
    b) Extrarenal losses: urine volume (decreased), urine sodium (decreased), specific gravity (increased)

F. Hyperkalemia in the cancer and BMT patient develops due to renal failure. This condition can develop due to tumor lysis following conditioning therapy. The presenting symptoms are neuromuscular in nature, with the primary symptom being weakness.
    1. Etiology
        a) Renal failure secondary to treatment
        b) Tumor lysis syndrome
    2. Diagnostic study: serum potassium (increased)

G. Hyperuricemia and hyperuricosuria present a major problem for BMT patients with leukemias, lymphomas, and multiple myeloma. During conditioning therapy, massive tumor lysis results in excessive production of uric acid. Uric acid nephropathy results from the precipitation of uric acid crystals in the concentrated, acidic urine of the renal medulla, distal tubules, and the collecting ducts. The sludge leads to obstruction nephropathy, causing inflammatory interstitial changes.
    1. Etiology: rapid tumor lysis
    2. Diagnostic studies
        a) Serum uric acid (elevated)
        b) Urine uric acid (elevated)

IV. Body fluids

A. Bone marrow

1. Indication: diagnosis of a disease status or reevaluation of disease

2. Sites

   a) Posterior iliac crest: the preferred site for *adults and children over the age of 3 months*

   b) Tibia: the preferred site for *children under the age of 3 months*

3. Positioning for the iliac crest technique: Position patient on a firm table in the lateral recumbent position with neck, knees, and hip flexed or in a prone position with a pillow under the pelvis to elevate the pelvis slightly.

4. Anesthesia: Anesthetize the skin, soft tissue, and periosteum with local anesthesia (e.g., 1% lidocaine).

5. Technique

   a) Always use sterile technique for bone marrow aspiration.

   b) Enter the ileum at the posterior superior iliac spine, which is a visible and palpable bony prominence superior and lateral to the intergluteal cleft. It is inferior and medial to the crest.

   c) Insert the needle with a boring motion using steady pressure. Direct the needle perpendicular to the surface of the bone.

   d) When the needle enters the marrow space, decreased resistance may be felt. The needle will become anchored in place.

6. Smear technique

   a) Eject marrow from the syringe onto a clean slide. This should be done quickly to prevent clotting.

   b) Position the slide at an angle for the excessive blood and plasma to drain to the bottom of the slide. Bone marrow spicules should be apparent.

   c) With another slide, pick up the marrow spicules and smear them onto another slide.

B. Thoracentesis

  1. Indications: diagnosis or removal of an abnormal collection of fluid within the pleural space

  2. Site

   a) Select the interspace to be tapped on the basis of dullness to percussion and the level of effusion on the erect chest x-ray.

   b) In the event of a small pleural effusion, position the patient, tilting the patient laterally toward the affected side to maximize yield.

  3. Positioning: The procedure can be performed with the patient sitting on the side of the bed and with the assistant standing in front of the patient.

  4. Anesthesia: Anesthetize the skin, soft tissue, and pleura in the interspace above the rib with local anesthesia (i.e., 1% lidocaine).

  5. Technique

   a) Clean and drape the chest wall.

   b) Attach a large-bore needle or intravenous catheter to a three-way stopcock and syringe.

   c) With the needle bevel down, insert the needle directly on the rib below the desired interspace, and walk the needle over the superior edge of the rib.

   d) Advance the needle. A pop or pressure change is felt on entering the pleural space.

   e) Advance the catheter 2 to 3 mm, and remove the stylet.

   f) Attach the syringe with a stopcock to the hub of the catheter, and slowly withdraw the desired volume of fluid.

   g) At the end of the procedure, withdraw the needle or catheter, and place a dressing over the thoracentesis to avoid pneumothorax.

6. Pleural fluid analysis (Table 6.1)
   a) Send fluid for laboratory studies, including electrolytes, glucose protein, cell count, differential, Gram's stain, and culture.
   b) Malignant effusions are usually exudative but may be transudative. Results of fluid analysis may be nonspecific.

Table 6.1 Evaluation of Pleural and Pericardial Fluid

Laboratory test	Transudate	Exudate
Specific gravity	< 1.016	> 1.016
Protein	< 3.0 g/dL	> 3.0 g/dL
Fluid-serum ratio	< 0.5	> 0.5
Lactate dehydrogenase	< 200 IU	> 200 IU
White blood cells	< 1000/µL (lymphs)	> 10,000/IµL
Red blood cells	< 10,000/µL	Variable; > 100,000/µL is suspicious
Glucose	Same as serum	Decreased
pH	> 7.2	< 7.0

C. Pericardiocentesis
   1. Indications: To remove pericardial effusion fluid for diagnostic or therapeutic purposes.
   2. Site: Select the site left of the xiphoid process, 1.0 cm inferior to the bottom rib.
   3. Positioning: The procedure can be performed with the patient lying at a 30-degree angle.
   4. Anesthesia
      a) Sedate the patient, unless contraindicated, and monitor the electrocardiogram during the procedure.
      b) Anesthetize the skin, soft tissue, and puncture site with local anesthesia (e.g., 1% lidocaine).
   5. Technique
      a) Clean and drape the chest wall.

    b) With needle bevel down, insert an 18- or 20-gauge
       needle left of the xiphoid process, 1.0 cm inferior
       to the bottom rib at approximately a 60-degree
       angle to the skin.
    c) Advance the needle. A pop or pressure change is
       felt on entering the pericardial space.
    d) While gently aspirating, advance the needle
       toward the patient's left shoulder until pericardial
       fluid is obtained.
    e) On entering the pericardial space, clamp the
       needle at the skin edge to prevent further
       penetration.
    f) Attach a 30-mL syringe with a stopcock to the hub
       of the needle. Slowly withdraw the desired volume
       of fluid.
    g) Fluid should be withdrawn slowly. Too rapid a
       withdrawal of pericardial fluid can result in shock
       or myocardial insufficiency.
    h) At the end of the procedure, withdraw the
       needle slowly. Place a dressing over the
       pericardiocentesis.

D. Lumbar puncture
  1. Indications: To remove cerebrospinal fluid (CSF)
    for diagnostic or therapeutic purposes (e.g., infection,
    disease involvement [malignancy], or instillation of
    intrathecal chemotherapy).
  2. Site: Select the desired interspace (e.g., L3–4 or
    L4–5) by drawing a line between the top of the
    iliac crest sites.
  3. Precautions:
    a) Platelet count: A platelet count of 50,000/μL
       is recommended prior to performing
       this procedure.
    b) Physical examination: Prior to lumbar puncture,
       perform a funduscopic examination. The presence
       of papilledema, retinal hemorrhage, or clinical

evidence of increased intracranial pressure is a contraindication to the procedure. A sudden drop in intraspinal pressure by rapid release of CSF may cause herniation. If lumbar puncture is performed, proceed with extreme caution.

4. Positioning: The procedure can be performed with the patient in a sitting lateral recumbent position with hips, knees, and neck flexed.

5. Anesthesia: Anesthetize the skin, soft tissue, and puncture site with local anesthesia (e.g., 1% lidocaine).

6. Technique
   a) Position and locate the desired intraspace.
   b) Clean the skin with povidone-iodine and 70% alcohol. Drape the patient.
   c) Use a spinal needle with a stylet. Puncture the skin midline just below the palpated spinal process, angling the needle slightly cephalad. Advance the needle several millimeters at a time. Withdraw the stylet, checking for CSF.
   d) Advance the needle. A pop or pressure change is felt on entering the dura. If resistance is met, withdraw the needle to the skin surface, and redirect the angle slightly.
   e) Attach the manometer to the needle hub of the needle. Once free flow of CSF occurs, attach the manometer and measure the CSF. Withdraw the desired volume of fluid for specimen collection.
   f) Collect four tubes of CSF; 1 to 2 mL of fluid is necessary per specimen. Cell count and Gram's stain can be done with 1 mL of fluid.
   g) At the end of the procedure, withdraw the needle slowly. Place a dressing over the lumbar puncture site.

7. CSF analysis (Table 6.2)
   a) Specimens: Send fluid for laboratory studies, including electrolytes, glucose, protein, cell count and differential, Gram's stain, and cultures. Label the tubes as follows: "#1 Culture," "#2 Chemistries," and "#3 Cell count." Send specimens to the laboratory immediately.
   b) Appearance: Record the color and clarity of the fluid. Note the presence of coagula, pellicles, or sediment. Time required for the formation will vary with different diseases.

Table 6.2 Cerebrospinal Fluid Laboratory Values

Condition	CSF pressure	Glucose level	Cytology	Predominant leukocyte
Disease related				
Tumor	Increased	Normal	Rare	Mononuclear
Meningeal carcinomatosis	Decreased	Normal	Rare	Mononuclear
Infectious related				
Bacterial meningitis	Increased	Decreased	None	Neutrophil
Cryptococcal meningitis	Increased	Increased Decreased Normal	None	Lymphocyte
Epidural abscess	Decreased	Normal	None	Lymphocyte

V. Microbiology

A. Organism staining: To identify microorganisms under the microscope, staining is a critical element. The three stains most commonly used are the Gram's stain, acid-fast stain, and India ink stain. The techniques that provide the best results are thin smears, allowing smears to dry before they are fixed (heating wet smears distorts the organisms and cells), and fixing smears with heat by quickly passing the slide through a flame. The slide should not be stained until it cools.

1. Gram's stain
   a) Place gentian violet on the slide for one minute, and wash with running water.
   b) Flood with iodine solution for one minute, and wash with running water.
   c) Decolorize with acetone/alcohol for three to four seconds, and wash with water.
   d) Stain with safranin for 30 seconds, and wash with water.

2. Acid-fast stain
   a) Place Kinyoun carbolfuchsin stain on slide for five minutes, and wash with water.
   b) Decolorize with acid alcohol for two minutes, and wash with water.
   c) Counterstain with 0.5% methylene blue for two minutes, and wash with water.

3. India ink capsule stain
   a) Mix one drop of test fluid with one drop of India ink.
   b) Cover with a coverslip.
   c) Ring with petrolatum.
   d) Look for a round organism against a dark background.

B. Culture techniques: If culturing is unavailable from the hospital laboratory, culturing should be done as follows:

1. Bacterial cultures
   a) Blood: The sample volume should equal 10% of the volume of the culture medium. When the patient is treated with penicillin, consider using penicillinase-containing broth for culture.
   b) Ear and nose: chocolate blood agar, followed by 5% sheep blood agar, followed by MacConkey agar. Place the swab in the transport medium.

c) Throat: 5% sheep blood agar, followed by MacConkey agar. Place the swab in the transport medium.

d) Skin: 5% sheep blood agar, followed by MacConkey agar, followed by thioglycollate broth. Place the swab in the transport medium.

e) Cavity fluids: Place in anaerobic culture containers.

2. Fungal cultures
   a) Use a scalpel to scrape the edges of the lesion in which fungus is suspected onto a glass slide.
   b) Cover scraping with 10% to 20% KOH or NaOH, and apply a coverslip.
   c) Warm for a few minutes.
   d) Examine for spore fragments.

3. Viral cultures
   a) Pharyngeal, nasopharyngeal, and rectal cultures: Send in viral culture media.
   b) Blood, bone marrow, CSF, and urine: Send in sterile containers.
   c) Specimens should be cultured and sent within one hour after collection.

VI. Liver functions and gastroenterology

A. Stool examination

1. Blood: occult blood guaiac method
   a) Purpose: to screen for the presence of blood in the stool
   b) Reagents: glacial acetic acid, guaiac, hydrogen peroxide
   c) Method: Place a small amount of stool on the filter paper. Serially apply two drops of each reagent in the following order: acetic acid, guaiac, and hydrogen peroxide.

d) Interpretation: A positive test result will be a purple or dark blue color on the filter paper. A negative test result is a green color on the filter paper.

2. Parasites
   a) Direct smear: Add a small amount of fecal material to a drop of saline mix, remove feces with an applicator stick, and cover. Examine the specimen under low power to locate the parasites and high power to identify the parasites.
   b) Preservatives: Specimens should be delivered to the laboratory immediately. Place in formalin if a delay in specimen delivery is anticipated.

B. Diarrhea
   1. Definition: watery, frequent loose stool caused by a shift in the intestinal water and electrolyte transport due to an increased osmolar load or active secretion of water into the intestinal lumen
   2. Etiology of acute diarrhea (self-limiting, < 14 days)
      a) Infectious
      b) Preparative regimen: total body irradiation (TBI), ifosfamide, and carboplatin
      c) Drugs: antacids, antimicrobial agents, chemotherapy conditioning regimen, cardiac medications, magnesium replacement secondary to cyclosporin A
   3. Etiology of chronic diarrhea (> 14 days)
      a) Infectious: fungal (e.g., *Candida*), parasitic (e.g., Giardia), viral (e.g., cytomegalovirus)
      b) Inflammatory (e.g., ulcerative enterocolitis)
      c) GVHD of the gut
      d) Pseudomembranous colitis: secondary to antibiotic therapy caused by *Clostridium difficile*.
      e) Secretory diarrhea: caused by an abnormal secretion of water and electrolytes into the intestinal lumen. It persists despite fasting.

      f) Osmotic diarrhea: caused by the accumulation of poorly absorbed solutes in the intestine. It usually stops with fasting.

  4. Stool evaluation

      a) Fecal leukocytes: The presence of white blood cells is indicative of bacterial infection.

      b) Occult blood (Hemoccult): Blood present in the stool may indicate bacterial infection or inflammation of the bowel.

      c) Sudan III: Screen for fecal fat malabsorption.

      d) Stool electrolytes: Secretory diarrhea tends to have an elevated stool sodium and a lower osmotic gap (< 100 mOsm/L). In malabsorption or viral illness, the stool tends to have a decreased sodium and increased osmotic gap (> 100 mOsm/L).

      e) Endoscopy evaluation with biopsy: Platelet count should be in the 50,000/L range. Coagulation parameters should be within the normal range before a biopsy is performed. Biopsies should be taken from the normal mucosa and the edges of the ulcerated mucosa. Endoscopy intubation should be done with caution to prevent laryngeal bleeding.

C. Constipation

  1. Definition: a decrease in the frequency of the stool, usually associated with painful or difficult passage of hard stool.

  2. Etiology

      a) Functional: idiopathic

      b) Electrolyte imbalance: hypokalemia, hypocalcemia

      c) Drugs: antacids, anticonvulsants, antihypertensives, diuretics, opiates, phenothiazines

  3. Diagnostic studies

      a) Abdominal plain films to determine bowel obstruction

b) Barium enema/large intestine study: The test provides both x-ray and fluoroscopic techniques to demonstrate the anatomy of the large intestine. Indications include to rule out obstruction, masses, and inflammatory changes. Normal outcome shows normal position, contour, filling, and patency of the large bowel. The procedure is as follows: Contrast agent (barium) is given in the form of an enema via the rectum. Under fluoroscopy, the colon is completely filled to the ileocecal junction. Contrast is maintained in the colon for several minutes while the x-rays are taken. A postevacuation film is taken to ensure that all the barium is expelled. The importance of forcing fluids after the procedure is stressed.

D. Hemorrhage

1. Definition: Minor gastrointestinal bleeding presenting as small hematemesis or bleeding. Resolution usually occurs with correction of thrombocytopenia and correction of abnormal clotting.
2. Etiology
   a) Acute GVHD
   b) Duodenal ulcer
   c) Small bowel ulcer
   d) Gastric erosion
3. Diagnostic study: upper endoscopy evaluation with biopsy
   a) Platelet count should be in the 50,000/L range.
   b) Coagulation parameters should be within the normal range before a biopsy is performed.
   c) Biopsies should be taken from the normal mucosa and the edges of the ulcerated mucosa.
   d) Endoscopy intubation should be done with caution to prevent laryngeal bleeding.

E. Abdominal pain
   1. Etiology
      a) Duodenal ulcer
      b) Gallbladder disease
      c) GVHD
      d) Hemorrhagic cystitis
      e) Liver disease, veno-occlusive disease,
         viral hepatitis
      f) Pancreatitis
   2. Diagnostic studies
      a) Abdominal x-rays to determine bowel obstruction.
         Films should be performed erect and supine.
      b) Upper and/or lower endoscopy with biopsy:
         Platelet count should be in the 50,000/L range.
         Coagulation parameters should be within the
         normal range before a biopsy is performed.
         Biopsies should be taken from the normal mucosa
         and edges of the ulcerated mucosa. Endoscopy
         intubation should be done with caution in the
         transplant patient to prevent laryngeal or rectal
         bleeding. Symptoms of bowel perforation are
         abdominal distention, bleeding, fever, and pain.
      c) Abdominal ultrasound: noninvasive procedure that
         produces sound waves from a handheld transducer.
         Food restriction usually applies six to 12 hours
         prior to the examination. Water is normally
         permitted. The patient will be required to change
         position during the scanning procedure. Breathing
         may need to be controlled during the imaging.
         Examination time is usually 30 to 60 minutes.

VII. Cytogenetics

A. Definition: Cytogenetics is the study of the origin,
   structure, and function of chromosomes. It has the
   ability to identify certain genes that are associated
   with chromosomal abnormalities. There are normally

23 pairs of chromosomes. A chromosome is divided into three parts: a short arm called p, a long arm called q, and a centromere.

B. Karyotype analysis:
   1. When chromosomes are stained, regions and bands are named from the centromere toward the telomere (the region at the end of each chromosomal arm). Chromosomal abnormalities are then identified according to the banding pattern.
   2. Commonly identified chromosomal alterations are referred to as translocations, duplications, deletions, or inversions. There are genes that are located close to the chromosomal rearrangement that cause the aberrant expression of the genes that control cell growth.
   3. If there are changes in the leukocyte, they will result in unregulated leukocyte proliferation, and subsequently leukemia will develop.

C. Application
   1. Abnormalities of the patient's karyotype classify disease and predict prognosis.
   2. Cytogenetic markers do not always predict remission; however, they are often indicative of remission duration.
   3. Cytogenetic abnormalities can be classified as primary and secondary. Primary abnormalities influence the patient's treatment and prognosis. Secondary abnormalities, when identified, are indicative of a poor prognosis.
   4. The presence of additions or deletions on chromosomes has a more favorable prognosis.

D. Cytogenetic specimen sampling
   1. Cytogenetic specimens are usually obtained from bone marrow aspirate specimens.

2. In the event that bone marrow aspirate is unavailable, cytogenetics can be obtained from peripheral blood.

VIII. Endocrinology

A. Gonadal dysfunction

1. Definition: damage that occurs to the germ cells resulting in substantial alteration of gonadotropin-releasing hormone levels

2. Etiology
   a) TBI
   b) Chemotherapy conditioning regimen

3. Diagnostic studies
   a) Measure pituitary luteinizing hormone (LH) and follicle-stimulating hormone (FSH).
   b) Males: elevation of FSH. Testosterone and LH are normal.
   c) Females: elevation of FSH and LH. Estrogen is usually low.
   d) Prepubescent girls: Delayed puberty will occur in 50% of the cases. The delay is related to the age at the time treatment occurs.
   e) Postpubertal females: anovulation with low estrogen levels and elevated FSH and LH levels
   f) Prepubescent boys: Delayed puberty occurs in 70% to 90% of the cases.
   g) Spermatogenesis may be impaired.

B. Growth hormone (GH)

1. Definition: Impaired growth velocity and GH secretion may occur after high-dose chemotherapy and TBI. This is caused by the decreased production of GH and growth factors like IGF-I, an insulin-like growth factor.

2. Etiology
   a) Chemotherapy
   b) TBI
   c) GVHD

      d) Chronic glucocorticosteroid

      e) Compromised nutrition

  3. Diagnostic studies

      a) GH secretion is pulsatile. Diagnosis of GH deficiency requires two, low normal stimulation readings. Screening tests are not considered stimulation tests. Patients must be euthyroid for the test to be valid.

      b) Stimulation test: GH secretion can be stimulated by arginine, clonidine, insulin-induced hypoglycemia, L-dopa, and glucagon.

      c) GH level interpretation:

         (1) Greater than 10 ng/mL effectively rules out GH deficiency.

         (2) 5 to 10 ng/mL may be indicative of partial deficiency.

         (3) Less than 5 ng/mL is indicative of an abnormal test.

      d) Other contributing factors in females: Low levels of estrogen can contribute to decreased growth.

      e) Other contributing factors in males: Low levels of estrogen can contribute to decreased growth.

C. Hypothalamic and pituitary function

  1. Definition: Hypothalamic-pituitary function is an uncommon occurrence after BMT; however, it can occur after conditioning regimens with TBI. The pituitary synthesizes at least six hormones: prolactin, adrenocorticotropic hormone (ACTH), GH, FSH, LH, and thyroid-stimulating hormone (TSH). All are important in normal physiology; however, ACTH and TSH are critical for survival. The pituitary can be involved in hypo- and hyperfunction.

  2. Etiology

      a) TBI

      b) Radiation therapy to the cranial cavity: adults, 7500 cGy; children, 2400 cGy

3. Diagnostic studies
   a) Adrenal capacity test (ACTH stimulation test) is used to evaluate adrenal insufficiency, usually secondary (ACTH deficiency) to adrenal suppression after long-term steroid use for GVHD prophylaxis regimens. With a normal pituitary adrenal axis, there will be a rise in serum cortisol intravenous ACTH. With low pituitary function, there will be no rise in ACTH after a single dose of intravenous ACTH.
   b) GH deficiency: Most of the growth-promoting effects of GH are mediated by IGF-I. GH secretion is episodic, and its serum half-life is short. Measurement of serum IGF-I is the screening test of choice. The diagnosis can be confirmed by measuring serum GH after the administration of oral glucose, 75 g, with sampling obtained every 30 minutes for two hours. The GH should be less than 2 ng/mL.

D. Thyroid abnormalities
   1. Definition: Hypothyroidism is the most common thyroid abnormality seen after BMT. Hyperthyroidism is rare after BMT and is primarily due to immunosuppression. See Table 6.3.
   2. Etiology
      a) TBI
      b) Chemotherapy (high dose)
   3. Diagnostic studies
      a) TSH assay is usually elevated, with normal thyroid hormones.
      b) Free thyroxine index or free thyroxine assay to confirm the diagnosis and to rule out hypothyroidism secondary to pituitary or hypothalamic involvement: The levels will usually be low.

Table 6.3 Thyroid Function Table

	Thyroxine (T4)	Triiodothyronine (T3)	T index	Free thyroxine (Free T4)	TSH
First-degree hypothyroidism	Low	Low	Low	Low	High
Second-degree hypothyroidism	Low	Low	Low	Low	Normal to low
Thyroxine-binding globulin deficiency	Low	High	Normal	Normal	Normal
Hyperthyroidism	High	High	High	High	Low

E. Parathyroid hormone disturbances

   1. Definition: Hyperparathyroidism has been reported in about 11% of the patients who have received neck irradiation and appears more frequent with low doses, less than 750 cGy.[5,6]

   2. Etiology
      a) TBI
      b) Local irradiation

   3. Diagnostic study: serum calcium

F. Adrenal disorders

   1. Definition
      a) The adrenal gland secretes more than 50 different steroids. Clinically the most important hormones of the adrenal cortex are cortisol, the major glucocorticoid, and aldosterone, the mineralocorticoid.

      b) The production of cortisol is controlled by ACTH, which in turn is modified by levels of serum cortisol, hypothalamic hormone, and corticotropin-releasing hormone. Glucocorticoids have diverse functions, including regulation of both protein and carbohydrate metabolism, suppression of inflammation, and regulation of calcium absorption.

c) The primary disorder of the adrenal gland seen in BMT patients is Cushing's syndrome, which results from high levels of glucocorticoids. It may be due to excessive pituitary production of ACTH, which leads to adrenal hyperplasia or sustained excessive administration of glucocorticoids of ACTH.

2. Etiology: sustained administration of glucocorticoids used for GVHD prophylaxis

3. Diagnostic studies
   a) The diagnosis is frequently entertained but rarely sustained, as diagnosis can be made by physical examination.
   b) Serum chemistries: potassium decreased, glucose increased, chloride decreased, cholesterol increased
   c) 24-hour urine cortisol increased to greater than 100 µg/24 h
   d) Overnight high-dose dexamethasone suppression test[7]: Measure baseline plasma cortisol level (A.M.). Give patient 8 mg of dexamethasone PO at 11 A.M. Measure cortisol level at 7 A.M. the following morning. Interpretation: Suppression of plasma cortisol level more than 50% of baseline indicates Cushing's disease.

IX. Radiology

A. Plain film
   1. Method: X-ray produced by electromagnetic images of high-speed electrons that penetrate dense tissue. Structures that absorb the x-rays appear white on plain films. X-rays magnify the object because of the distance between the object and the film. As the distance increases, so does the magnification.

2. Applications of chest films: Chest films are obtained to look for pathology in the thorax, including the heart and mediastinum. The chest x-ray may also be used to check for placement of apheresis or central venous catheters.

a) Silhouette sign is used to describe the blurring of the normally sharp borders between air containing lung and intrathoracic structures. Lower lobe processes silhouette posterior structures, such as the diaphragm and descending aorta.

b) Central line placement: Central venous catheters are usually placed with the tip at the junction of the superior vena cava and right atrium. Some extension into the right atrium is acceptable. If the catheter is noted to curve to the left on posteroanterior film or ventrally or anteriorly on lateral film, the catheter may be positioned in the right ventricle.

c) Consolidation: Any lobe may be involved, and fissures may not be displaced.

d) Volume loss pattern: Right upper lobe and right middle lobe are common locations. Compensatory hyperinflation may develop in remaining aerated areas.

3. Application of abdominal x-rays: Abdominal x-rays are useful in evaluating obstruction or mass effect. The following types of films should be obtained:

a) Supine: Provides useful information concerning bowel distention.

b) Lateral decubitus: Is used for the diagnosis of free air or enterocolitis.

c) Chest x-ray: May also need to be included to exclude a pulmonary pathology, which can mimic an abdominal process.

4. Advantages
   a) Availability
   b) Portable
   c) Inexpensive
5. Disadvantages
   a) Radiation exposure
   b) Operator dependent

B. Computed tomography (CT) scan
   1. Method: Combination computer and thin x-ray beam passing through the body at different angles. The x-ray is directed at and moves around the stationary body part.
   2. Application: Can be used to image intracranial disease, abdominal and chest disease, and bowel disease.
   3. Procedure precautions
      a) IV access is necessary if contrast will be used.
      b) If IV contrast is used, adequate hydration is necessary because contrast dye is nephrotoxic.
      c) Assess prior history of IV contrast dye allergy. If a contrast dye allergy exists, premedicate the patient with prednisone, 50 mg PO 12 hours and 6 hours prior to the scan, and diphenhydramine, 50 mg prior to the scan.
      d) The length of the procedure is approximately 30 to 90 minutes, depending on the extent of the body that is scanned.
   4. Advantages
      a) Availability
      b) Cheaper than magnetic resonance imaging (MRI)
      c) CT-guided biopsy
      d) Wide field of view
   5. Disadvantages
      a) Radiation exposure
      b) Not sensitive to cutaneous manifestations

c) Not sensitive to white matter

d) Limited scanning planes

C. Magnetic resonance imaging (MRI)

1. Method: An imaging technique that does not use ionizing radiation. Images are created by reemission of absorbed energy in the form of radio signals by atomic nuclei stimulated radio waves in a magnetic field.

2. Applications

a) Central nervous system: Better than CT scan for evaluating brain stem, posterior fossa, and spinal cord defects. Able to evaluate demyelinating disorders, focal seizures. MRI may not be able to reveal calcifications that are consistent with disease recurrence or metastatic disease.

b) Mediastinal lymphadenopathy

c) Cardiac: Able to image flowing blood and myocardium.

d) Abdomen: more sensitive than CT scan for evaluating hepatic disease

e) Skeletal: Able to detect avascular necrosis of the femoral head that may be a result of GVHD therapy. Able to detect marrow replacement by leukemic infiltrates.

3. Advantages

a) No radiation exposure

b) Multiple imaging planes

c) Sensitive to the presence of abnormal tissue

4. Disadvantages

a) Sensitive to motion

b) Confined space, which can lead to claustrophobia, usually requiring sedation

c) Unable to perform scan in a patient with a metal implantable device

d) If critical care equipment is required to support the patient (e.g., ventilator), it may be difficult to perform the scan.

D. Bone scan
  1. Method: An injection of an isotope, usually technetium 99m, to image the bony skeleton. The patient is injected with the isotope and a waiting period must elapse. This is necessary to obtain proper isotope concentration levels.
  2. Applications: useful in evaluating skeletal pain, metastatic disease
  3. Advantage: sensitive to the presence of bony disease
  4. Disadvantages
     a) Radiation exposure
     b) Length of procedure

E. Muga scan/rest heart wall motion
  1. Method: An isotope is injected to tag red blood cells, which emit radiation to detect regional wall motion, primarily of the left ventricle, and to determine quantitative data (e.g., ejection fraction and left ventricular function).
  2. Application: to determine cardiac function prior to conditioning regimen therapy or to assess toxicity of therapy
  3. Advantage: sensitive test to determine cardiac function
  4. Disadvantage: radiation exposure

X. Immunology

A. B-cell antibody deficiency and serum immunoglobulins
  1. Three months after transplant, B lymphocytes have not repopulated. These immature B-cells are not capable of producing quantities of normal IgG. This deficiency results in an increased susceptibility to infection.
  2. Normal B-cell function recovery occurs six months to one year after transplant.[8]

3. Serum IgG levels are low for three months after transplant. IgG and IgM have reached normal levels by one year; however, IgA levels remain low often until two years.

4. Diagnostic studies
   a) Serum antibody levels for IgG (reference value, 700 to 1500 mg/dL)[9]
   b) Serum antibody levels for IgM (reference value, 25 to 170 mg/dL)[9]
   c) Serum antibody levels for IgA (reference value, 60 to 360 mg/dL)[9]
   d) Antibody titers to protein vaccines (e.g., tetanus, diphtheria)
   e) Antibody titer to polysaccharide vaccines (e.g., Pneumovax)

B. T-cell mediated deficiency
   1. T-cell function is abnormal after engraftment and in patients experiencing chronic GVHD. Cellular immunity is impaired for as long as two years after transplant.
   2. There is usually an increased number of T cells in circulating blood early post-transplant and then a decline toward the normal range three months post-transplant.
   3. Chronic GVHD patients experience impaired immunity until resolution of symptoms.
   4. Diagnostic studies
      a) WBCs with total lymphocyte count
      b) T-cell lymphocytes [9,10]: CD4 levels are decreased (normal, 10% to 40%). CD8 levels are normal or high (normal, 17% to 38%). Reversal of the normal CD4/CD8 ratio occurs initially after transplant. The ratio returns to normal in healthy patients; however, they will remain elevated in patients experiencing chronic GVHD.

C. Monocyte function
1. Monocytes and macrophages are similar to granulocytes in their ability to locate, ingest, and kill microorganisms; however, their microbicidal potency is reduced.
2. Monocytes are particularly important in the killing of mycobacteria, viruses, fungi, and protozoa.
3. Lymphocyte-mediated cytokines known as lymphokines, resulting from the development of delayed hypersensitivity, activate monocytes and enhance phagocytosis.
4. Monocytes in the peripheral blood return to normal rapidly after transplant.
5. The monocyte antigen activity returns to normal when the monocyte level returns to normal.
6. Diagnostic study: WBCs with differential to include monocyte count

D. Use of immune globulin therapy
1. There are several uses for immune globulin therapy in the BMT patient.
2. Passive immune therapy with intravenous immune globulin after transplant has been shown to decrease the risk of bacterial infection, gram-negative sepsis, interstitial pneumonitis, and acute GVHD.
3. Intravenous immune globulin provides antibody levels with a half-life of three to four weeks.
4. Intravenous immune globulin replaces IgG; however, it contains only small amounts of IgA and IgM.
5. Dosage[11]
   a) 500 mg/kg weekly from day of transplant to day 80–100 post-transplant
   b) 200 mg/kg on day of transplant and every 21 days until day 100

References

1. Klump TR. Immunohematologic complications of bone marrow transplantation. *Bone Marrow Transplant*. 1991;8:159–170.

2. Bosi A, Vannucchi AM, Grosi A. Serum erythropoietin levels in patients undergoing autologous bone marrow transplantation. *Bone Marrow Transplant*. 1991;7:421–425.

3. First LR, Smith BR, Lipton J, et al. Isolated thrombocytopenia after allogeneic bone marrow transplant and chronic thrombocytopenia syndromes. *Blood*. 1985;65:368–374.

4. deAlarcon PA. Pattern of response of megakaryocyte colony stimulating activity in the serum of patients undergoing bone marrow transplantation. *Exp Hematol*. 1988;16:316–319.

5. Chisholm DJ. Endocrine complications. In: Atkinson K, ed. *Clinical Bone Marrow Transplantation*. Cambridge, England: Cambridge University Press; 1994:498–504.

6. Redman JR, Bajorunas DR. Therapy related thyroid and parathyroid dysfunction in patients with Hodgkin's disease. In: Redman MJ, *Hodgkin's Disease: The Consequences of Survival*. Philadelphia: Lea & Febiger; 1989:222.

7. Tyrell JB, et al. An overnight high dose dexamethasone suppression test for rapid differential diagnosis of Cushing's syndrome. *Ann Intern Med*. 1986;104:180.

8. Small TN, Keever CA, Weiner–Fedus S, et al. B cell differentiation following autologous conventional or T cell depleted bone marrow transplantation. *Blood*. 1990;76:1647–1656.

9. Bing DH. Plasma proteins: immunoglobulins. In: Hoffman R, Benz EJ, Shattil SJ, et al., eds., *Hematology: Basic Principles and Practice*. New York: Churchill Livingstone, Inc; 1991.

10. Parkman R. Transplantation biology. In: Hoffman R, Benz EJ, Shattil SJ, et al., eds. *Hematology: Basic Principles and Practice*. New York: Churchill Livingstone; 1991.

11. Sullivan KM, Kopecky KJ, Jocom J, et al.
Immunomodulatory and antimicrobial efficiency of intravenous
immunoglobulin in bone marrow transplantation. *N Engl J Med.*
1990;323:705–712.

Bibliography

Anasetti C, Rybka W, Sullivan KM, et al. Graft versus host
disease is associated with autoimmune like thrombocytopenia.
Blood. 1989;73:1054–1058.

Anderson KC, Soiffer R, Delage R, et al. T cell depleted autologous
bone marrow transplantation therapy: analysis of immune deficiency
and late complications. *Blood.* 1990;76:235–244.

Aucouturier P, Barra A, Intrator L, et al. Long lasting IgG subclass
and antibacterial polysaccharide antibody deficiency after allogeneic
bone marrow transplantation. *Blood.* 1987;70:779–785.

Barnes HV. Pleural effusion. In: Spivak JL, Barnes HV, eds. *Manual
of Clinical Problems in Internal Medicine.* 4th ed. Boston: Little,
Brown and Co; 1990:514.

Chisholm, DJ. Endocrine complications. In: Atkinson K, ed.
Clinical Bone Marrow Transplantation. Cambridge University Press,
Cambridge, England; 1994: 498–504.

Devuyst O, Lambert M, Scheiff JM, et al. High amylase activity
in pleural fluid and primary bronchogenic adenocarcinoma.
Eur Respir J. 1990;3:1217.

Dodds A. Hematological complications. In: Atkinson K, ed.
Clinical Bone Marrow Transplantation. Cambridge, England:
Cambridge University Press; 1994:534–538.

Flier JS, Moses AC. Diabetes in acromegaly and other endocrine
disorders. In: DeGroot LJ, ed. *Endocrinology.* Philadelphia:
WB Saunders; 1989:1389–1399.

Frohman LA. Endocrine and reproductive disorders. In: Wyngaarden JB, Smith LH, Bennett JC, eds. *Cecil Textbook of Medicine*. 19th ed. Philadelphia: WB Saunders; 1992:1194–1395.

Heimpel H, Arnold R, Hertzel WD, et al. Gonadal function after bone marrow transplantation in the adult male and female patients. *Bone Marrow Transplant*. 1991;8(suppl 1):21–24.

Kjeldsberg CR, Knight JA. *Body Fluids*. 2nd ed. Chicago: American Society of Clinical Pathologists, 1986.

Kleine TO, Hackler R, Meyer-Rienecker H. Classical and modern methods of cerebrospinal fluid analysis. *Eur J Clin Chem Biochem*. 1991;29:705.

Light RW. Pleural disease. *Di M*. 1992;38:1.

Sanders JE. Endocrine problems in children after bone marrow transplant for hematological malignancies. *Bone Marrow Transplant*. 1991;8(suppl 1)2–4.

Savdie E. Renal complications. In: Atkinson K, ed. *Clinical Bone Marrow Transplantation*. Cambridge, England: Cambridge University Press; 1994:458–466.

Schouten HC, Maragos D, Vose J, et al. Diabetes mellitus or an impaired glucose tolerance as a potential complicating factor in patients treated with high dose therapy and autologous bone marrow transplantation. *Bone Marrow Transplant*. 1990;6:333–335.

Sheridan JF, Tutschka PJ, Sedmak DD, Copelan EA. Immunoglobulin G subclass deficiency and pneumococcal infection after allogeneic bone marrow transplantation. *Blood*. 1990;75:1583–1586.

Speicher CE. *The Right Test: A Physician's Guide to Laboratory Medicine*. Philadelphia: WB Saunders Co; 1993:73–77.

Witherspoon RP. Immunological reconstruction after allogeneic marrow, autologous marrow or autologous peripheral blood stem cell transplantation. In: Atkinson K, ed. *Clinical Bone Marrow Transplantation*. Cambridge, England: Cambridge University Press; 1994:62-72.

C H A P T E R 7

Formulary

I. Drugs common to bone marrow and stem cell transplants[1-5]

Disclaimer: Drug information is constantly evolving because of ongoing research and clinical experience and is often subject to interpretation. While great care has been taken to ensure the accuracy of the information presented, the reader is advised that the authors, editors, reviewers, contributors, and publisher cannot be responsible for the continued currency of the information or for any errors or omissions in the formulary or for any consequences arising therefrom. Because of the dynamic nature of drug information, readers are advised that decisions on drug therapy must be based on the independent judgment of the clinician, changing information about a drug (e.g., as reflected in the literature and the manufacturer's most current product information), and changing medical practices.

A. Antibacterial/Antiprotozoal agents

Drug	Supplied as	Dose and route	Special considerations
Amikacin sulfate (Amikin) Class: aminoglycoside	Injection: 50, 250 mg/mL	<u>Children & adults</u>: 15 mg/kg/24 h divided q8 h Maximum (max) dose: 1.5 g/24 h <u>Infusion rate</u>: Infant: 1–2 h Children & adults: 30–60 min	<u>Therapeutic levels</u>: peak: 20–30 mg/L; trough: 5–10 mg/L Adjust dose for renal impairment. Side effects (SE): ototoxicity, nephrotoxicity, rash, fever, eosinophilia, headache; ototoxicity effects are synergistic when used with furosemide (Lasix)
Amoxicillin (Amoxil, Larotid, Trimox, Wymox Utimox) Class: amino derivative	Drops: 50 mg/mL (15, 30 mL) Suspension (Susp): 125, 250 mg/5 mL (80, 100, 150, 200 mL) Caps: 250, 500 mg Chewable tablets (tab): 125 mg	<u>Children</u>: 20–40 mg/kg/24 h divided q8 h <u>Adults</u>: 250–500 mg per dose q8 h by mouth (PO)	Renal elimination, achieves serum levels about twice those achieved with ampicillin SE: rash, diarrhea
Amoxicillin-Clavulanate potassium (Augmentin)	Tab: 125 & 250 mg Chewable tab: 125 & 250 mg Susp: 125 & 250 mg/5 mL	<u>Children</u>: 20–40 mg/kg/24 h divided q8 h <u>Adults</u>: 250–500 mg per dose q8 h PO Max dose: 1.5 g/24 h	β-lactamase inhibitor extends activity of amoxicillin to include β-lactamase producing

Class: amino derivative	(31.25 & 62.5 mg clavulanate) (75, 150 mL)		strains of *Haemophilus influenzae*, *Branhamella catarrhalis*, some *Staphylococcus aureus*.
Ampicillin (Omnipen, Polycillin, Principen)	Drops: 100 mg/mL (20 mL) Susp: 125, 250 mg/mL (8, 100, 150, 200 mL) 500 mg/mL (100 mL)	<u>Children:</u> mild to moderate infection: 50–100 mg/kg/24 h divided q6 h PO, intramuscularly (IM), intravenously (IV) Max dose: 2–4 g/24 h renal dose for creatinine	Has penicillin cross-reactivity; rash commonly seen 5–10 d after starting; may cause interstitial nephritis; clearance < 10–15 mL/min
Class: amino derivative	Capsules (caps): 250, 500 mg Injection: 125, 250, 500 mg; 1, 2 g vials	Severe infection: 200–400 mg/kg/24 h divided q4–6 h IM or IV Max dose: 10–12 g/24 h	
Ampicillin/Sulbactam (Unasyn) Class: amino derivative	Injection: 1.5, 3.0 g	Mild to moderate infection: 100 mg/kg/24 h divided q6 h Severe infection: 200 mg/kg/24 h divided q6 h	May cause false positive urinary glucose levels SE: diarrhea, rash, nausea/vomiting (N/V), candidiasis, fatigue, malaise, headache, chest pain, flatulence, and others
Ancef (see cefazolin sodium, p. 295)			

Drug	Supplied as	Dose and route	Special considerations
Aztreonam (Azactam) Class: β-lactam	Injection: 2 g	<u>Children:</u> 90–120 mg/kg divided q6–8 h <u>Adults:</u> 500 mg – 1 g divided q8–12 h Severe infection: 2 g q6–8 h	Provides good gram-negative coverage; avoid β-lactamase production (imipenem, cefoxitin)
Bacitracin, neomycin & polymyxin B (Neosporin) Class: topical antibacterial	Ointment: <u>Ophthalmic:</u> bacitracin 400 U, neomycin sulfate 3.5 mg, & polymyxin B sulfate 10,000 U/g <u>Topical:</u> bacitracin 400 U, neomycin sulfate 3.5 mg, & polymyxin B sulfate 5000U/g	<u>Topical:</u> Apply 1–3 times per d <u>Ophthalmic:</u> Apply q3–4 h for 7 d	For short-term treatment of superficial skin or ocular infection
Bactrim (see co-trimoxazole, p. 301)			
Bactroban (see mupirocin, p. 307)			
Bicillin C-R (see penicillin G benzathine & penicillin G procaine)			
Carbenicillin disodium (Geopen, Pyopen)	Injection: 1, 2, 10 g	<u>Children & adults:</u> mild infection: 50–200 mg/kg/24 h divided q4–6 h	May cause platelet destruction; unpredictable

Drug	Dosage Forms	Dosing	Comments
Class: amino derivative		Severe infection: 400–500 mg/kg/24 h divided q4–6 h Max dose: 40 g/24 h	interaction with gentamycin; may cause anaphylaxis, hyponatremia, hypokalemia, metabolic alkalosis, rash, & elevated level of aspartate aminotransferase (AST); adjust dose with renal failure; use with caution in penicillin-allergic patient; contains 4.7 mEq of sodium (Na) per g.
Cefaclor (Ceclor) Second generation	Caps: 250, 500 mg Susp: 125, 250 mg/mL (75, 150 mL)	Infants & children: Mild infection: 40 mg/kg/24 h divided q8 h PO Adults: 250–500 mg per dose divided q8 h PO Max dose: 4 g/24 h	Use with caution in patients with penicillin allergy or renal impairment. May cause positive reaction to Coombs' test or urine glucose test
Cefadroxil (Duricef, Ultracef) First generation	Susp: 125, 250, 500 mg/5 mL (50, 100 mL) Tab: 1 g Caps: 500 mg	Infants & children: 30 mg/kg/24 h divided q12 h PO Adults: 1–2 g/24 h divided q12 h PO Max dose: 2 g/24 h	Use with caution in patients with penicillin allergy. May cause headache (H/A), rash, N/V, positive reaction to Coombs' test, pseudomembranous colitis, transient neutropenia, anemia
Cefazolin sodium (Ancef, Kefzol) First generation	Injection: 0.25, 0.5, 1, 5, 10 g	Infants & children: 25–100 mg/kg/24 h divided q6–8 h IV/IM Adults: 1–6 g/24 h divided q6–8 h	Use with caution in patients with penicillin allergy or renal impairment. May cause leukopenia, thrombocytopenia, elevated liver enzymes, phlebitis

Drug	Supplied as	Dose and route	Special considerations
Cefixime (Suprax) Third generation	Tab: 200, 400 mg Susp: 100 mg/5mL	<u>Infants & children:</u> 8 mg/kg/24 h divided q12–24 h <u>Adults:</u> 400 mg/24 h divided q12–24 h	Use with caution in patients with penicillin allergy or renal impairment. SE: diarrhea, abdominal cramps, N/V, H/A
Cefoperazone sodium (Cefobid) Third generation	Injection: 1, 2 g	<u>Infants & children:</u> 100–200 mg/kg/24 h divided q12 h IM/IV <u>Adults:</u> 2–4 g/24 h divided q12 h IM/IV Max dose: 12 g/24 h	Use with caution in patients with penicillin allergy or renal impairment. Contains 1.5 mEq of Na per g; may cause disulfiram-like reaction with alcohol intake (ETOH).
Cefotaxime sodium (Claforan) Third generation	Injection: 0.5, 1, 2, 10 g	<u>Infants & children:</u> (< 50 kg): 50–200 mg/kg/24 h divided q4–6 h IV/IM <u>Adults:</u> (50 kg): 2–12 g/24 h divided q4–12 h IV/IM Max dose: 12 g/24 h	Use with caution in patients with penicillin allergy or renal impairment. May cause leukopenia, thrombocytopenia, eosinophilia, positive reaction to Coombs' test, elevated liver enzyme levels, elevated blood urea nitrogen (BUN)/creatinine level; contains 2.2 mEq of Na per g

Cefotetan disodium (Cefotan) Third generation	Injection: 1, 2 g	<u>Infants & children:</u> 40–80 mg/kg/24 h divided q12 h IV/IM <u>Adults:</u> 2–4 g/24 h divided q12 h IV/IM Max dose: 6 g/24 h	Use with caution in patients with penicillin allergy or renal impairment. Contains 3.5 mEq of Na per g
Cefoxitin sodium (Mefoxin) Second generation	Injection: 1, 2 g	<u>Infants & children:</u> 80–160 mg/kg/24 h divided q4–6 h IV/IM <u>Adults:</u> 4–12 g/24 h divided q6–8 h IV/IM Max dose: 12 g/24 h	Use with caution in patients with penicillin allergy or renal impairment. Contains 2.3 mEq of Na per g
Cefprozil (Cefzil) Second generation	Tab: 250, 500 mg Susp: 25 mg/mL (50, 100 mL) 50 mg/mL (50, 100 mL)	<u>Infants & children:</u> 30 mg/kg/24 h divided q12 h <u>Adults:</u> 250–500 mg divided q12–24 h	Use with caution in patients with penicillin allergy or renal impairment. SE; diarrhea, abdominal cramps, N/V, H/A
Ceftazidime (Fortaz, Tazidime, Tazicef) Third generation	Injection: 1, 2 g	<u>Infants & children:</u> 90–150 mg/kg/24 h divided q8 h IV/IM <u>Adults:</u> 2–6 g/24 h divided q8–12 h IV/IM Max dose: 6 g/24 h	Use with caution in patients with penicillin allergy or renal impairment. Contains 2.3 mEq of Na per g

Drug	Supplied as	Dose and route	Special considerations
Ceftizoxime sodium (Cefizox) Third generation	Injection: 1, 2 g	Infants & children: 150–200 mg/kg/ 24 h divided q8 h IV/IM Adults: 2–12 g/24 h divided q8–12 h IV/IM Max dose: 12 g/24 h	Use with caution in patients with penicillin allergy or renal impairment. Contains 2.6 mEq of Na per g
Ceftriaxone sodium (Rocephin) Third generation	Injection: 0.25, 0.5, 1, 2, 10 g	Infants & children: 50–75 mg/kg/24 h divided q12–24 h IV/IM Adults: 1–4 g/24 h divided q12 h IV/IM Max dose: 12 g/24 h Meningitis: 100 mg/kg/24 h divided q12 h	Use with caution in patients with penicillin allergy or renal impairment. Contains 2.6 mEq of Na per g
Cefuroxime sodium (Zinacef, Kefurox) Second generation	Injection: 0.75, 1.5, 7.5 g	Infants & children: 50–100 mg/kg/ 24 h divided q6–8 h IV/IM Adults: 2.25–9 g/24 h divided q6–8 h IV/IM Max dose: 12 g/24 h Meningitis: 200–240 mg/kg/24 h divided q6–8 h	Use with caution in patients with penicillin allergy or renal impairment. Contains 2.4 mEq of Na per g
Cefuroxime Axetil (Ceftin) Second generation	Tab: 125, 250, 500 7.5 g	< 12 y: 125–250 mg PO bid > 12 y: 250–500 mg PO bid	Use with caution in patients with penicillin allergy or renal impairment.

Drug	Preparations	Dosing	Comments
Cephalexin (Keflex) First generation	Tab: 1 g Caps: 250, 500 mg Susp: 125, 250/5 mL (100, 200 mL) Drops: 100 mg/mL (10 mL)	<u>Infants & children:</u> 25–50 mg/kg/24 h divided q6–12 h PO <u>Adults:</u> 1–4 g/24 h divided q6–12 h IV/IM Max dose: 4 g/24 h	Some cross-reactivity with penicillin; frequent gastrointestinal (GI) disturbance
Cephalothin sodium (Keflin) First generation	Injection: 1, 2, 4 g	<u>Infants & children:</u> 80–160 mg/kg/24 h divided q4–6 h IV/deep IM <u>Adults:</u> 2–12g/24 h divided q4–6 h IV/IM Max dose: 12 g/24 h	Use with caution in patients with penicillin allergy. Frequent GI disturbance; contains 2.8 mEq of Na per g
Cephradine (Velosef, Anspor) First generation	Susp: 125 & 250 mg/5 mL (100, 200 mL) Caps: 250 & 500 mg Injection: 0.25, 0.5, 1, 2, 4 g	<u>Infants & children:</u> PO: 25–50 mg/kg/24 h divided q6 h IV/IM: 50–100 mg/kg/24 h divided q6 h <u>Adults:</u> PO: 1–4 g/24 h divided q6 h IV/IM: 2–8 g/24 h divided 6 h Max oral dose: 4 g/24 h Max parenteral dose: 8 g/24 h	Use with caution in patients with penicillin allergy. Frequent GI disturbance; contains 2.8 mEq of Na per g

Drug	Supplied as	Dose and route	Special considerations
Ciprofloxacin hydrochloride (Cipro) Class: anti-infective	Tab: 250, 500, 750 mg Injection: 200 mg/20 mL Opthalmic solution: 3.5 mg/mL (2.5, 5.0 mL)	<u>Children</u>: 20–30 mg/kg/24 h IV/PO divided q12 h <u>Adults</u>: Oral: 250–750 mg per dose divided q12 h Max dose: 2 g/24 h IV: 200–400 mg per dose divided q12 h	SE: N/V, renal failure, GI bleeding, restlessness; can cause cartilage arthropathy in children; used with reservation in children < 16 y of age
Clarithromycin (Biaxin Filmtabs) Class: anti-infective	Tab: 250, 500 mg	<u>Children</u>: 15 mg/kg/24 h PO divided q12 h <u>Adults</u>: 250–500 mg per dose divided q12 h	SE: diarrhea, N/V, bad taste, dyspepsia, abdominal cramping; may increase carbamezide, theophylline levels; contraindicated in patients sensitive to erythromycin
Clindamycin (Cleocin T, Cleocin, others) Class: lincomycins	Caps: 75, 150, 300 mg Oral liquid: 75 mg/5 mL (100 mL) Injection: 150 mg/mL (contains 9.45 mg of benzyl alcohol per mL) Topical solution: 1% (3960 mL) Gel: 1% (7.5, 3 g)	<u>Children</u>: 20–30 mg/kg/24 h divided q6 h PO; 25–40 mg/kg/24 h divided q6–8 h IM/IV <u>Adults</u>: 150–450 mg per dose divided q6–8 h PO; 600–3600 mg/24 h IM/IV divided q6–12 h. Max dose: 4.8 g/24 h PO Topical: apply bid	Pseudomembranous colitis may occur up to several weeks after cessation of therapy. May cause Stevens-Johnsons syndrome, diarrhea, rash, pancytopenia

Co-trimoxazole
(trimethoprim [TMP]
and sulfamethoxazole
[SMX], Bactrim,
Septra, TMP-SMX)

Class: sulfonamide

Tab (regular strength):
80 mg TMP & 400 mg SMX
Tab (double strength):
160 mg TMP & 800 mg SMX
Susp: 40 mg TMP & 200 mg
SMX per 5 mL
Injection: 16 mg of TMP per mL
& 80 mg of SMX per mL

Doses based on mg TMP:
Pneumocystis carinii pneumonia
(PCP) prophylaxis
Children: 8–10 mg/kg/24 h
divided bid3 times per wk PO
Adults: 1 double strength tab divided
bid 3 times per wk
Minor infections:
Children: 8–10 mg/kg/24 h
divided q12 h
Adults: (> 40 kg) 160 mg per dose q12 h
Severe infection & PCP:
20 mg/kg/24 h IV divided q6–8 h

May cause bone marrow suppression,
blood dyscrasias; use with reservation
in patients with absolute neutrophil
count (ANC) < 1000/mL or platelets
< 60,000; discontinue if rash
develops; has been associated with
Stevens-Johnsons syndrome; may also
cause crystalluria, glossitis, renal or
hepatic injury, GI irritation allergy,
or hemolysis in glucose-6-phosphate
dehydrogenase (G6PD); reduce dose
in renal impairment

Dapsone
(Avlosulfon)

Class: anti-infective

Tab: 25, 100 mg

PCP prophylaxis:
Children: 1 mg/kg/24 h qd or
3 times per wk PO
Adults: 100 mg/24 h qd or
3 times per wk PO

May be used for PCP prophylaxis
in bone marrow transplant (BMT)
patients who cannot take TMP-SMX
due to low blood counts; may cause
hemolysis in patients with G6PD
deficiency; SE: hypersensitivity
(discontinue for rash), N/V, H/A,
blurred vision, peripheral neuropathy,
tinnitus. Do not use in patients
with hypersensitivity to TMP-SMX.

Drug	Supplied as	Dose and route	Special considerations
Dicloxacillin sodium Class: penicillinase-resistant	Caps: 125, 250, 500 mg Susp: 62.5 mg/5 mL (80, 100, 200 mL)	<u>Children:</u> (< 40g) Mild/moderate infection: 12.5–25 mg/kg/24 h divided q6 h PO Severe infection: 50–100 mg/kg/24 h divided q6 h PO <u>Adults:</u> (> 40 kg) 125–500 mg/dose divided q6 h PO	Give 1–2 h before meals or 2 h after. Do not use in patients with known penicillin allergy. SE: rash, fever, eosinophilia, serum sickness-like reaction, neutropenia, thrombocytopenia, N/V, diarrhea, elevated liver function test (LFT) results
Doxycycline (Vibramycin) Class: tetracycline/antiprotozoal	Caps: 50, 100 mg Tab: 50, 100 mg Syrup: 50 mg/5 mL (30 mL) Susp: 25 mg/5 mL (60 mL) Injection: 100, 200 mg	<u>Initial:</u> < 45 kg: 5 mg/kg/24 h divided bid PO or IV for 1 d to max of 200 mg/d. 45 kg: 200 mg/24 h divided bid PO or IV for 1 day <u>Maintenance:</u> < 45 kg: 2.5–5 mg/kg/24 h divided qd bid PO or IV. 45 kg: 100–200 mg/24 h divided qd bid PO or IV	Use with caution in patients with hepatic and renal impairment. Avoid use in children < 8 y because of tooth enamel hypoplasia and discoloration. Infuse IV over 1–4 h. SE: GI upset, photosensitivity, hemolytic anemia, hypersensitivity reaction
Erythromycin (E.E.S., E-Mycin, Ery-tab, Erythrocin, Ilotycin, Pediamycin) Class: erythromycins	<u>Erythromycin:</u> Caps: 125, 250 mg Tab: 250, 333, 500 mg Topical: 1.5%, 2% (60 mL) Ophthalmic ointment: 0.5% (3.75 g)	<u>Oral:</u> Children: 30–50 mg/kg/24 h divided q6–8 h; max: 2 g/24 h Adults: 1–4 g/24 h divided q6 h	Take after meals. Use with caution in liver disease. May produce elevated digoxin, theophylline, carbamazepine, cyclosporin, methylprednisolone levels; treatment of choice for legionella pneumonia.

E.E.S.:

Susp: 200, 400 mg/5 mL
(60, 100, 200 mL)

Drops: 100 mg/2.5 mL (50 mL)

Tab: 200, 400 mg

Erythromycin lactobionate:

Inj: 500, 1000 mg

Erythromycin estolate:

Tab: 500 mg

Chewables: 125, 250 mg

Drops: 100 mg/mL (10 mL)

Caps: 125, 250 mg

Susp: 125, 250 mg/5 mL

Erythromycin stearate:

Tab: 125, 250, 500 mg

Injection: 250, 500, 1000 mg

Erythromycin gluceptate:

Injection: 250, 500, 1000 mg

Parenteral:

Children: 20–50 mg/kg/24 h divided
q6 h IV or continuous infusion

Adults: 15–20 mg/kg/24 h divided
q6 h IV or continuous infusion

Dental prophylaxis:

20 mg/kg (max 1 g) PO 1 h
before and 10 mg/kg (max 0.5 g)
PO q6 h after procedure

Ophthalmic:

Apply 0.5 inch ribbon to affected
eye bid-qid

Gentamicin sulfate
(Garamycin)

Class: aminoglycoside

Injection: 10, 40 mg/mL

Ophthalmic ointment:
0.3% (3.5 g)

Drops: 0.3% (5 mL)

Topical ointment: 0.1%

Parenteral: IM or IV

Children: 6–7.5 mg/kg/24 h divided q8 h

Adults: 3–5 mg/kg/24 h divided q8 h

Max dose: 300 mg/24 h

Intrathecal/intraventricular:

Therapeutic levels: 4–10 µg/mL (peak);
<0.5–2 µg/mL (trough) Follow renal
function closely; may cause proximal
tubule dysfunction and ototoxicity

Adjust dose for creatinine clearance

Drug	Supplied as	Dose and route	Special considerations
Gentamicin sulfate (*Continued*)	Intrathecal injection: 2 mg/mL	> 3 mo: 1–2 mg daily Adults: 4–8 mg daily Ophthalmic ointment: apply q6–8 h Ophthalmic drops: 1–2 gtt q4 h	< 80 mL/min/1.73 m²: 2.5 mg/kg.
Imipenem-Cilastatin (Primaxin) Class: β-lactam	Injection: 500 mg/13 mL	Children: < 12 y 60–100 mg/kg/d divided q6–8 h Adults: 250–1000 mg per dose divided q6–8 h Max dose: 4 g/d Dose adjustment for renal dysfunction | Creatinine clearance (mL/min/1.73 m²)	Frequency	% decrease in dose
---	---	---
30–70	q6 h	50
20–30	q8 h	63
5–20	q12 h	75		SE: N/V, diarrhea, rash, pseudomembranous colitis, eosinophilia, neutropenia, positive Coombs' test results, seizures, rash, hypotension, emergence of resistant strains of Pseudomonas aeruginosa
Isoniazid (INH, Nydrazid, Laniazid)	Tab: 50, 100, 300 mg Susp: 10 mg/mL Syrup: 50 mg/mL Injection: 100 mg/mL	Prophylaxis: Infants & children: 10 mg/kg/ 24 h qdPO or 20–40 mg/kg per dose PO 2 times per wk (after 1 mo	Use with caution in patients with liver dysfunction. Follow LFT results monthly. Should not be used alone as treatment for tuberculosis (TB).

Class: antitubercular

of qd therapy); treat for 12 mo
Adults: 5 mg/kg/24 h qd PO
(usual dose 300 mg) for 12 mo
Treatment:
Infants & children: 10–20 mg/kg/24 h
qd PO OR 20–40 mg/kg/dose 2 times
per wk for 9 months with rifampin
Adults: 5 mg/kg/24 h qd PO OR
15 mg/kg/24 h 2 times per wk
for 9 months with rifampin
Max dose: 300 mg
Max single 2 times per wk dose: 900 mg

Supplemental pyridoxine 1–2 mg/kg/
24 h is recommended. May cause false
positive urine glucose test results;
increases serum concentrations of
carbamazepine, diazepam, phenytoin,
& prednisone. SE: peripheral
neuropathy, optic neuritis, seizures,
encephalopathy, psychosis

Kanamycin
(Kantrex)

Caps: 500 mg
Injection: 37.5, 250,
333 mg/mL

Class: aminoglycoside

Infants & children: 15–30
mg/kg/24 h divided q8–12 h IV/IM
Max dose: 1.5 g/24 h
Adults: 15 mg/kg/24 h divided
q8–12 h IV/IM
Max dose: 1.5 g/24 h

Therapeutic levels:
Peak: 15–30 µg/mL
Trough: no > 5–10 µg/mL
Use with caution in patients
with renal dysfunction. Also has
ototoxicity; PO poorly absorbed, and
used to treat bacterial overgrowth

Keflex
(see cephalexin, p. 299)

Kefzol
(see cefazolin sodium,
p. 295)

Drug	Supplied as	Dose and route	Special considerations
Mefoxin (see cefoxitin sodium, p. 297)			
Methicillin sodium (Staphcillin) Class: penicillinase-resistant	Injection: 1, 4, 6 g	<u>Infants > 1 mo & children:</u> 100–400 mg/kg/24 h divided q4–6 h IV <u>Adults:</u> 4–12 g/24 h divided q4–6 h IV Max dose: 12 g/24 h	Has allergic cross-reactivity with penicillin SE: hematuria, nephritis, reversible bone marrow depression, phlebitis at infusion site, eosinophilia, rash.
Metronidazole (Flagyl) Class: anti-infective, anti-protozoal	Tab: 250, 500 mg Susp: 100 mg/mL or 50 mg/mL Injection: 500 mg or 5 mg/mL ready to use	<u>Anaerobic infection:</u> Infants, children & adults: Loading dose: 15 mg/kg IV Maintenance: 7.5 mg/kg/dose divided q6 h IV Max dose: 4 g/24 h <u>Giardiasis:</u> Children: 15 mg/kg/24 h divided tid PO for 10 d Adults: 500–750 mg/24 h divided tid PO for 10 d <u>Clostridium difficile:</u> 0.75–2 g/24 h divided tid-qid PO	Instruct to refrain from alcohol use; potentiates anticoagulants. SE: N/V, urticaria, dry mouth, leukopenia, vertigo

Mezlocillin (Mezlin) Class: penicillinase-resistant	Injection: 1, 2, 3, 4 g	Infants & children: 50–75 mg/kg per dose divided q4–6 h IV Adults: 1–4 g per dose divided q4–6 IV Max dose: 24 g/24 h	Contains 1.85 mEq of Na per g. SE: Hypersensitivity, N/V, eosinophilia, leukopenia, neutropenia, anemia, elevated levels of BUN, creatinine & liver enzymes.
Mupirocin (Bactroban) Class: topical antibacterial	Ointment: 2% (15 g)	Apply small amount to affected area tid.	May cause local irritation, burning
Nafcillin sodium (Unipen, Nafcil, Naftopen) Class: penicillin	Tab: 500 mg Caps: 250 mg Oral solution: 250 mg/5 mL	Infants & children: PO: 50–100 mg/kg/24 h divided q6 h IV: 100–200 mg/kg 24 h divided q6 h Adults: PO: 250–1000 mg q4–6 h IV: 500–2000 mg q4–6 h Max: 12 g/24 h	Allergic cross-reactivity with penicillin; poor absorption PO; high incidence of phlebitis with IV route; contains 2.9 mEq of Na per g
Neomycin sulfate (Mycifradin) Class: aminoglycoside	Tab: 500 mg Susp: 125 mg/5 mL Injection: 500 mg	Infants & children: 50–100 mg/kg/24 h divided q4–6 h PO Adults: 500–2000 mg divided q6–8 h PO Bowel prep: 90 mg/kg/24 h	Potent aminoglycoside; IV administration should be avoided. Follow for renal toxicity and ototoxicity. Do not use in ulcerative colitis or bowel obstruction. Oral absorption is limited but may accumulate.

Drug	Supplied as	Dose and route	Special considerations
Nitrofurantoin (Furadantin, Macrodantin) Class: nitrofurans	Tab: 50, 100 mg Caps: 25, 50, 100 mg Susp: 25 mg/5 mL	<u>Children</u>: 5–7 mg/kg/24 h divided q6 h PO Prophylaxis: 1–2 mg/kg qhs <u>Adults</u>: 50–100 mg per dose divided q6 h PO Prophylaxis: 50–100 mg qhs Max dose: 400 mg/day	Contraindicated in patients with G6PD deficiency, children < 1 mo, renal disease. SE: N/V, anorexia, H/A, dizziness, interstitial pneumonitis/ fibrosis, hepatotoxicity, rash, exfoliative dermatitis, hemolytic anemia.
Omnipen (see ampicillin, p. 293)			
Oxacillin sodium (Bactocil, Prostaphlin) Class: penicillinase-resistant	Caps: 250, 500 mg Oral solution: 250 mg/5 mL Injection: 0.25, 0.5, 1, 2 g	<u>Children</u>: 50–100 mg/kg/24 h divided q6 h PO <u>Adults</u>: 500–1000 mg/dose divided q4–6 h PO	SE: hypersensitivity reaction, N/V, leukopenia, elevated serum glutamic-oxaloacetic transaminase (SGOT) level
Penicillin G preparations/potassium & sodium Class: penicillin G-related	<u>Potassium:</u> Tab: 250,000, 400,000, 500,000, 800,000 Solution: 200,000, 400,000, U/5 mL (100, 200 mL) Injection: 0.2, 0.5, 1, 5, 10, 20 million U	<u>Children</u>: 100,000–300,000 U/ kg/24 h divided q4–6 h IM/IV 40,000–80,000 U/kg/24 h divided q6 h PO <u>Adults</u>: 100,000–250,000 U/kg/ 24 h divided q4–6 h IV/IM 300,000–1.2 million U/24 h	SE: anaphylaxis, hemolytic anemia, interstitial nephritis, confusion, myoclonus, positive Coombs' test result 1 mg = approximately 1600 U Contains 1.7 mEq of Na or K per 1 million U

	Sodium: Injection: 5 million U	divided q6 h	
Penicillin V potassium (Pen•Vee K, V-Cillin K) Class: penicillin G-related	Tab: 250, 500 mg Susp: 50 mg/mL (100 mL)	Children: 25–50 mg/kg/d divided q6–8 h Max dose: 3 g/24 h Adults: 1–2 g/24 h divided q6–8 h Pneumococcal prophylaxis: < 5 y: 125 mg PO bid > 5 y: 250 mg PO bid	SE: hypersensitivity reaction, N/V, diarrhea, fever, rash, anaphylaxis, acute interstitial nephritis, convulsions, positive Coombs' test results, hemolytic anemia
Pentamidine Isethionate (Pentam 300, Nebupent) Class: antiprotozoal	Injection: 300 mg (Pentam) Inhalation: 300 mg (Nebupent)	IV (or IM): Trypanosoma gambiense: 4 mg/kg/24 h qd for 10 d P. carinii: 4 mg/kg/24 h qd for 10 d PCP prophylaxis: 4 mg/kg per dose IV q2 wk OR > 5 y 300 mg in 6 mL H₂O via Respirgard jet nebulizer q2–4 wk	Infuse IV slowly over 1 h to reduce risk of hypotension. Inhaled difficult to administer to very young children SE: hypoglycemia, transient hypotension, tachycardia, N/V, mild liver toxicity, megaloblastic anemia, granulocytopenia, hypocalcemia, renal toxicity, pancreatitis, fever, rash.
Pen•Vee K (see penicillin V potassium, this page)			

Drug	Supplied as	Dose and route	Special considerations
Piperacillin sodium (Pipracil) Class: extended-spectrum penicillin	Injection: 2, 3, 4 g	<u>Children > 12 y:</u> 200–300 mg/kg/24 h divided q4–6 h IV <u>Adults:</u> 3–4 g per dose q4–6 h IV Max dose: 24 g/24 h	Similar to penicillin; should not be used in patients with known hypersensitivity SE: fever, rash, eosinophilia, exfoliative dermatitis, serum sickness-like reaction, positive direct Coombs' test result, hemolytic anemia, thrombocytopenia, prolonged bleeding time, diarrhea, interstitial nephritis, hypokalemia, elevated LFT levels, seizures, thrombophlebitis
Polycillin (see ampicillin, p. 293)			
Primaxin (see imipenem-cilastatin, p. 304)			
Pyrimethamine (Daraprim) Class: antiprotozoal anti-toxoplasmosis	Tab: 25 mg	<u>Children:</u> Initial dose: 2 mg/kg/d qd for 3 d Maintenance: consult Infectious Disease Service <u>Adults:</u> 25 mg qd with sulfadiazine for 3–4 wk (depending on response)	SE: Megaloblastic anemia, hypersensitivity, leukopenia, thrombocytopenia, folic acid deficiency, atrophic glossitis, rash, ataxia, tremors, seizures, N/V, fatigue, shock

Rifampin (Rifadin)	Caps: 150, 300 mg	Causes red discoloration of body
	Liquid: 10 mg/mL (1%)	fluids. SE: N/V, H/A, diarrhea, rash,
Class: antitubercular	Susp: 15 mg/mL	pruritus, stomatitis, eosinophilia,
		drowsiness, fatigue, ataxia, confusion,
	Anti-TB:	fever, hepatitis, blood dyscrasias,
	10–20 mg/kg per dose up to max dose	flulike syndrome
	of 600 mg per dose PO qd or 2 times	
	per wk	
	H. influenzae & legionella:	
	0–1 mo: 10 mg/kg/24 h PO qd for	
	4 d	
	> 1 mo: 20 mg/kg/24 h PO qd	
	Max dose: 600 mg/24 h qd	
	Meningococcal prophylaxis:	
	Children: 20 mg/kg/d q12 h for 2 d	
	Adults: 600 mg q12 h for 2 d	
Rocephin		
(see ceftriaxone sodium		
p. 298)		
Septra		
(see co-trimoxazole p.301)		
Silver sulfadiazine	Topical cream: 10 mg/g	Use with caution in BMT patient
(Silvadene)	(20 g, 40 g)	with large body surface area
		(BSA) involvement because of
Class: Topical	Apply 1–2 times per d with	granulocytopenia; may accumulate
antibacterial/antifungal	sterile gloves.	in patients with impaired renal or
		hepatic function. SE: pain, rash
		itching, hemolytic anemia, interstitial
		nephritis, allergic reaction

Drug	Supplied as	Dose and route	Special considerations
Sulfacetamide sodium (Bleph-10, Sodium Sulamyd) Class: topical ophthalmicantibacterial	Ointment: 10% (3.5 g) Solution: 10% (5 mL, 10 mL)	<u>Ointment:</u> Apply to lower conjuctival sac 1–4 times per d <u>Solution:</u> Instill 1–2 gtt q2–3 h	Inactivated by purulent exudates SE: local irritation, stinging, burning, local irritation, Stevens-Johnson syndrome.
Sulfadiazine (Microsulfon) Class: sulfonamide; antitoxoplasmosis	Tab: 500 mg	<u>Toxoplasmosis:</u> Children: 25 mg/kg q6 h for 3–4 wk with pyrimethamine Adults: 1 g q6 h for 3–4 wk with pyrimethamine	Contraindicated in patients with known sulfa allergy
Sulfisoxazole (Gantrisin) Class: sulfonamide-related	Susp: 100 mg/mL (480 mL) Tab: 500 mg	<u>Children:</u> > 2 mo 120–150 mg/kg/d divided q6 h Max dose: 6 g/d <u>Adults:</u> 4–8 g/24 h divided q6 h	Contraindicated in patients with known sulfa allergy. SE: thrombocytopenia, leukopenia, hemolytic anemia, hypersensitivity reaction, jaundice, kernicterus, nephrotoxicity
Suprax (see cefixime, p. 296)			
Tazidime (see ceftazidime, p. 297)			

Tetracycline hydrochloride (Sumycin, Tetracyn) Class: tetracycline; antiprotozoal	Caps: 100, 250, 500 mg Injection: 250, 500 mg (IV)	<u>Children</u> > 8 y 25–50 mg/kg/d divided qid PO Max dose: 3 g/d IV: 20–30 mg/kg/24 h divided q8–12 h PO <u>Adults</u>: 250–500 mg divided qid PO IV: 250–500 mg per dose divided q6–12 h	SE: N/V, diarrhea, stomatitis, glossitis, candidal superinfection, pseudomembranous colitis, rash, fever, hypersensitivity reactions, photosensitivity, liver toxicity, Fanconi's-like syndrome, thrombophlebitis, injury to growing bones and teeth, pseudotumor cerebri, renal damage
Ticarcillin disodium (Ticar) Class: penicillin derivative	Injection: 1, 3, 6, 20, 30 g	<u>Children</u>: 200–300 mg/kg/24 h divided q4–6 h IV Max dose: 24–30 g/d <u>Adults</u>: 200–300 mg/kg/24 h divided q4–6 h IV Max dose: 24–30 g/d	Contraindicated in patients with known penicillin allergy; contains 5.2–6.5 mEq of Na+. SE: may cause inhibition of platelet aggregation, bleeding, diathesis, hypernatremia, hypocalcemia, allergy, rash, increased SGOT level
Ticarcillin and clavulanate (Timentin) Class: penicillin derivative	Injection: 3.1 g (3.0 g ticarcillin and 1 g clavulanate)	Dosing same as ticarcillin Max dose: 18 g/24 h	Similar to ticarcillin except β-lactamase inhibitor broadens spectrum to include *S. aureus* and *H. influenzae*

Drug	Supplied as	Dose and route	Special considerations
Tobramycin sulfate (Nebcin) Class: aminoglycoside	Injection: 10, 40 mg/mL Ophthalmic ointment: 0.3% (3.5 g) Ophthalmic solution: 0.3% (5 mL)	<u>Children:</u> 6–7.5 mg/kg/24 h divided q8 h IV <u>Adults:</u> 3–5 mg/kg/24 h divided q8 h IV <u>Ophthalmic:</u> Apply thin ribbon of ointment to affected eye bid-tid; or 1–2 gtt q4 h	Therapeutic levels: Peak: 6–10 µg/mL Trough: < 2 µg/mL SE: ototoxicity, nephrotoxicity, myelotoxicity, allergy; ototoxic effects synergistic with furosemide (Lasix); higher doses may be needed in the neutropenic patient
Trimethoprim and sulfamethoxazole (see co-trimoxazole, p. 301)			
Vancomycin (Vancocin) Class: anti-infective, other	Injection: 500, 100 mg Caps: 125, 250 mg Solution: 1, 10 g (reconstitute to 500 mg/6 mL)	<u>Children:</u> 10 mg/kg/24 h divided q8–12 h <u>Adults:</u> 2 g/24 h divided 12 h <u>Gut decontamination:</u> 125 mg caps, 1–4 times per d PO <u>C. difficile colitis:</u> Children: 40–50 mg/kg/24 h divided q6 h PO Max dose: 2 g/24 h Adults: 0.5–2 g/24 h divided q6 h PO	Therapeutic levels: Peak: 25–40 µg/mL Trough: < 10 µg/mL SE: ototoxicity, nephrotoxicity, allergy; "red man syndrome" may occur with rapid infusion (increase infusion time to 2–3 h) Diphenhydramine is used as a premed to treat red man syndrome.

B. Antidiarrheal agents

Drug	Supplied as	Dose and route	Special considerations
Diphenoxylate hydrochloride with atropine sulfate (Lomotil)	Solution: diphenoxylate hydrochloride 2.5 mg and atropine sulfate 0.025 mg per 5 mL (60 mL) Tab: diphenoxylate hydrochloride 2.5 mg and atropine sulfate 0.025 mg	Children: 0.3–0.4 mg/kg/24 h in 2–4 divided doses < 2 y: Not recommended 2–5 y: 2.5 mg 3 times per d 5–8 y: 2.5 mg 4 times per d 8–12 y: 2.5 mg 5 times per d Adults: 15–20 mg/d in 3–4 divided doses	Use with caution in patients with intestinal infection, *C. difficile.* SE: N/V, abdominal discomfort, paralytic ileus, pancreatitis, sedation, dizziness, pruritus, urticaria, H/A, tachycardia, blurred vision, dry mouth, euphoria, respiratory depression, hyperthermia, urinary retention
loperamide hydrochloride (Imodium) Class: antidiarrheal	Caps: 2 mg	2–5 y: 1 mg 3 times per d 6–8 y: 2 mg 2 times per d 8–12 y: 2 mg 3 times per d Max dose: should not exceed recommended daily dose Adults: Initial dose of 4 mg then 2 mg after each unformed stool Max dose: 16 mg/24 h	Use with caution in patients with intestinal infection, *C. difficile.* SE: N/V, abdominal discomfort, constipation, tiredness, drowsiness, dizziness, dry mouth

Drug	Supplied as	Dose and route	Special considerations
Octreotide acetate (Sandostatin) Class: antidiarrheal	Injection: 50, 100, 500, 1,000 µg/mL	200–300 µg 3–4 times per d (IV/SQ) OR 450–1000 µg/24 h by continuous IV No data available in children	SE: N/V, diarrhea, abdominal pain, H/A, dizziness, fatigue, flushing, edema, hypoglycemia

C. Antiemetic agents

Drug	Supplied as	Dose and route	Special considerations
Chlorpromazine hydrochloride (Thorazine) Class: phenothiazine, antiemetic	Tab: 10, 25, 50, 100, 200 mg Syrup: 10 mg/5 mL (120 mL) Suppository: 25, 100 mg Oral concentration: 30 mg/mL (120 mL), 100 mg/mL (60 and 240 mL) Injection: 25 mg/mL	<u>Children:</u> (> 6 mo) As antiemetic: 0.5–1 mg/kg per dose divided q4–6 h PO 0.5–1 mg/kg per dose q6–8 h IV Max dose: < 5 y: 40 mg/d 5–12 y: 75 mg/d <u>Adults:</u> As antiemetic: 10–25 mg per dose divided q4–6 h PO 25–50 mg per dose divided q4–6 h IV	SE: drowsiness, lowered seizure threshold, extrapyramidal symptoms, jaundice, hypotension, arrhythmias, agranulocytosis May potentiate effects of narcotics Monitor vital signs closely.

Compazine
(see prochlorperazine maleate, p. 320)

Dimenhydrinate
(Dramamine)

Class: antihistamine, antivertigo

Tab: 50 mg
Injection: 50 mg/mL (1 mL)

Children: 5 mg/kg/24 h divided q6 h PO/IV
Max dose: 300 mg/d
Adults: 50 mg divided q6 h PO 50–100 mg divided q6 h IV
Max dose: 400 mg/d

SE: drowsiness, H/A paradoxical excitement, blurred vision, tinnitus, dry mouth, dizziness, hypotension, anorexia, urinary frequency

Diphenhydramine hydrochloride
(Benadryl)

Class: antihistamine

Caps: 25, 50 mg
Elixir: 2.5 mg/mL (5, 10, 120 mL)
Injection: 50 mg/mL (1, 10 mL)

Children: 5 mg /kg/d divided q6–8 h PO/IV
Max dose: 300 mg/d
Adults: 25–50 mg q2–6 h PO/IV
Max dose: 400 mg/d

Generally not effective alone as antiemetic, but may potentiate phenothiazines; may also prevent extrapyramidal symptoms (EPS) when used in combination with phenothiazines.
SE: sedation, dizziness, hypotension, paradoxical excitement, N/V, dry mucous membranes, urinary retention, blurred vision, palpitations, insomnia, tremor

Drug	Supplied as	Dose and route	Special considerations
Droperidol (Inapsine) Class: anesthetic adjunct, antiemetic	Injection: 2.5 mg/mL (2 mL)	<u>Children:</u> 0.088–0.165 mg/kg per dose IV q6 h <u>Adults:</u> As premedication: 2.5–10 mg 30 min prn: 0.088–0.165 mg/kg per dose IV q6 h Max dose: 10 mg/d	Neuroleptic malignant syndrome can occur within wk of administration and can be life-threatening. SE: hypotension, tachycardia, dystonic reaction, akathisia, oculogyric crisis, anxiety, hyperactivity, drowsiness, dizziness, hallucinations, chills, laryngospasm, bronchospasm
Hydroxyzine (Vistaril) Class: antihistamine, sedative/hypnotic	Injection: 5, 10, 20, 25, 30, 40, 50, 75, 100 mg Tab: 25, 50, 100 mg	<u>Children:</u> 2–4 mg/kg/d divided q6–8 h PO 1 mg/kg per dose divided q4–6 h IV <u>Adult:</u> 25–100 mg per dose q6 h PO/IV	SE: Drowsiness, dry mouth, dizziness, ataxia, weakness, H/A, hypotension
Metoclopramide hydrochloride (Reglan) Class: parasympathomimetics; antiemetic	Injection: 5 mg/mL (2, 10 mL) Syrup: 1 mg/mL Tab: 10 mg	<u>Children:</u> GI hypomotility: PO/IV: 0.1 mg/kg per dose up to 4 times per d. Max dose: 0.5 mg/kg/d	SE: diarrhea, weakness, restlessness, drowsiness, skin rash, insomnia, dry mouth, extrapyramidal reaction, depression, hypotension, tachycardia, urticaria

Ondansetron hydrochloride
(Zofran)

Class: antiemetic

Injection: 2 mg/mL (20 mL);
32 mg (single-dose vial)
Tab: 4, 8 mg

Antiemetic:
1–2 mg/kg 30 min before chemo
and then q2–4 h IV
<u>Adults</u>: GI hypomotility: PO/IV:
10 mg 30 min before meals (ac)
& at bedtime
Antiemetic:
1–2 mg/kg 30 min before & q2–4 h IV

<u>Children</u>:
10–20 kg: 2 mg PO/IV
20–40 kg: 4 mg PO/IV
> 40 kg: 8 mg PO/IV
<u>Adults</u>:
< 70 kg: 8 mg PO/IV
Single dose: 24 or 32 mg may be
given 30 min prior to chemotherapy.
Multiple dose: 4 and 8 h after
first dose; no more than 2 subsequent
doses within 24 h period

Small number of patients may
experience tachyphylaxis with
multiple doses. SE: constipation,
diarrhea, abdominal cramping,
dizziness, dry mouth, rash, weakness

Phenergan
(see promethazine
hydrochloride, p. 320)

Drug	Supplied as	Dose and route	Special considerations
Prochlorperazine maleate (Compazine) Class: phenothiazine, antiemetic	Caps (sustained release): 10, 15, 30, 75 mg Tab: 5, 10, 25 mg Syrup: 5 mg/mL (120 mL) Suppository (supp): 2.5, 5, 25 mg (12 to box) Injection: 5 mg/mL (2, 10 mL)	<u>Children:</u> (10 kg) 0.4 mg/kg/24 h PO/per rectum (PR) 0.1–0.15 mg/kg per dose q6–8 h <u>Adults:</u> 5–10 mg q6–8 h POPR Sustained release: 10 mg q12 h Max dose: 40 mg/d 5–10 mg q3–4 h IV Max dose: 40 mg/24 h	SE: akathisia, dystonia, hypotension, pigmentary retinopathy, tardive dyskinesia, constipation, increased sweating, orthostatic hypotension, nasal congestion, extrapyramidal symptoms, tachycardia, metallic taste
Promethazine hydrochloride (Phenergan, Provigan) Class: antihistamine, Phenothiazine, antiemetic	Injection: 25, 50 mg/mL (1 mL) Supp: 12.5, 25, 50 mg Syrup: 6.25 mg/ 5 mL 25 mg/5 mL with 7% alcohol Tab: 12.5, 25, 50 mg	<u>Children:</u> 0.25–1.0 mg/kg per dose q4–6 h prn PO/IV <u>Adults:</u> 12.5–25 mg q4–6 h prn PO/IV	Drowsiness, thickening of bronchial secretions, H/A, fatigue, increased appetite, weight gain, nervousness, dizziness, diarrhea, dry mouth
Scopolamine hydrobromide (Transdermal Scop) Class: parasympatholytic, antivertigo agent	Patch: 1.5 mg delivers 0.5 mg over 3 d Injection: 0.43 mg/0.5 mL	<u>Children:</u> 6 μg/kg per dose q6–8 h IV prn Max dose: 0.3 mg per dose > 12 y: 1 patch q3 d <u>Adults:</u> 0.3–0.65 mg per dose q4–6 h IN prn Patch: 1 patch q3 d	SE: constipation; decreased sweating; sweating, dry mouth, nose, and throat; local irritation; difficulty swallowing; increased sensitivity to light.

Tigan
(see trimethobenzamide
hydrochloride, this page)

**Trimethobenzamide
hydrochloride**

Caps: 100, 250 mg
Supp: 100, 200 mg
Injection: 100 mg/mL

Children: IV/IM: not recommended
Oral: 13–40 kg: 100–200 mg
3–4 times per d
Rectal: < 13 kg: 100 mg 3–4 times
per d or 15–20 mg/kg/day divided
q6–8 h 14–40 kg: 100–200 mg
3–4 times per d
Adults: Oral: 250 mg 3–4 times per d
IM/IV: 200 mg 3–5 times per d

Not approved for IV administration
SE: sedation, extrapyramidal symptoms,
hypersensitivity skin reactions,
hypotension, blurred vision, dizziness,
seizures, blood dyscrasias, diarrhea,
mood changes, hepatotoxity

Class: antiemetic

Thorazine
(see chlorpromazine
hydrochloride, p. 316)

Zofran
(see ondansetron,
hydrochloride, p. 319)

D. Antifungal agents

Drug	Supplied as	Dose and route	Special considerations
Amphotericin B (Fungizone) Class: antifungal	Injection: 50-mg vial	Prophylaxis: 0.1–0.25 mg/kg/d Emperic dose: Initial: 0.25 mg/kg/d until desired dose of 1–1.5 mg/kg/d is achieved Critically ill patient: may initiate with 1–1.5 mg/kg/d with close observation Cumulative dose: 1.5–2 g over 6–10 wk	SE: fevers, rigors; premedication with acetaminophen and diphenhydramine is required; extremely nephrotoxic: other nephrotoxins should be avoided if possible; other SE: H/A, anemia, hypokalemia, hypomagnesemia, anorexia, malaise, generalized pains, bone marrow depression, flushing
Amphotericin B lipid complex (Abelcet, ABCD) Class: antifungal	Injection: 5 mg (20 mL)	<u>Children and adults:</u> 5 mg/kg/d	SE: similar to that of amphotericin B; is less nephrotoxic; increased risk of hypotension, cardiac arrest, respiratory failure
Clotrimazole (Gyne-Lotrimin, Lotrimin, Mycelex) Class: antifungal	Cream: Topical: 1% (30 g) Vaginal 1% (45 g) Solution, topical: 1% (30 mL) Tab, vaginal: 100 mg (7 s) Troche: 10 mg	<u>Children > 3 y & adults:</u> Oral: 10 mg troche dissolved 5 times per d Topical: apply 2 times per d <u>Adults:</u> Vaginal cream: 5 g (1 applicator)/24 h Vaginal tablet: 1 (100 mg)/24 h for 7 d	SE: abnormal LFT levels, N/V, local burning, irritation, bad taste

Fluconazole
(Diflucan)

Class: antifungal

Tab: 50, 100, 200 mg
Injection: 2 mg/mL
(100, 200 mL)

Children: 3–8 mg/kg/d q24 h PO/IV
Doses up to 12 mg/kg/d have been
used in immunocompromised
children.

Adults:

Prophylaxis: 200 mg/d PO/IV

Coccidioidal/cryptococcal infection:
400 mg load, then 200 mg/d IV

Acute systemic candidal infections:
400 mg load, then 200 mg/d IV

Oral/esophageal candidiasis (in
immunocompromised patients):
200 mg/d

SE: Use with caution in patients
with known hepatic or renal
dysfunction.

For creatinine clearance (mL/min)
50, give 100% of dose
21–50, give 50% of dose
11–20, give 25% of dose
Other SE: H/A, nausea, rash,
abdominal pain, elevated levels of
ALT, alanine Transaminase (ALT),
and alkaline phosphatase. Do not
administer to patients on cisapride
or terfenadine.

Itraconazole
(Sporanox)

Class: antifungal

Caps: 100 mg

Children: No data available

Adults:

Prophylaxis: 200 mg/d PO

Treatment: 200–400 mg/d

Max dose: 600 mg/d

SE: N/V, diarrhea, edema,
fatigue, fever, H/A, rash, pruritis
Instruct patient to take with
carbonated beverage. Do not
administer to patients on cisapride
or terfenadine.

Ketoconazole
(Nizoral)

Tab: 200 mg

Children: 3.3–6.6 mg/kg/d

Adults: 200–400 mg/d

Dose reduction should be considered
in patients with liver disease.

Drug	Supplied as	Dose and route	Special considerations
Ketoconazole (continued) Class: antifungal			Do not administer to patients on cisapride or terfenadine. SE: N/V, pruritus, abdominal pain
Miconazole nitrate (Monistat) Class: antifungal	Cream: Topical: 2% (30 g) Vaginal, as nitrate: 2% Lotion: 2% (30 mL) Vaginal supp: 100, 200 mg Injection: 10 mg/mL divided q8 h	Children: IV: 20–40 mg/kg/d divided q8 h Topical: Apply 1–2 times per d Adults: IV: initial 200 mg, then 1.2–3.6 g/d Topical: apply 1–2 times per d Vaginal: 1 applicator of cream (100 mg) qhs for 7 d OR 200-mg suppository qhs for 3 d	Use with caution in patients with hepatic dysfunction. SE: Fever, chills, rash, itching, N/V, anemia, thrombocytopenia IV form not commonly used in bone marrow transplantation (BMT) setting
Nystatin (Mycostatin, Nilstat) Class: topical antifungal	Cream, topical: 100,000 U/g (15 g) Ointment: 100,000U/g (15 g) Powder: 100,000 U/g (15 g) Susp: 100,000 U/mL (60 mL) Tab/pastille: 500,000 U Vaginal tablet: 100,000 U (15s, 30s)	Oral candidiasis: treatment & prophylaxis Infants: 200,000 U 4 times per d Children and adults: 400,000–600,000 U 4 times per d OR Troche: 200,000–400,000 U 4–5 times per d Mucocutaneous infections: Children and adults: Topical cream	Have patient swish and swallow oral form. SE: N/V, abdominal cramping, diarrhea

Troche: 200,000 U

or ointment to affected areas, moist
areas are best treated with powder

Vaginal infections:

Adults: vaginal tablets: insert
1 tablet/d at hs for 2 wk

E. Antihypertensive agents/diuretics

Drug	Supplied as	Dose and route	Special considerations
Bumetanide (Bumex) Class: loop diuretics	Tab: 0.5, 1, 2 mg Injection: 0.25 mg/mL (1% benzyl alcohol)	<u>Children:</u> 0.015 mg/kg every day (qd) to 0.1 mg/kg qd PO <u>Adults:</u> 0.5–2 mg/24 h PO as single dose PO; may give second and third doses at 4–5 h intervals to max dose of 10 mg/24 h IV: 0.5–1 mg over 1–2 min may give second and third doses at 2–3 h intervals, not to exceed max 10 mg IV	Safety and efficacy in children < 18 y has not been established. Half-life is 2 times longer in infants < 6 mo. SE: muscle cramps, dizziness, hypotension, H/A, encephalopathy, hypokalemia, hypochloremia, hyponatremia, hypophosphatemia, hypocalcemia, metabolic alkalosis
Captopril (Capoten) Class: antihypertensive angiatensin converting enzyme (ACE) inhibitor	Caps: 0.5, 1 mg Tab: 12.5, 25, 50, 100 mg	<u>Infants > 2 mo & children:</u> Initial dose: 0.5 mg/kg; titrate dose in twofold increments to max dose of 6 mg/kg/d in 1–4 divided doses or 75 mg/d	Use with caution in patients with underlying renal dysfunction or those on other nephrotoxins. SE: neutropenia, agranulocytosis, proteinuria, rash, loss of taste

Drug	Supplied as	Dose and route	Special considerations
Captopril (continued)		<u>Adults:</u> Initial dose: 25 mg 2–3 times per d; may increase at 1–2 week intervals up to 150 mg 3 times per d.	
Chlorothiazide (Diuril) Class: thiazide diuretic	Tab: 250 mg Susp: 50 mg/mL (237 mL) Injection: 500 mg/20 mL	<u>Children:</u> Oral: < 6 mo: 30 mg/kg/d divided bid > 6 mo: 20 mg/kg/d divided bid IV: 20–40 mg/kg/d in 2 divided doses <u>Adults:</u> Oral: 500–2000 mg/d divided bid IV: 250–1000 mg per dose	SE: hypokalemia, hyperuricemia, prerenal azotemia, hypochloremic alkalosis, hyperglycemia, hyperlipidemia, rarely blood dyscrasias Commonly used 30 min prior to loop diuretics in patients with low urine output
Clonidine (Catapres) Class: antihypertensive: alpha 2 agonist	Tab: 0.1, 0.2 mg Transdermal patch (Catapres TTS): 1, 2, 3 (0.1, 0.2, 0.3 mg/d) 7-d patches	<u>Oral:</u> Children: 5–10 µg/kg/d divided q8–12 h; gradually increase at 5–7 d intervals to 25 µg/kg/d in divided doses q6 h Max dose: 0.9 mg/d	Safety and efficacy in children < 12 y has not yet been established SE: dry mouth, drowsiness, dizziness, constipation, N/V, abnormal LFT levels, nervousness, agitation, depression, H/A, orthostatic hypotension, rash, weakness, fatigue, nocturia

Diltiazem hydrochloride
(Cardizem, Cardizem
CD, Dilacor XR)

Class: calcium
channel blocker

Caps (sustained release):
Cardizem CD: 120, 180, 240,
300 mg
Cardizem SR: 60, 90, 120 mg
Injection: 5 mg/mL
Tab: 30, 60, 90, 120 mg

Adults:
Oral: Initial short-acting dose is
30–60 mg PO tid OR 180–240 mg
once daily. Maximum anti-
hypertensive effect is usually after
14 d of therapy. Adjust dose
accordingly up to max dose of 360
mg/d. **IV*** (requires infusion pump):
Initial bolus: 0.25 mg/kg actual body
weight (wt) over 2 min (average dose
= 20 mg) **Repeat** bolus (after 15 min
if no response): 0.35 mg/kg actual
body wt (average dose = 25 mg)
Continuous infusion: 15 mg/h not
recommended; initial infusion rate of
10 mg/h; rate may be increased in 5 mg/h
increments up to 15 mg/h
* Start oral approximately 3 h after
bolus if possible:

3 mg/h IV = 120 mg/d PO
5 mg/h IV = 180 mg/d PO
7 mg/h IV = 240 mg/d PO
11 mg/h IV = 360 mg/d PO

Use with caution in renal or hepatic
impairment. SE: H/A, dizziness,
bradycardia, atrioventricular
(A-V) block, edema, electrocardiogram
(ECG) abnormality, asthenia, angina,
abnormal dreams, depression, achieved
insomnia, nervousness

Drug	Supplied as	Dose and route	Special considerations
Enalapril maleate (Vasotec) Class: ACE inhibitor	Tab: 2.5, 5, 10, 20 mg	<u>Children:</u> Safety in children not yet established; consult renal service before using <u>Adults:</u> 5 mg qd intially PO up to 40 mg/24 h	Use with extreme caution in patients with renal impairment. Use only after other agents have failed to achieve control. SE: renal failure, nausea, diarrhea, H/A, hypotension, rash, neutropenia, anemia, loss of taste, hyperkalemia, cough, muscle cramps, impotence
Furosemide (Lasix) Class: loop diuretic	Tab: 20, 40, 80 mg Injection: 10 mg/mL Liquid: 10 mg/mL (60 mL) 8 mg/mL	<u>Oral:</u> Infants & children: 2 mg/kg per dose 6–8 h prn; may increase by 1–2 mg/kg per dose Adults: 20–80 mg/24 h qd or bid May increase 20–40 mg up to 600 mg/24 h <u>Parenteral:</u> Infants & children: 1 mg/kg per dose q6–12 h IV prn; may increase by 1 mg/kg per dose Adults: 20–80 mg per dose Max single dose: 6 mg/kg	SE: Ototoxicity may occur in presence of renal disease, especially when used with aminoglycosides. Use with caution in hepatic disease. Other SE: hypokalemia, alkalosis, dehydration, hyperuricemia, increased calcium excretion; prolonged use in premature infants may result in nephrocalcinosis

Hydralazine hydrochloride (Apresoline)	Caps: 5 mg Tab: 10, 25 mg Injection: 20 mg/mL (1 mL)	<u>Children:</u> Oral: 0.25–1 mg/kg 3–4 times per d Max dose: 7 mg/kg/d IV (hypertensive crisis): 0.1 mg/kg per dose 4–6 times per d <u>Adults:</u> Oral: 10–75 mg 4 times per d IV (hypertensive crisis): 10–50 mg per dose 3–4 times per d	SE: H/A, palpitations, tachycardia, anorexia, N/V, diarrhea, orthostatic hypotension, dizziness, edema, SLE-like syndrome, peripheral neuritis, weakness
Class: antihypertensive			
Hydrochlorothiazide (HydroDIURIL)	Tab: 25 mg	< 6 mo: 3 mg/kg/d divided bid > 6 mo: 2 mg/kg/d divided bid <u>Adults:</u> 25–100 mg/d in 1–3 divided doses Max dose: 200 mg/d	<u>Children:</u> SE: Hypokalemia, hypotension, hyperglycemia, prerenal azotemia
Class: thiazide diuretic			
Labetalol hydrochloride (Trandate, Normodyne)	Tab: 100 mg Injection: 5 mg/mL (20 mL)	<u>Children:</u> Oral: Initial: 4 mg/kg/d divided bid IV: Intermittent bolus of 0.3–1 mg/kg per dose Continuous IV infusion:	SE: Dyspnea, congestive heart failure (CHF), dizziness, irregular heartbeat, orthostatic hypotension, N/V, reduced peripheral tone, stuffy nose, weakness
Class: β blocker			

Drug	Supplied as	Dose and route	Special considerations
Labetalol hydrochloride *(continued)*		0.4–1 mg/kg/h; max dose of 3 mg/kg/h Adults: Oral: 100 mg bid; may increase prn q2–3 d by 100 mg until desired effect achieved; usual dose 200–400 mg bid Max dose: 2.4 g/d IV: 20 mg or 1–2 mg/kg (whichever is lower) intravenous push (IVP) over 2 min; may give 40–80 mg at 10 min intervals up to 300 mg Continuous IV infusion: may start at 2 mg/min; titrate to response up to 300 mg total dose	
Nifedipine (Adalat, Procardia, Procardia XL) Class: calcium channel blocker	Caps: 10, 20 mg (may be punctured for sublingual administration)	Children: 0.25–0.5 mg/kg per dose Adults: Initial: 10 mg 3–4 times per d Maintenance: 10–30 mg 3–4 times per d Max dose: 180 mg/d	SE: H/A, dizziness, giddiness, light-headedness, flushing, heat sensation, weakness, nausea, heartburn, muscle cramps, tremor, palpitations, dyspnea, cough, nasal congestion, sore throat, hypotension

Spironolactone
(Aldactone)

Class: potassium-sparing diuretic

Tab: 25, 50, 100 mg	
Suspension: 2 mg/mL	

Children: 1.0–3.3 mg/kg/24 h divided bid-qid PO

Adults:
25–100 mg/24 h divided bid-qid PO
Max dose: 200 mg/24 h

Contraindicated in acute renal failure; may potentiate other ganglionic blocking agents and other antihypertensives SE: hyperkalemia, GI upset, rash, gynecomastia

Verapamil
(Calan, Calan SR, Isoptin, Verelan)

Class: calcium channel blocker

Injection: 5 mg/2 mL (2 mL)
Tab: 40, 80, 120 mg
Tab (sustained release [SR]): 240 mg

Children: dose recommendations for treatment of supraventricular tachycardia (SVT) only
Adults: 80 mg 3 times per d or 240 mg/d (SR); range: 240–480 mg/d (no edema, evidence of benefit at doses 360 mg/d)

Use with caution in hepatic or renal impairment. SE: rash, bradycardia, second or third degree heart block, CHF, hypotension, peripheral dizziness, constipation, nausea, tiredness

F. Antiviral agents

Drug	Supplied as	Dose and route	Special considerations
Acyclovir (Zovirax) Class: antiviral	Caps: 200, 800 mg Injection: 500 mg/10 mL Ointment: 5% (15 g)	Herpes simplex virus (HSV) & HSV prophylaxis: Children and adults: 250 mg/m^2 q8 h IV OR Adults: 200 mg PO 5 times per d OR 400 mg PO tid HSV encephalitis:	Adjust dose for diminished renal function. Maintain adequate urine output and hydration. SE: nephrotoxicity, H/A, lethargy, tremulousness, delirium, seizures, N/V, rash, sore throat, insomnia, bone marrow depression, elevated liver enzymes levels

Drug	Supplied as	Dose and route	Special considerations
Acyclovir (*continued*)		Children: 1500 mg/m²/d divided q8 h for 10 d	
		Adults: 10 mg/kg per dose q8 h for 10 d	
		Topical HSV treatment:	
		1/2 inch ribbon to affected area 6 times per d	
		Treatment of varicella zoster virus (VZV) infection:	
		Children: 10–20 mg/kg per dose up to 800 mg 4 times per d PO	
		Adults: 600–800 mg per dose 5 times per d OR 1000 mg q6 h PO	
		IV (adults and children): 1500 mg/m² d divided q8 h OR 10 mg/kg per dose q8 h	
		Cytomegalovirus (CMV) prophylaxis:	
		Adults and children: 1500 mg/m²/d divided q8 h OR 10 mg/kg per dose q8 h IV (only until ganciclovir can be tolerated)	

Foscarnet sodium
(Foscavir)

Class: antiviral

Injection: 24 mg/mL
(250, 500 mL)

CMV prophylaxis:
Children and adults:
90–120 mg/kg/d IV
Maintenance dosing based on
creatinine clearance (mL/min/kg)

Very nephrotoxic and may be additive
to other nephrotoxins
SE: fever, N/V, anemia, H/A, seizures

Creatinine clearance	Equivalent to 90 mg/kg	Equivalent to 120 mg/kg
≥ 1.4	90	120
1.2–1.4	78	104
1–1.2	75	100
0.8–1	71	94
0.6–0.8	63	84
0.4–0.6	57	76

Ganciclovir
(Cytovene)

Class: antiviral

Injection: 500 mg

CMV prophylaxis:
Adults and children:
5–6 mg/kg per dose qd 3–5 times
per week
CMV infection: Initial (with normal
renal function):
5 mg/kg q12 h IV
Maintenance: 5 mg/kg/d IV OR
6 mg/kg 5 d per week

Dose adjustments or interruption of
therapy may be required in patients
with low blood counts or renal
dysfunction. SE: granulocytopenia,
thrombocytopenia, H/A, confusion,
rash, fever, abnormal LFT levels,
elevated creatinine

G. Anxiolytic/Analgesics

Drug	Supplied as	Dose and route	Special considerations
Amitriptyline hydrochlorine (Elavil, Endep) Class: tricyclic antidepressant	Tab: 10, 25 mg	<u>Children: > 6 y</u> Initial dose: 0.5 mg/kg/d; increase by 0.5 mg/kg/d q1–2 wk; range: 0.5–5 mg/kg/d in 1–2 divided doses <u>Adolescents:</u> 1–5 mg/kg/d in 1–2 divided doses <u>Adults:</u> 150–300 mg/d qd	Effective adjunct to long-term analgesia for neuropathic pain SE: sedation, weakness, fatigue, tremor, anxiety, impaired cognitive function, seizures, dry mouth, blurred vision, constipation, urinary retention, postural hypotension, tachycardia, sudden death
Chloral hydrate (Noctec) Class: sedative/hypnotic	Caps: 500 mg Syrup: 100 mg/mL	<u>Children:</u> Sedation, anxiety: 15–25 mg/kg per dose OR 25 mg/kg/d in 3 divided doses Hypnotic: 50 mg/kg per dose <u>Adults:</u> Sedation, anxiety: 250 mg 3 times per d Hypnotic: 500–1000 mg at hs OR 30 min prior to procedure Max dose: 2 g/24 h	Effective short-term sedation prior to procedures SE: N/V, diarrhea, flatulence, sedation, disorientation, ataxia, excitement, rash, dizziness, H/A, urticaria, fever, leukopenia, eosinophilia
Codeine (Various brands)	Tab: 15, 30, 60 mg Injection: 15, 30, 60 mg/mL Oral solution: 15 mg/mL	<u>Children:</u> 0.5–1.0 mg/kg per dose q4–6 h PO, <u>Adults:</u>	SE: central nervous system (CNS) and respiratory depression, constipation Do not administer IV.

Class: opioid analgesic, antitussive	Elixir: 120 mg of acetaminophen & 12 mg of codeine per 5 mL Tab: (all contain 300 mg Tylenol/tab) Tylenol #1 – 7.5 mg codeine Tylenol #2 – 15 mg codeine Tylenol #3 – 30 mg codeine Tylenol #4 – 60 mg codeine	30–60 mg per dose q4–6 h	Do not use in children < 2 y of age.
Diazepam (Valium) Class: benzodiazepine sedative	Tab: 2, 5 mg Injection: 5 mg/mL (2 mL)	<u>Children:</u> Sedation: 0.12–0.8 mg/kg/d divided q6–8 h PO OR 0.04–0.3 mg/kg per dose q2–4 h Max dose: 0.6 mg/kg within 8 h period Status epilepticus: Infants ≥ 1 mo & children < 5 yr: 0.05–0.5 mg/kg per dose q15–30 min IV to max dose of 5 mg; repeat in 2–4 h if needed. Children > 5 yr: 0.05–0.3 mg/kg per dose q15–30 min to max dose of 10 mg; repeat in 2–4 h prn OR 1 mg q2–5 min to max dose of 10 mg	In children, do not exceed 1–2 mg/min IVP: for adults: 5 mg/min SE: decreased repiratory rate, apnea, cardiac arrest, drowsiness, confusion, dizziness, ataxia, hypotension, bradycardia, cardiovascular collapse, laryngospasm, phlebitis

Drug	Supplied as	Dose and route	Special considerations
Diazepam *(continued)*		<u>Adults:</u> Anxiety: Oral: 2–10 mg 2–4 times per d IV: 2–10 mg; may repeat in 3–4 h prn Skeletal muscle relaxation: Oral: 2–4 mg 2–4 times per d IV: 5–10 mg; may repeat in 2–4 h Status epilepticus: 5–10 mg IV q10–20 min; up to 30 mg/8 h; may repeat in 2–4 h Transdermal: Initial: 25 µg/24 h patch If patient is taking opiates; convert to fentanyl equivalent. To convert from oral to IV, the previous 24 h analgesic requirement should be calculated and converted.	
Fentanyl citrate (Sublimaze, Duragesic)	Injection: 0.05 mg/mL (2, 5, 10, 20 mL) Transdermal patch: 25, 50, 75, 100 µg	<u>Children:</u> Sedation for minor procedures: IV: 1–2 µg/kg per dose, may repeat at 30–60 min intervals	Give IV injection over 3–5 min: may cause apnea SE: bradycardia, hypotension, respiratory depression,

| Class: opioid analgesic | Lozenge: 200, 300, 400 μg | Transmucosal: 5 μg/kg, fearful children may require 5–15 μg/kg | orthostatic hypotension, rash, itching |

Continuous analgesia/sedation:

Initial IV bolus: 1–2 μg/kg then 1 μg/kg/h; titrate upward; usual dose 1–3 μg/kg/h

Transdermal: Not recommended for children

Adults:

Sedation/pain control for procedures:

IV: 0.5–2 μg/kg per dose

Transmucosal: 5 μg/kg, suck 20–40 min before procedure

Continuous analgesia/sedation:

Initial IV bolus: 1–2 μg/kg then 1 μg/kg/h; titrate upward; usual dose 1–3 μg/kg/h

Transdermal:

Initial: 25 μg/24 h patch

If patient is taking opiates, convert to fentanyl equivalent (Table 7.1 and 7.2). To convert from oral to IV, the previous 24 h analgesic requirement should be calculated and converted.

Table 7.1 Equianalgesic Doses of Opioid Agonists

Drug	Equianalgesic dose (mg)	
	IM	**PO**
Codeine	130	200
Hydromorphone	1.5	7.5
Levorphanol	2	4
Meperidine	75	—
Methadone	10	20
Morphine	10	60
Oxycodone	15	30
Oxymorphone	1	10 (PR)

Table 7.2 Corresponding Doses of Oral/Intramuscular Morphine and Duragesic

Oral 24–hour morphine (Mg/d)	IM 24–hour morphine (mg/d)	Duragesic dose (µg/h)
45–134	8–27	25
135–224	28–37	50
225–314	38–52	75
315–404	53–67	100
405–494	68–82	125
495–584	83–97	150
585–674	98–112	175
675–764	113–127	200
765–854	128–142	225
855–944	143–157	250
945–1034	158–172	275
1035–1124	173–187	300

Drug	Supplied as	Dose and route	Special considerations
Hydromorphone hydrochloride (Dilaudid) Class: opioid analgesic	Tab: 2, 4 mg Injection: 2 mg/mL 4 mg/mL	<u>Young children:</u> Oral: 0.05–0.1 mg/kg/d q6 h Max dose: 5 mg per dose <u>Older children & adults:</u> 1–4 mg per dose q4–6 h (PO or IV) Continuous infusion: Begin at 0.25 mg/h and titrate for comfort (no more than 4 incremental increases of 0.25–1 mg/h in a 24 h period).	SE: CNS and respiratory depression, N/V, constipation, hypotension, bradycardia, peripheral vasodilation, histamine release, increased intracranial pressure, miosis, biliary or urinary tract spasm, drowsiness, sedation, antidiuretic hormone (ADH) release
Lidocaine and prilocaine (EMLA Cream) prilocaine Class: topical anesthetic	Topical cream: lidocaine 2.5% & prilocaine 2.5% (5, 30 g with 2 Tegaderms)	<u>Children & adults:</u> Apply thick layer of cream to intact skin and cover with occlusive dressing. Minor procedures: Apply 2.5 g to site for 60 min. Painful procedures: Apply 2 g/10 cm^2 for at least 2 h.	SE: Contact dermatitis, burning, stinging, angioedema, urticaria
Lorazepam (Ativan)	Tab: 0.5, 1, 2 mg Injection: 2 mg/mL (1, 10 mL); 4 mg/mL (1. 10 mL)	<u>Infants & children:</u> Oral/IV: 0.05 mg/kg per dose (range 0.02–0.09 mg/kg) q4–8 h	SE: confusion, CNS depression, sedation, drowsiness, lethargy, hangover effect, dizziness,

Drug	Supplied as	Dose and route	Special considerations
Class: benzodiazepine sedative/hypnotic			bradycardia, circulatory collapse,
Lorazepam *(continued)*		<u>Adults:</u> Oral/IV: 1–10 mg/d (anxiety, insomnia) in 2–3 divided doses Premedication (premed): 0.044 mg/kg IV 15–30 min prior to procedure or chemotherapy <u>Status epilepticus:</u> Infants & children: 0.1 mg/kg IV over 2–5 min; may repeat second dose of 0.05 mg/kg IV in 10–15 min if needed Adolescents: 0.07 mg/kg IV over 2–5 min; may repeat in 10–15 min Adults: 4 mg per dose IV over 2–5 min; may repeat in 10–15 min; max dose: 8 mg	transitory hallucinations, diplopia, ataxia, nystagmus, constipation, dry mouth, nausea, vomiting, urinary incontinence or retention, respiratory depression, hypertension or hypotension
Meperidine hydrochloride (Demerol)	Tab: 50 mg Syrup: 10 mg/mL Injection: 25 mg/0.5 mL, 50 mg/0.5 mL, 100 mg/0.5 mL	<u>Children:</u> 1–1.5 mg/kg per dose q3–4 h prn OR may repeat once for rigors Max dose: 100 mg per dose	SE: tachycardia, CNS and respiratory depression, N/V, constipation, hypotension, bradycardia, peripheral vasodilatation, histamine release,

Class: opioid analgesic	**Adults:** 50–150 mg per dose q3–4 h prn Rigors: 25–50 mg IV; may repeat 1–2 times prn	increased intracranial pressure, miosis, biliary or urinary tract spasm, drowsiness, sedation, ADH release, physical and psychologic dependence
Midazolam hydrochloride Injection: 1 mg/mL, 5 mg/mL (Versed) Class: benzodiazepine	**Children:** Preoperative (preop) sedation: 0.08 mg/kg per dose Sedation for procedures: Begin with 0.035 mg/kg IV over 2 min; repeat prn Max dose: 0.2 mg/kg **Adults:** Preop sedation: 0.07–0.08 mg/kg Sedation for procedures: begin with 0.035 mg/kg IV over 2 min Max initial IV dose: 2.5 mg	Pediatric doses not well established SE: respiratory depression, hypotension, bradycardia, hiccups, N/V, amnesia, dizziness
Morphine sulfate (Duramorph, MS Contin) Tab: 15, 30 mg Controlled release tab: (MS Contin): 30, 60, 100 mg Supp: 5, 10, 20 mg Solution: 10 mg/5 mL, 20 mg/5 mL, 20 mg mL Injection: 2 mg/mL, 4 mg/mL, 5 mg/mL, 8 mg/mL, 10 mg/mL, 15 mg/mL Class: opioid analgesic	**Infants & children:** Oral: immediate release: 0.2–0.5 mg/kg per dose q4–6 h prn Controlled release: 0.3–0.6 mg/kg per dose q12 h (ATC) IV: 0.1–0.2 mg/kg per dose q2–4 h prn Usual max dose: 15 mg per dose IV: continuous infusion: 0.025–2 mg/kg/h; postoperative	Doses should be titrated to appropriate effect. Oral doses are approximately 50% as effective as parenteral. SE: CNS and respiratory depression, N/V, constipation, hypotension, bradycardia, peripheral vasodilation, histamine release, increased intracranial pressure, miosis, biliary or urinary tract spasm,

Drug	Supplied as	Dose and route	Special considerations
Morphine sulfate (*continued*)	Injection (preservative-free): 1 mg/mL (2, 10 mL); 0.5 mg/mL (10 mL) Patient controlled analgesia (PCA) injection: 1 mg/mL (30 mL syringe); 5 mg/mL (30 mL syringe)	(postop) pain: 0.01–0.04 mg/kg/h Sedation for procedures: 0.05–1 mg IV before procedures <u>Adolescents: ≥ 12 y</u> Sedation/analgesia for procedures: 3–4 mg IV and repeat in 5 min <u>Adults:</u> Oral: 10–30 mg q4 h prn Controlled release: 15–30 mg q8–12 h; titrate up to effect IV: 2.5–15 mg q2–4 h prn IV: continuous infusion: Initial: 0.8–10 mg/h; adjust to maintenance dose of 0.8–80 mg/h	drowsiness, sedation, ADH release, physical and psychologic dependence
Trazodone hydrochloride (Desyrel) Class: antidepressant	Tab: 50, 100 mg	<u>Children:</u> not recommended for patients < 18 y <u>Adults:</u> For sleep: initial 50 mg qhs; may increase to 150 mg qhs Antidepressant: Initial 150 mg/d in 3 divided doses, increase by 50 mg/d q3–4 d Max dose: 400 mg/d	SE: sedation, postural hypotension, arrhythmias, priapism, dizziness, weakness, H/A, insomnia, confusion, agitation, seizures, dry mouth, blurred vision, N/V

H. Coagulation agents

Drug	Supplied as	Dose and route	Special considerations
Aminocaproic acid (Amicar) Class: antihemorrhagic/ hemostatic	Tablet: 500 mg Syrup: 250 mg/mL (480 mL) Injection: 250 mg/mL	<u>Children:</u> Oral/IV: Loading: 100–200 mg/kg Maintenance: 100 mg/kg per dose q6 h <u>Adults:</u> Oral: 5 g during First 1 h; followed by 1–1.25 g/h for 8 h or until bleeding stops Max daily dose: 30 g IV: 4–5 g in 250 mL of diluent during First hour followed by continuous infusion of 1–1.25 g/h in 50 mL diluent; continue for 8 h or until bleeding stops	Contraindicated in disseminated intravascular coagulation (DIC) SE: GI irritation, dizziness, tinnitus, malaise, H/A, rash, hypotension, bradycardia, arrhythmia, nasal congestion
AquaMEPHYTON (see phytonadione, p. 344)			
Heparin sodium Class: anticoagulant	Injection: 10, 100, 1000, 5000, 10,000, 20,000 40,000 U/mL Respository injection:	<u>Infants & children:</u> Initial: 50 U/kg IV bolus Maintenance: 10–25 U/kg/h as continuous infusion OR 100 U/kg per dose q4 h IV	For therapeutic heparin; adjust dose to give clotting time of 20–30 min or partial thromboplastin time (PTT) of 1.5–2.5 times control value. SE: allergy, bleeding, alopecia, thrombocytopenia

Drug	Supplied as	Dose and route	Special considerations
Heparin sodium (*continued*)	20,000 U/mL	*Adults:* Initial: 5000–10,000 U IV bolus Maintenance: 20,000–40,000 U IV/24 h as constant infusion OR 5000–10,000 U q4 h IV *Veno-occlusive disease (VOD) prophylaxis:* 100–150 U/kg/24 h as continuous IV infusion; start with conditioning regimen and continue until about d 30 *Heparin line flush:* Peripheral IV: 1–2 mL of 10 U/mL q4 h Central lines: 2–5 mL of 100 U/mL each lumen q24 h	<u>Antidote:</u> Protamine sulfate (1 mg/100 U heparin in previous 4 h)
Phytonadione (AquaMEPHYTON, Vitamin K)	Tab: 5 mg Injection: 10 mg/mL Injection (neonates): 1 mg/0.5 mL	*Vitamin K deficiency:* Infants & children: Oral: 2–5 mg/24 h IV: 1–2 mg per dose as a single dose Adults: Oral: 5–25 mg/24 h IV: 10 mg (usually given for 3 d)	Hypersensitivity reactions resembling anaphylaxis have been reported with IV administration. Use IV only when necessary. SE: GI upset with oral administraton

Thrombin, topical (Thrombinar, Thrombogen Thrombostat) Class: hemostatic agent	Powder: 5000 U	Use 1000–2000 U/mL of solution; apply directly to site of bleeding. Use 100 U/mL for bleeding from mucosal surfaces or skin.	Do not inject: for topical use only. SE: Rash, allergic reaction, fever
Urokinase (Abbokinase) Class: thrombolytic	Injection: 5000 U	Withdraw full dose into TB syringe and gently instill into clotted CVL; never force (CVL) line instillation. Attach 10-mL syringe and aspirate urokinase using milking technique. If clot is not aspirated, return urokinase to CVL and wait additional hour. If unsuccessful again, repeat dose. If patency restored, flush catheter with 3 mL NS.	If catheter remains clotted, consider drug precipitate; central venous catheter study may be warranted.

I. BMT conditioning agents

Drug	Supplied as	Dose and route	Special considerations
Busulfan (Myleran) Class: alkylating agent	Tab: 2 mg	Conventional dose: 2–4 mg/kg BMT dose: 14–16 mg/kg (consult protocol)	SE: myelosuppression with nadir of 14–21 d; N/V, pulmonary fibrosis, hyperpigmentation, hyperuricemia, hepatic dysfunction, dizziness, blurred vision, seizures Dose-limiting toxicity: stomatitis, VOD

Drug	Supplied as	Dose and route	Special considerations
Carboplatin (Paraplatin) Class: alkylating agent	Injection: 50, 150, 400 mg	Conventional dose: 300–400 mg/m^2 BMT dose: 1500–2000 mg/m^2 (consult protocol)	SE: N/V, nephrotoxicity, neutropenia, leukopenia, thrombocytopenia; nadir between 14 and 21 d; anemia, peripheral neuropathy, ototoxicity, abnormal LFT levels, hypocalcemia, hypomagnesemia, rash, urticaria, alopecia, pain, asthenia Dose-limiting toxicity: peripheral neuropathy, hepatotoxicity, nephrotoxicity, ototoxicity
Carmustine (BCNU) Class: alkylating agent	Injection: 100 mg	Conventional dose: 240–300 mg/m^2 BMT dose: 250–1000 mg/m^2 (consult protocol)	SE: pancytopenia, N/V, pain, thrombophlebitis, myelosuppression with nadir at 28 d, hepatotoxicity, flushing, pulmonary fibrosis, renal failure, dermatitis, pneumonitis Solution contains 10% ethanol; patients may experience "hangover" following administration. Dose-limiting toxicity: pneumonitis, VOD

Chlorambucil
(Leukeran)

Class: alkylating agent

Tab: 2 mg

Conventional dose: 2 mg/m^2
BMT dose: 6 mg/kg
(consult protocol)

SE: leukopenia, thrombocytopenia, anemia, sterility, N/V, weakness, seizures, rash, pulmonary fibrosis pneumonitis, hyperuricemia, hepatotoxicity
Dose-limiting toxicity: neurological toxicity

Cisplatin
(Platinol)

Class: alkylating agent

Injection: 1 mg/mL (50 mL)
Powder: 10 mg

Conventional dose: 40–80 mg/m^2
BMT dose: 150–240 mg/m^2
(consult protocol)

SE: severe renal toxicity, myelosuppression, N/V, ototoxicity, hypomagnesemia, hypocalcemia, hypophosphatemia, peripheral neuropathy, optic neuritis, anaphylactoid reaction, papilledema, bradycardia, arrhythmias, elevated LFT levels, phlebitis, hyperuricemia, mild alopecia
Dose-limiting toxicity: nephrotoxicity, ototoxicity

Cyclophosphamide
(Cytoxan)

Class: alkylating agent

Tab: 25, 50 mg
Injection: 500 mg

Conventional dose: 500–1500 mg/m^2
BMT dose: 6000–7500 mg/m^2
OR 100–120 mg/kg

SE: N/V, anorexia, diarrhea, mucositis, hemorrhagic cystitis, hematuria, syndrome of inappropriate antidiuretic hormone (SIADH),

Drug	Supplied as	Dose and route	Special considerations
Cyclophosphamide (*continued*)			immunosuppression, sterility, pulmonary fibrosis, alopecia, myocardial necrosis, secondary cancer Dose-limiting toxicity: hemorrhagic cystitis, myocarditis, pneumonitis
Cytarabine (ara-C, cytosine arabinoside) Class: antimetabolite	Injection: 100, 500 mg	Conventional dose: 1–3 g/m^2 BMT dose: 4–36 g/m^2 (consult protocol)	SE: N/V, diarrhea, myelosuppression, acral dermatitis, oral and anal inflammation with ulceration, hepatic dysfunction, anorexia, diarrhea, alopecia, fever, somnolence, H/A, conjunctivitis, ataxia, peripheral neuropathy, cerebellar toxicity, possible hemorrhagic cystitis, lung damage Dose-limiting toxicity: cerebellar effects, pneumonitis
Etoposide (VP-16, VePesid) Class: plant alkaloid	Injection: 20 mg/mL (5mL)	Conventional dose: 240–500 mg/m^2 BMT dose: 450 mg/m^2 or 60 mg/kg (consult protocol)	SE: fevers, chills, rash, skin desquamation, tachycardia, myelosuppression, N/V, H/A, hepatotoxicity, peripheral neuropathy, somnolence, fatigue, anaphylaxis,

Ifosfamide
(Ifex)

Class: alkylating agent

Injection: 1, 3 g

Conventional dose: 5–12 g/m^2
BMT dose: 18 g/m^2
(consult protocol)

secondary acute myelogenous leukemia (AML), hematuria, mucositis
Granulocyte nadir about 7–14 d, platelet nadir 9–16 d
Dose-limiting toxicity: skin desquamation, mucositis

SE: hemorrhagic cystitis, N/V, dysuria, myelosuppression, (leukocyte nadir, 7–14 d), alopecia, CNS toxicity (somnolence, confusion, depressive psychosis, hallucination, dizziness, seizures), renal tubular acidosis, elevated LFT levels, phlebitis, fever, stomatitis, cardiotoxicity.
Dose-limiting toxicity: renal insufficiency

Melphalan
(Alkeran)

Class: alkylating agent

Injection: 50 mg
Tab: 2 mg

Conventional dose: 40 mg/m^2
BMT dose: 100–180 mg/m^2
(consult protocol)

SE: leukopenia, anemia, thrombocytopenia, agranulocytosis, N/V, hemolytic anemia, diarrhea, severe mucositis, rash, pruritus, secondary leukemia
Dose-limiting toxicity: mucositis

Drug	Supplied as	Dose and route	Special considerations
Mitomycin C (MTC) Class: plant antibiotic	Injection: 5, 20 mg	Conventional dose: 10 mg/m^2 BMT dose: 90 mg/m^2 (consult protocol)	SE: moderate N/V, mucositis, myelosuppression with nadir at 21–36 d, discolored fingernails, extremity tingling, interstitial pneumonitis or fibrosis, elevated creatinine level, hemolytic uremic syndrome, elevated LFT levels Dose-limiting toxicity: hepatic toxicity
Mitoxantrone hydrochloride (Novantrone) Class: plant antibiotic	Injection: 2 mg/mL (20, 25, 30 mg vials)	Conventional dose: 14 mg/m^2 BMT dose: 75 mg/m^2 (consult protocol)	SE: myelosuppression, N/V, CHF, hypotension, urticaria, rash, dyspnea, mucositis Dose-limiting toxicity: mucositis, CHF
Thiotepa (TESPA, TSPA) Class: alkylating agent	Injection: 15 mg	Conventional dose: 12–30 mg/m^2 BMT dose: 1135 mg/m^2 (consult protocol)	SE: leukopenia, anemia, thrombocytopenia, N/V, stomatitis, alopecia, H/A, dizziness, rash, hematuria Dose-limiting toxicity: mucositis

J. Electrolytes

Drug	Supplied as	Dose and route	Special considerations
Calcium chloride (27% calcium) Class: calcium replacement	Injection: 100 mg/mL (10%) (1.36 mEq calcium/mL) Each g of salt contains 13.6 mEq = 270 mg of calcium	<u>Maintenance/hypocalcemia:</u> <u>Infants & children:</u> 200–300 mg/kg/24 h PO as 2% solution divided q6 h <u>Adults:</u> 4–8 g/24 h PO as 2% solution divided q6 h <u>Cardiac arrest:</u> <u>Infants & children:</u> 20 mg/kg per dose (0.2 mL/kg per dose) IV q10 min <u>Adults:</u> 250–500 mg per dose (2.5–5 mL per dose) IV q10 min Do not exceed 1 mL/min with IV infusion.	May cause GI irritation, phlebitis; use IV with extreme caution; causes vasodilatation, hypotension, bradycardia, ventricular fibrillation (VF), arrhythmias, syncope, muscle weakness, lethargy, coma, mania, erythema, low magnesium, hypercalcemia, hypercalciuria Has acidifying effect; give only 2–3 d then change to another calcium salt; treat IV infiltrate with hyaluronidase
Calcium glubionate (Neo-Calglucon) (6% calcium) Class: calcium replacement	Syrup: 1.8 g/5mL Each 5 mL contains 5.6 mEq = 115 mg of calcium	<u>Maintenance for hypocalcemia:</u> <u>Infants & children:</u> 600–2000 mg/kg/24 h PO divided qid <u>Adults:</u> 6–18 g/24 h divided qid	Administer before meals for best absorption. SE: GI irritation, diarrhea, hypercalcemia, hypercalciuria, dizziness, H/A, constipation

Drug	Supplied as	Dose and route	Special considerations
Calcium gluconate (9.4% calcium) Class: calcium replacement	Tab: 500, 650, 1000 mg Injection: 100 mg/mL Each g of salt contains 4.5 mEq = 90 mg of calcium	Maintenance for hypocalcemia: Infants: IV: 200–500 mg/kg/24 h divided q6 h PO: 400–800 mg/kg/24 h divided q6 h Children: PO/IV: 200–500 mg/kg/24 h divided q6 h Adults: PO/IV: 5–15 g/24 h divided q6 h Cardiac arrest: Infants & children: 100 mg/kg per dose (1 mL/kg per dose) IV q10 min Adults: 500–800 mg per dose (5–8 mL per dose) IV q10 min	SE: vasodilatation, hypotension, bradycardia, cardiac arrest, VF, muscle weakness, lethargy, coma, mania, erythema, tissue necrosis, elevated amylase, decreased serum magnesium, hypercalcemia, hypercalciuria
Calcium lactate (13% calcium) Class: calcium replacement	Tab: 325, 650 mg Each 325 mg contains 2.1 mEq = 42.2 mg of calcium	Infants/children: 400–500 mg/kg/24 h PO divided q4–8 h Adults: 1.5–3 g PO q8 h Max dose: 9 g/24 h	SE: nausea, diarrhea, hypercalcemia, hypercalciuria, GI upset; take with meals
Magnesium gluconate Class: magnesium replacement	Tab: 500 mg	Children: 3–6 mg of elemental magnesium per kg per 24 h divided tid-qid Max dose: 400 mg/24 h	SE: diarrhea, hypotension, hypermagnesemia, respiratory depression Easy to crush and mix with water

Magnesium oxide

Class: magnesium replacement

Tab: 400, 420, 500 mg
Caps: 140 mg

Adults:
200–400 mg of elemental magnesium per 24 h divided tid-qid

Children:
3–6 mg of elemental magnesium per kg per 24 h divided tid-qid
Max dose: 400 mg/24 h

Adults:
200–400 mg elemental magnesium per 24 h divided tid-qid

SE: diarrhea, hypotension, hypermagnesemia, respiratory depression

Easy to crush and mix with water

Magnesium sulfate

Class: magnesium replacement

Oral solution: 50%
Injection: 100 mg/mL (0.8 mEq/mL)
125 mg/mL (1 mEq/mL)
250 mg/mL (4 mEq/mL)
500 mg/mL (2 mEq/mL)

Laxative:
Children: 0.25 g/kg per dose POq4–6 h
Adults: 10–30 g per dose PO q4–6 h
Hypomagnesemia or hypocalcemia:
IV/IM: 25–50 mg/kg per dose q4–6 h for 3–4 doses; repeat prn
PO: 100–200 mg/kg/24 h divided qid
Maintenance: 0.25–0.50 mEq/kg/24 h
OR 30–60 mg/kg/24 h
Max dose: 1 g/24 h

Rapid IV infusion may cause hypotension, respiratory depression, hypermagnesemia. Use with caution in renal insufficiency. Calcium gluconate (IV) should be available as antidote.

Drug	Supplied as	Dose and route	Special considerations
Phosphorus supplements			
K Phosphate (Neutra Phos-K)	Caps: phosphorus (P): 250 mg = 8 mmol potassium (K): 14.25 mEq Injection: P:94 mg = 3 mmol/mL K:4.4 mEq Powder: 75 g	Hypophosphatemia: 5–10 mg/kg per dose IV over 6 h Maintenance: Children: IV: 15–45 mg/kg/24 h PO: 30–90 mg/kg/24 h Adults: IV: 1.5–2 g/24 h PO: 3–4.5 g/24 h	SE: tetany, hyperphosphatemia, hyperkalemia, hypocalcemia; IV may cause hypotension, renal failure, or myocardial infarction; PO may cause N/V, abdominal pain, and diarrhea Reconstitution of 1 bottle of Neutra Phos or Neutra Phos K Powder in 1 gal of water provides concentration equivalent to reconstitution of 1 capsule in 75 mL water.
Sodium phosphate (Neutra Phos)	Solution: P:128 mg = 4.1 mmol/mL Na:4.9 mEq/mL Injection: P:94 mg = 3 mmol/mL Na:4 mEq/mL	Max infusion rate: 0.2 mmol/kg/h of phosphate; when potassium salt is used, rate may be limited by max potassium infusion rate	
Sodium and K phosphate	Caps: P:250 mg = 8 mmol K:7 mEq Na:7 mEq Powder: 67.5 g		
Potassium supplements (many brand names)	Potassium chloride: 40 mEq K = 3 g KCl Sustained-release caps: 8, 10 mEq Tab: 2.5, 4, 13.4 mEq Sustained-release tab: 8, 10, 20 mEq	Starting dose should be determined by considering maintenance, losses, and desired replacement. See Chapter 8. Children: 1–4 mEq/kg/24 h as required to maintain normal serum K	SE: hyperkalemia, N/V, abdominal discomfort, cardiac arrhythmias, hypotension, paresthesias, mental confusion, muscle weakness

Class: potassium replacement	Powder: 15, 20, 25 mEq Solution: 10% (6.7 mEq/5 mL) 15% (10 mEq/5 mL) 20% (13.3 mEq/5 mL) Injection: 2 mEq/mL <u>Potassium gluconate:</u> 40 mEq K = 9.4 g K gluconate Tab: 2, 5 mEq Elixir: 20 mEq/15 mL <u>Potassium acetate-bicarbonate-citrate:</u> 40 mEq K = 4.1 g Elixir: 500 mg of each salt per 5 mL (15 mEq/5 mL) <u>Potassium acetate:</u> Injection: K 2 mEq and acetate 2 mEq/mL (20 mL)	<u>Adults:</u> 10–15 mEq per dose tid-qid Max infusion rate: < 0.5–1 mEq/kg/h Max peripheral IV concentration: < 40 mEq/L
Sodium bicarbonate Class: bicarbonate replacement	Tab: 324 mg = 3.9 mEq Solution: 1 mEq/mL Injection: 324 mg = 3.9 mEq	<u>Cardiac arrest:</u> Assure adequate ventilation before administration: Infants: Use 1:1 dilution of 1 mEq/mL NaHCO₃ or 0.5 mEq/mL at a dose of 1 mEq/kg IVP; may repeat	Use of IV NaHCO₃ should be reserved for documented metabolic acidosis and for hyperkalemia-induced cardiac arrest. SE: Metabolic alkalosis, hypernatremia, hypokalemia, hypocalcemia, edema, tissue necrosis,

Drug	Supplied as	Dose and route	Special considerations
Sodium bicarbonate *(continued)*		with 0.5 mEq/kg in 10 min prn; infusion rate should not exceed 10 mEq/min Children and adults: initial IVP: 1 mEq/kg; may repeat with 0.5 mEq/kg in 10 min once as indicated _Metabolic acidosis:_ mEq bicarbonate needed = 0.4 times wt (kg) x base deficit (mEq/L); give one-half calculated dose, then reevaluate If acid-base status not available: Children and adults: 2-5 mEq/kg IV over 4–8 h _Urine alkalinization:_ (Oral) Children: 1–10 mEq (84–840 mg)/kg/d in divided doses; dose should be titrated to desired urinary pH _Adults:_ Initial: 48 mEq (4 g), then 12–24 mEq (1–2 g) q4 h; dose should be titrated to desired urinary pH; doses up to 16 g/d have been used	cerebral hemorrhage (especially with rapid injection), intracranial acidosis (especially with inadequate ventilation), gastric distension, flatulence

K. Immune regulators

Drug	Supplied as	Dose and route	Special considerations
Granulocyte colony-stimulating factor (filgrastim, Neupogen) Class: blood formation	Injection: 300 μg/mL (1, 1.6 mL)	<u>Children and adults:</u> 5–10 μg/kg/d (~ 150–300 μg/m-d) once daily until absolute neutrophil count (ANC) is approximately 7000–10,000/mL Dose escalations at 5 μg/kg/d may be required in some individuals when response is inadequate (IV or SQ). (Refer to individual protocols.)	SE: medullary bone pain, especially in lower back, iliac crests, sternum, splenomegaly, fever, rash, hypersensitivity
Granulocyte-macrophage colony-stimulating factor (Sargramostim, Leukine, Prokine) Class: blood formation	Injection: 250, 500μg	<u>Children:</u> (No dosing for children has been FDA approved.) 250 μg/m²/d IV over 2 h to begin 2–4 h after marrow infusion, or not less than 24 h after chemotherapy; if toxicity is noted, then cut dose in half <u>Adults:</u> 250 μg/m²/d IV over 2 h to begin 2–4 h after marrow infusion, or not less than 24 h after chemotherapy (refer to individual protocols)	SE: "first-dose" reaction with fever, hypotension, tachycardia, rigors, N/V, flushing, dyspnea; also may cause asthenia, H/A, bone pain, myalgia, rash, malaise, diarrhea, elevated LFT levels, pericardial effusion, fluid retention, stomatitis, polydipsia, GI hemorrhage

Drug	Supplied as	Dose and route	Special considerations
Cytomegalovirus immune globulin Class: immune regulator		CMV prophylaxis: 100–150 mg/kg/wk IV until d 100 Treatment of CMV disease: 100–150 mg/kg/d for 3–5 d; may repeat as indicated	SE: hypersensitivity reaction may occur (premedicate with subsequent doses); fever, rash, hives, chills, flushing
Intravenous immune globulin (IVIG; various brands) Class: immune regulator		Prophylaxis: (generalized/CMV): 250–500 mg/kg IV qwk until day 100 Treatment of CMV disease: 500 mg/kg/d IV for 5–7 d; may repeat as indicated Platelet alloimmunization: 500–2000 mg/kg/d IV for 3–5 d administered just before transfusion; may repeat as indicated	SE: hypersensitivity reaction may occur (pre-medicate with subsequent doses); fever, rash, hives, chills, flushing

L. Immunosuppressants

Drug	Supplied as	Dose and route	Special considerations
Antithymocyte globulin (ATG, ATGAM) Class: immunosuppressant	Injection: 50 mg/5mL	<u>Conditioning agent:</u> 10–30 mg/kg/d for 1–3 doses pretransplant (refer to individual protocol) <u>Treatment of steroid-resistant graft-versus-host disease (GVHD):</u> 10–20 mg/kg/d for 5–7 d; may repeat once at 7–14 d <u>Test dose:</u> must give 1:1000 intradermal test dose prior to first dose	Have SQ epinephrine at bedside for test dose. SE: allergic reaction, serum sickness (fever, chills, rash, arthralgias, myalgias), leukopenia, thrombocytopenia
Azathioprine (Imuran) Class: immunosuppressant	Injection: 5 mg/mL Tab: 50 mg	<u>Chronic GVHD:</u> 1–3 mg/kg/d PO	SE: bone marrow depression, N/V, anorexia, diarrhea, rash, fever, alopecia, hepatotoxicity, aphthous stomatitis, retinopathy, arthralgias
Cyclosporin A (Sandimmune, Neoral) Class: immunosuppressant	Caps: 25, 100 mg Solution: 100 mg/mL (50 mL) Injection: 50 mg/mL	<u>Children and adults:</u> IV: 1.5 mg/kg IV q12 h starting day -1; continue until conversion to PO Oral: Conversion to oral is 1:3 or 1:4. Reduce dose with renal	Dose adjustments based on biweekly levels (see center-specific protocol) SE: renal failure, neurologic toxicity (ataxia, seizures, cortical blindness, H/A), burning in hands and feet,

Drug	Supplied as	Dose and route	Special considerations
Cyclosporin A (*continued*)		impairment (adults).	hirsutism, gingival hyperplasia, hepatic dysfunction; hemolytic uremic syndrome, hypertrichosis, hypertension. lymphoproliferative disorder

Creatinine (mg/dL) / Cyclosporin A Reduction:

Creatinine (mg/dL)	Cyclosporin A Reduction
> 1.5	25%
> 1.75	75%
> 2.0	Hold until creatinine < 2.0 mg/dL, then resume at 20% to 25% of prior dose

Drug	Supplied as	Dose and route	Special considerations
FK-506 (tacrolimus) Class: immunosuppressant	Caps: 1, 5 mg Injection: 5 mg/mL (1 mL)	<u>Children and adults:</u> IV: 0.01–0.1 mg/kg/d by continuous IV infusion starting day −1; continue until conversion to PO Oral: Conversion to oral is 1:4. Adjust dose for renal and liver impairment based on therapeutic levels.	Dose adjustments based on biweekly levels; 10–60 ng/mL for 24 h CI; 0.5–2 ng/mL for oral dosing (see center-specific protocol) SE: nephrotoxicity with hyperkalemia, elevated creatinine level, hypertension, neurotoxicity (insomnia, tremors, H/A, photophobia, hyperesthesia, confusion, seizure, coma) dysarthria, N/V, abdominal pain, diabetes, lymphoproliferative disorder

Methotrexate sodium
(Mexate)

Class: antimetabolite

Tab: 2.5 mg
Injection: 25 mg/mL

GVHD prophylaxis:
Day 1: 15 mg/m2 IV
Days 3, 6, 11*: 10 mg/m2 IV
*Day 11 dose is eliminated in
some regimens.
CNS prophylaxis:
10–12 mg given intrathecally before
BMT and intermittently thereafter
(see individual protocol)

Doses may be held due to severe
mucositis or elevations in creatinine
or bilirubin levels. SE: Mucositis,
N/V, hepatotoxicity, rash

Methylprednisolone
(Depo-Medrol, Medrol,
Solu-Medrol)

Class:
immunosuppressant

Injection: As acetate (Depo-
Medrol): 40 mg/mL (1 mL)
As sodium succinate
(Solu-Medrol): 40, 125, 500 mg
Tab (Medrol): 4, 16 mg

GVHD prophylaxis:
0.5–1 mg/kg/d divided q6–12 h
(see individual protocol)
Treatment of GVHD:
2–10 mg/kg/d divided q6–12 h
Tapered by 10% qwk once
control is obtained

SE: increased appetite, muscle
weakness, osteoporosis, fractures,
Cushing's syndrome, pituitary-adrenal
axis suppression, growth suppression,
glucose intolerance, acne, edema,
hypertension, hypokalemia, alkalosis,
cataracts, glaucoma, peptic ulcer, N/V,
H/A, vertigo, seizures, psychosis,
pseudotumor cerebri, skin atrophy,
striae H2 blocker is indicated.

Drug	Supplied as	Dose and route	Special considerations
Muromonab-CD3 (Orthoclone OKT3) Class: immunosuppressant	Injection: 1 mg/mL	Refractory GVHD: Children: Dose recommendation not available Adults: 5 mg/d IV	Premedication with methylprednisolone 1 mg/kg IV prior to dose, and hydrocortisone 100 mg 30 min after infusion are highly recommended. SE: first-dose anaphylaxis, fever, chills, rash, severe pulmonary edema; CPR may be required
Prednisone (Deltasone, Orasone) Class: immunosuppressant	Tab: 1, 2.5, 5, 10, 20, 50 mg Solution: 5 mg/mL Syrup: 5 mg/mL	Treatment of GVHD: 2–10 mg/kg/d divided q6–12 h Tapered by 10% qwk once control is obtained	Patients are generally converted from IV methylprednisolone to PO prednisone once GVHD is under control and patient can tolerate PO. SE: see methylprednisolone. Ensure patient is on H_2 blocker.

M. Premedications

Drug	Supplied as	Dose and route	Special considerations
Acetaminophen (Tylenol, Tempra, Panodol, others)	Tab: 325, 500 mg Chewable: 80 mg Drops: 80 mg/0.8 mL Elixir: 160 mg/5 mL	Children: 10–15 mg/kg per dose q4 h OR 0–3 mo: 40 mg per dose 4–11 mo: 80 mg per dose	Contraindicated in patients with known G6PD deficiency; overdose (OD) can cause hepatotoxicity

Class: antipyretic/ analgesic	Syrup: 160 mg/5 mL	12–24 mo: 120 mg per dose 4–5 y: 240 mg per dose 6–8 y: 320 mg per dose 9–10 y: 400 mg per dose 11–12 y: 480 mg per dose Adults: 325–650 mg q4 h Max dose: 5 doses per 24 h	
Diphenhydramine hydrochloride (Benadryl) Class: antihistamine	Caps: 25, 50 mg Elixir: 2.5 mg/mL (5, 10, 120 mL) Injection: 50 mg/mL (1, 10 mL)	Children: 5 mg/kg/d divided q6–8 h PO/IV Max dose: 300 mg/d Adults: 25–50 mg q2–6 h PO/IV Max dose: 400 mg/d	SE: sedation, dizziness, hypotension, paradoxical excitement, N/V, dry mucous membranes, urinary retention, blurred vision, palpitations, insomnia, tremor
Hydrocortisone (Solu-Cortef) Class: anti-inflammatory glucocorticoid	Tab: 5 mg Injection: 100 mg	Children: 0.8–4 mg/kg per dose prior to blood products, antithymosite globulin (ATG), Ampho B (may be added to bag) IV Adults: 100–500 mg/kg per dose prior to blood products, ATG, Ampho B (may be added to bag) IV	SE: euphoria, insomnia, H/A, hypertension, edema, acne, cataracts, peptic ulcer, immunosuppression, hypokalemia, hyperglycemia, dermatitis, Cushing's syndrome, skin atrophy

Formulary **363**

N. Urinary tract medications

Drug	Supplied as	Dose and route	Special considerations
Allopurinol (Zyloprim) Class: genitourinary agents	Tab: 100, 300 mg Susp: 10, 20 mg/mL	Children and adults: 10 mg/kg/24 h divided tid-qid OR 300 mg/m²/24 h divided q6 h Max dose: 600 mg/24 h	Decrease dose with renal impairment. SE: rash, neuritis, GI disturbances, hepatotoxicity
Oxybutynin chloride (Ditropan) Class: urinary antispasmodic	Tab: 5 mg Syrup: 1 mg/mL (473 mL)	Children: 1–5 y: 0.2 mg/kg per dose 2–4 times per day > 5 y: 5 mg 2 times per d Max dose: 5 mg 3 times per d Adults: 5 mg 2–3 times per d Max dose: 5 mg 4 times per d	SE: Dry mouth, decreased sweating, urinary hesitancy, retention, hot flushes, fever, tachycardia, palpitations, blurred vision, drowsiness, weakness, dizziness, insomnia, N/V, constipation, rash
Phenazopyridine hydrochloride (Pyridium) Class: urinary analgesic	Tab: 100, 200 mg Caps: 50 mg	Children: 12 mg/kg/d in 3 divided doses PO hemolytic anemia, acute Adults: 200 mg tid PO	SE: methemoglobinemia, renal failure, H/A, skin pigmentation, vertigo, rash, hepatitis

Sodium 2-mercaptoethane sulfonate (mesna, Mesnex) Class: uroprotectant	Injection: 100 mg/mL (2, 4, 10 mL)	Children and adults: Ifosfamide: 20%–100% weight per weight dose at time of administration and 4 and 8 h after each dose (refer to individual protocol) Cyclophosphamide: 20% to 100% w/w of dose prior to administration and 3, 6, 9, and 12 h after each dose (refer to individual protocol)	SE: diarrhea, N/V, H/A, (w/w) of malaise, rash, bad taste, limb pain, hypotension

O. Miscellaneous medications

Drug	Supplied as	Dose and route	Special considerations
Albumin (human) (5%/25%) (normal serum albumin) Class: protein/volume replacement	Injection: 5% (5 g/dL) 25% (25 g/dL) Each contains 130–160 mEq of Na per L	Hypoproteinemia: 0.5–1 g/kg per dose IV over 2–4 h OR by continuous IV infusion (in TPN solution); repeat q1–2 d or as calculated to replace losses Hypovolemia: 0.5–1 g/kg per dose IV; repeat prn as rapidly as necessary Max dose: 6 g/kg/24 h	

Drug	Supplied as	Dose and route	Special considerations
Digoxin (Lanoxin) Class: digitalis glycoside	Tab: 0.125, 0.25 mg Pediatric elixir: 50 µg/mL (60 mL) Injection (pediatric): 0.1 mg/mL Injection (adult): 0.25 mg/mL	<table><tr><th>Age</th><th colspan="2">Total Digoxin dose (µg/kg)</th><th colspan="2">Daily maintenance dose (µg/kg)</th></tr><tr><th></th><th>PO</th><th>IV</th><th>PO</th><th>IV</th></tr><tr><td>1 mo–2 y</td><td>35–60</td><td>30–50</td><td>10–15</td><td>7.5–12</td></tr><tr><td>2–5 y</td><td>30–40</td><td>25–35</td><td>7.5–10</td><td>6–9</td></tr><tr><td>5–10 y</td><td>20–25</td><td>15–30</td><td>5–10</td><td>4–8</td></tr><tr><td>>10 y</td><td>10–15</td><td>8–12</td><td>2.5–5</td><td>2–3</td></tr></table> Loading doses are administered in divided doses with approximately 50% of total dose given as the first dose; additional fractions of the loading dose (generally 25% fractions) are administered at 4–8-h intervals IV or 6–8-h intervals PO, until a therapeutic response is attained, toxic effects occur, or the total digitalizing dose has been administered. Adults: Total Digoxin dose: 0.75–1.5 mg PO 0.5–1 mg IV Daily maintenance dose: 0.125–0.5 mg PO 0.1–0.4 mg IV	Therapeutic concentration: 0.8–2.0 µg/L Decrease dose for renal insufficiency. SE: anorexia, N/V, sinus bradycardia, AV block, sinoatrial block, atrial or nodal arrhythmias, bigeminy, trigeminy, atrial tachycardia, H/A, fatigue, lethargy, neuralgia, vertigo, disorientation, hyperkalemia with acute toxicity, feeding intolerance, blurred vision, halos, diplopia, photophobia, flashing lights

Drug	Formulation	Dose	Notes / SE
Dopamine hydrochloride (Inotropin) Class: sympathomimetic	Injection: 40–80, 160 mg/mL Prediluted in D5W: 800, 1600 μg/mL	Low dose: (renal dose) 2–5 μg/kg/min IV Intermediate dose: 5–15 μg/kg/min IV High dose: 20 μg/kg/min IV (decreases renal perfusion) Max recommended dose: 20–50μg/kg/min IV	Correct hypovolemic states. SE: Tachyarrhythmias, ectopic beats, hypertension, vasoconstriction, vomiting
Folic acid (Folvite) Class: blood formation	Tab: 1 mg Injection: 1 mg/mL Oral solution: 1 mg/mL	Children: 0.5–1.0 mg/24 h qd Adults: 1–3 mg/24 h divided qd-tid	Normal levels: serum > 4 ng/mL; whole blood > 50 ng/mL SE: allergic reaction with pruritus
Leucovorin calcium (Folinic acid) Class: blood formation	Tab: 5 mg Injection: 50 mg	Children and adults: 10–15 mg/m² IV on days of methotrexate dosing (refer to individual protocol)	SE: Rash, pruritus, erythema, urticaria, wheezing, thrombocytosis
Medroxyprogesterone acetate (Provera, Depo-Provera) Class: progestin	Tab: 10 mg (Provera) Injection: 100 mg/mL (5 mL) (Depo-Provera)	Adolescents and adults: (BMT setting) Oral: 10 mg/d PO; may increase by 10 mg/d increments for breakthrough bleeding prn; continue until platelet recovery	Assure adequate platelet count before administering IM. SE: Weight gain, mood swings, breakthrough bleeding, cholestatic jaundice, melasma, depression, urticaria, acne, thromboembolic disorders, dizziness,

Drug	Supplied as	Dose and route	Special considerations
Omeprazole (Prilosec) Class: proton pump inhibitor	Caps: 20 mg	Injection: (IM): 100 mg IM prior to BMT offers 3 mo of protection. Adults: 20 mg PO qd	nervousness SE: H/A, diarrhea, N/V, abdominal pain, dizziness, rash, constipation, cough, asthenia, back pain
Ranitidine hydrochloride (Zantac) Class: histamine antagonist	Tab: 150 mg Oral solution: 15 mg/mL Injection: 25 mg/mL	Children: Oral: 2–3 mg/kg per dose q12 h IV: 1 mg/kg per dose q8 h Adults: Oral: 150 mg per dose q12 h IV: 50 mg per dose q8 h Dosing interval with renal failure: (creatinine clearance < 50 mL/min) Oral: administer q24 h IV: administer q18–24 h	SE: H/A, dizziness, sedation, malaise, mental confusion, constipation, N/V, rash, hepatitis, gynecomastia, bradycardia, tachycardia, arthralgias

II. Special drug monitoring

A. Cyclosporin A (Sandimmune, Neoral)
1. Pharmacokinetics and metabolism are highly variable. Neoral is a microemulsion formula of cyclosporin A developed to improve absorption and bioavailability in order to reduce variability.
2. Cyclosporin A is extensively metabolized in the liver and intestine by the cytochrome P-450 mechanism. Numerous interactions with other drugs undergo the same route of metabolism.
3. The most common adverse effect is nephrotoxicity, which is dose and concentration dependent.
4. Trough levels of cyclosporin A should be measured frequently (i.e., twice weekly).
5. A variety of methods exists for measurement of cyclosporin A levels: high-performance liquid chromatography (HPLC), radioimmunoassay (RIA), and fluorescent polarization immunoassay (FPIA). Each assay provides a different target concentration.
6. The polyclonal FPIA correlates with renal insufficiency. See p. 345 for dosing in renal insufficiency.
7. Each transplant center will determine a target concentration range based upon the type of assay used. If the trough dose is elevated, the dose of cyclosporin A should be decreased by 20%–25%.
8. Low trough levels may be a risk for the development of GVHD. Dose should be increased if the trough level is lower than the target concentration.

B. FK-506/Tacrolimus (Prograf)
1. FK-506 is a macrolide antibiotic with immuno-suppressant efficiency comparable to cyclosporin A.
2. Pharmacokinetics and metabolism are highly variable. Metabolism is via the cytochrome P-450 mechanism.

3. Two assays are available for measurement of drug levels: enzyme-linked immunoabsorbent assay (ELISA) and microparticle enzyme immunoassay (MEIA).
4. As with cyclosporin A, numerous drug interactions exist.
5. Trough levels should be monitored frequently.
6. Hepatic dysfunction will prolong drug half-life and slow clearance.

C. Aminoglycoside antibiotics
1. Specific immunoassays are available to measure drug levels.
2. Trough levels must be monitored at least every 48 hours.
3. Clearance of the drug is decreased in patients with impaired renal function.
4. The risk of ototoxicity and nephrotoxicity increases if the trough concentration > 2 mg/L (5 mg/L with amikacin).
5. Dehydration will increase the risk of toxicity.
6. The risk of toxicity increases with longer duration of treatment.

D. Vancomycin
1. Peak and trough concentrations should be monitored regularly. Peak concentration samples are collected 30 to 60 minutes after the end of the infusion. The exact time of the infusion and specimen collection should be noted.
2. Trough concentrations should not exceed 5 to 10 mg/L.
3. The relationship of peak/trough levels to toxicity is not clear.

III. Antiemetic management

A. There are three categories of emesis related to
   chemotherapy: anticipatory nausea/vomiting,
   acute chemotherapy-induced emesis, and delayed
   nausea/vomiting.[6]

B. In the BMT setting, anticipatory nausea and
   vomiting may occur in patients previously treated with
   chemotherapy. Medications having amnesic effect may
   be effective in combination with antiemetic drugs.

C. Acute chemotherapy-induced emesis is multifactorial.
   Patient-related factors include advancing age, poor
   general health, and metabolic disturbances.[6] The variable
   related to chemotherapy is the emetic potential. Each
   chemotherapeutic agent exhibits some potential for
   inducing emesis, ranging from very low to very high
   potential. Table 7.3 summarizes the emetic potential
   of many chemotherapeutic agents in current use.

Table 7.3 Emetic Potential of Chemotherapeutic Agents

Emetic potential	Chemotherapeutic agent
VERY HIGH (> 90%)	Cisplatin
	Cyclophosphamide (high dose)
	Cytarabine
	Dacarbazine
	Mechlorethamine hydrochloride
	Streptozocin
HIGH (60%–90%)	Carboplatin
	Carmustine
	Cyclophosphamide (standard dose)
	Dactinomycin
	Daunorubicin
	Doxorubicin
	Lomustine
MODERATE (30%–60%)	Etoposide
	5-Fluorouracil
	Idarubicin hydrochloride
	Ifosfamide
	Mitomycin
	Mitoxantrone
	Procarbazine hydrochloride
	Topotecan hydrochloride
LOW (0%–30%)	Adriamycin
	Bleomycin
	Busulfan
	Cytarabine
	Docetaxel
	Hydroxyurea
	Melphalan
	Methotrexate
	6-Mercaptopurine
	Taxol
	Thioguanine
	Thiotepa
	Vinblastine sulfate
	Vincristine sulfate

D. Delayed emesis occurs more than 24 hours after chemotherapy administration and may significantly affect the patient's level of nutrition and hydration. In cases of delayed emesis, antiemetic agents should be used as long as necessary. The addition of drugs such as dexamethasone, diphenhydramine, lorazepam, and metoclopramide may be useful in controlling delayed emesis and promoting oral intake.

E. Numerous antiemetic medications are available, with a wide range of cost. The use of serotonin antagonists, such as granisetron and ondansetron, should be reserved for use with chemotherapeutic agents of moderate to very high emetic potential. Often, combinations of standard antiemetic medications can provide excellent relief at lower cost.

IV. Pain and sedation

A. Proper assessment of pain is essential to achieving effective intervention. Assessment of pain should address onset, duration, location, radiation, quality, intensity, pattern, aggravating factors, and alleviating factors. Intensity of pain may be described by use of a numeric scale in adolescents and adults. In children, the use of a visual scale may be helpful.

B. In BMT pain is generally the result of the underlying disease. The toxicities inherent in the transplant process limit the choice of analgesic agents, since some agents can compound these toxicities.

C. Nonsteroidal anti-inflammatory drugs (NSAIDs) are an excellent choice for mild to moderate pain in the general public. These agents should, however, be used very cautiously in the BMT patient because of their antiplatelet effect and their potential for nephrotoxicity.

D. Care should also be taken when using acetaminophen in the BMT patient. This agent has an antipyretic effect, which may delay recognition of infection. Additionally, there is a potential for hepatotoxicity with aceta-minophen.

E. Propoxyphene, 65 mg, or codeine is an excellent choice for mild to moderate analgesia in the BMT patient. These agents demonstrate no significant hepatic or renal toxicity.

F. Opioids, particularly morphine or fentanyl, are the agents of choice for management of severe pain in the BMT patient. Opioids should be used in adequate doses on a regular (not prn) schedule. Sustained-release morphine or transdermal fentanyl can be used with "on demand" immediate-release morphine or oxycodone-hydrochloride for use with breakthrough pain. Meperidine is not useful in this setting, because of its short duration of action and poor effect when taken orally.

G. Adjuvant medications may be utilized for treatment of specific types of pain. Tricyclic antidepressants are useful in management of "burning" neuropathy. Certain anticonvulsants, such as carbamazepine, clonazepam, and valproic acid, are useful in management of lancinating or "stabbing" neuropathy.

H. Herpes zoster is a common complication in the post-transplant setting. Management of herpetic pain can utilize corticosteroids, topical capsaicin, antidepressants, or carbamazepine.

I. Nonpharmacologic methods of pain management should always be used in combination with medication. These methods include counterirritant cutaneous stimulation, transcutaneous electrical nerve stimulation [TENS], massage, distraction, guided imagery, biofeedback, hypnosis, and relaxation therapy.

J. Sedation is often required in BMT for use with painful

procedures (bone marrow biopsy, central line placement, etc.). In these situations sedative agents with an amnesic effect are desirable. Lorazepam and midazolam hydrochloride are two benzodiazepine medications with excellent sedative and amnesic effect. These drugs do not cause severe respiratory or cardiovascular depression in most patients. Additionally, midazolam affords fast recovery since it is not metabolized to an active metabolite.

V. Antimicrobial selection

A. Fever in an immunocompromised patient may be the first indication of bacterial, fungal, or viral infection.

B. Unfortunately, a documented source of infection is found in less than two-thirds of cases of neutropenic fever.

C. When fever develops in the BMT patient, it is important to rule out reaction to blood products or medications. A diagnostic work-up should be initiated, including the following:
   1. Throat culture
   2. Sputum culture (if possible)
   3. Peripheral blood culture (2)
   4. Central line culture
   5. Urine culture
   6. Wound culture (if applicable)
   7. Chest x-ray

D. Most infections are related to gram-positive or gram-negative bacteria, especially *P. aeruginosa*, *Escherichia coli*, *Klebsiella pneumoniae*, *S. aureus*, or *Staphylococcus epidermidis*.

E. After cultures are obtained, empiric antibiotic therapy should be initiated. To aid in the choice of antibiotics, the primary pathogens of each transplant center should be known.

F. Monotherapy is not advisable for empiric treatment in

a neutropenic patient. A combination of two or three broad-spectrum agents will provide good coverage of common pathogens. These agents should be administered at the maximum dose individualized for the patient.

G. It is especially important to provide coverage for gram-negative organisms, since early morbidity and mortality is seen with gram-negative infection.[7]

H. There are many options of empiric antibiotic combinations, such as semisynthetic penicillin plus aminoglycoside, third-generation cephalosporin plus aminoglycoside, and semisynthetic penicillin plus third-generation cephalosporin.

I. If there is no response to antibiotic therapy and no documented bacterial infection, an antifungal agent should be added to the combination. As the duration of neutropenia increases, the risk of fungal infection also increases.

J. Most fungal infections are *Candida* species, but other species may be seen in the BMT setting, especially *Aspergillus* in patients with GVHD on steroids.

K. Empiric therapy options for fungal infection include the following:
   1. Amphotericin B, 0.5–1.0 mg/kg/d
   2. Fluconazole, 400 mg on day 1 and 200 mg for 4 weeks for systemic *Candida*
   3. Fluconazole, 200 mg on day 1 and 100 mg for 2 weeks for esophageal *Candida*

L. In the BMT setting, HSV, cytomegalovirus (CMV), and VZV can be seen as primary infection or as a reactivation of a prior infection.

M. The goal of treatment in the case of viral infection is to prevent dissemination of the virus.

N. HSV can be treated with acyclovir or famciclovir. Topical acyclovir should not be used as the only agent in the BMT patient.

O. CMV may cause retinitis, hepatitis, pneumonia, or suppression of the bone marrow. It can be treated with ganciclovir or forcarnet sodium in combination with IVIG.

P. VZV is generally treated with acyclovir. Vidarabine may also be used but must be initiated within 72 hours of the onset of symptoms and has severe side effects.

VI. Drugs in renal failure

A. If certain essential drugs cannot be discontinued in the case of renal failure, doses must be adjusted to avoid additional nephrotoxicity, as well as toxic drug levels. Dose adjustments can be made by decreasing the dose or by lengthening the interval between doses.

B. Cyclosporine doses should be decreased in the case of renal insufficiency. Dose reduction is based on serum creatinine levels, as follows:
   1. Serum creatinine, 2.2: 50% dose reduction
   2. Serum creatinine, 3.0: 75% dose reduction
   3. Serum creatinine, 4.0: discontinue temporarily

C. In the event of renal failure, the dose interval of amphotericin B should be increased to 1 to 3 times weekly rather than daily dosing.

References

1. *Physicians' Desk Reference*. Montvale, NJ: Medical Economics Co Inc; 1996.

2. Children's Hospital of Boston. *Hospital Formulary*. Hudson, Ohio: Lexi-Comp Inc; 1996.

3. University of Arizona Medical Center. *Drug Formulary*. Hudson, Ohio: Lexi-Comp Inc; 1996.

4. Johnson K, ed. *The Harriet Lane Handbook*. 13th ed. St Louis: Mosby; 1993.

5. Sanford JP, Gilbert DN, Gerberding JL, Sande MA, et al., eds. *The Sanford Guide to Antimicrobial Therapy*. 24th ed. Dallas: Antimicrobial Therapy Inc, 1996.

6. Clayton BD, Frye CB. Nausea and vomiting. In: Herfinadal ET, Gourley DR, eds. *Textbook of Therapeutics: Drugs and Disease Management*. 6th ed. Baltimore: Williams and Wilkins; 1996.

7. McIntyre WJ, Parr MD. Infections in the immunosuppressed patient. In: Herfindal ET, Gourley DR, eds. *Textbook of Therapeutics: Drug and Disease Management*. 6th ed. Baltimore: Williams and Wilkins; 1966.

Bibliography

Beam TR. Principles of anti-infective chemotherapy. In: Smith CM, and Reynard AM, eds. *Essentials of Pharmacology*. Philadelphia: WB Saunders; 1995.

Fischer DS, Knobf MT, Durivage HJ. *The Cancer Chemotherapy Handbook*. St Louis: Mosby; 1993.

Gambertoglio JG. Drug use in renal disease. In: Knoben JE, Anderson PO, eds. *Handbook of Clinical Drug Data*. Hamilton, Ill: Drug Intelligence Publications; 1993.

Italian Group for Antiemetic Research. Dexamethasone, granisetron, or both for the prevention of nausea and vomiting during chemotherapy for cancer. *N Engl J Med*. 1995;332(1):1–5.

Melocco T, Kerr S, McKenzie C. Drug toxicity and interactions posttransplant. In: Atkinson K, ed. *Clinical Bone Marrow Transplantation: A Reference Textbook*. Cambridge, United Kingdom: Cambridge University Press; 1995.

Reisner-Keller LA. Pain management. In: Herfindal ET, Gourley DR, eds. *Textbook of Therapeutics: Drug and Disease Management*. 6th ed. Baltimore: Williams and Wilkins; 1996.

Sanford JP, Gilbert DN, Sande MA. *Guide to Antimicrobial Therapy*. Dallas: Antimicrobial Therapy Inc; 1995.

Smith CM. Sensory pharmacology. In: Smith CM, Reynard AM, eds. *Essentials of Pharmacology*. Philadelphia: WB Saunders; 1995.

Tett S. Therapeutic drug monitoring in bone marrow transplant patients. In: Atkinson K, ed. *Clinical Bone Marrow Transplantation: A Reference Textbook*. Cambridge, United Kingdom: Cambridge University Press; 1994.

Therapeutic Data

Management of patients undergoing stem cell and bone marrow transplantation (BMT) requires complex medical interventions. This chapter outlines important therapeutic data necessary for the care of such patients. This includes transfusion therapy, nutritional support, ideal and adjusted body weight calculations, nutritional requirements, and fluid balance calculations. Finally, information crucial to caring for pediatric patients, such as growth charts, surface area calculations, Tanner staging, and normal blood values in children, is also provided.

I. Transfusion therapy

A. Table 8.1 outlines marrow donor-recipient red blood cell incompatibility.

Table 8.1 Marrow Donor-Recipient Red Blood Cell Incompatibility

Recipient Type	Donor Type	Transplant incompatibility	Transfuse: red blood cells	Plasma
A	O	Minor	O	A,AB
A	B	Major	O	AB
A	AB	Major	A,O	A,AB
B	O	Minor	O	B,AB
B	A	Major	O	B,AB
B	AB	Major	B,O	B,AB
O	A	Major	O	A,AB
O	B	Major	O	AB
O	AB	Major	O	AB
AB	O	Minor	O	AB
AB	A	Minor	A,O	AB
AB	B	Minor	B,O	AB

1. The ABO and Rh blood types of both the patient and the bone marrow donor are important considerations in red cell transfusion of the marrow transplant recipient.
2. The genes for red cell antigens are not located on the same chromosomes as those controlling the human leukocyte antigen (HLA) type.
3. Patients who are undergoing major ABO incompatibility are at risk of acute hemolytic transfusion reactions due to isoagglutinins produced by the donor lymphocytes in the transplanted marrow.
4. These donor-type isoagglutins may cause hemolysis of recipient red blood cells, including transfused cells.
5. Rarely, the donor and the recipient may be incompatible for other red cell antigens.
6. For transfusion of recipients of ABO-incompatible marrow, the transfusion support guidelines must be followed as soon as the transplant conditioning regimen is started (See B. transfusion support).

B. Transfusion support
1. Transfusion support is required during the period of pancytopenia post transplant for a period of four to 12 weeks.
2. Pretransplant: Optimal product management pretransplant is to use leukocyte-poor red cells and platelets from unrelated donors.
3. Donations from family member: should be avoided to minimize the risk of allosensitization to donor specific antigens, which could lead to marrow rejection.
4. Post-transplant: Blood products should be leukocyte depleted (filtered) and irradiated.
5. Irradiation, gamma type (15 to 25 Gy), is used to inactivate viable T cells in the blood product to prevent transfusion-induced graft-versus-host disease (GVHD). When immunocompetent

allogeneic lymphocytes are transfused into a severely immunocompromised host, there is a likelihood of developing post-transfusion GVHD.

6. Leukocyte depletion is performed to
   a) Reduce the potential of HLA alloimmunization, therefore resulting in less platelet refractoriness.
   b) Reduce the transmission of cytomegalovirus (CMV) and nonhemolytic febrile reactions.

II. Blood and blood products

A. Red blood cell transfusions

1. Indications
   a) Cytomegalovirus (CMV)-negative blood products: CMV-negative red cells are only given to CMV-negative recipients, regardless of the CMV status of the donor. Seropositive patients should receive CMV untested red cells. Red cell transfusions should be leukocyte depleted (filtered) and irradiated.
   b) Patients usually need red cell support for six to 12 weeks post-transplant. This can be prolonged if delayed engraftment, hemolysis, or bleeding develops.

2. Administration
   a) If there is no history of a nonhemolytic febrile reaction, no premedication is required.
   b) If there is a history of a nonhemolytic febrile reaction, premedicate with prophylactic diphenhydramine, 25 to 50 mg IV, and acetaminophen, 650 mg PO.
   c) Do not administer any medications or IV fluids without 0.9% normal saline solution, since hemolysis of the cells will occur.
   d) Rate: A unit of packed red cells can be administered as rapidly as the patient is able to tolerate the fluid volume.

     e) Red cells should be leukocyte depleted to prevent the potential of HLA alloimmunization and the transmission of CMV.

B. Platelet transfusions
  1. Indications
    a) CMV-negative products: CMV-seronegative recipients require CMV-negative platelets.
    b) Platelet concentrations are needed to maintain a platelet count greater than 10,000 to 15,000 µL. Patients undergoing procedures such as a central line insertion, gut biopsy, or lumbar puncture should have a platelet concentration of 50,000 to 100,000/L at the time of the procedure. Post-transfusion platelet counts can be obtained as early as 10 minutes after the completion of the platelet transfusion.
  2. Types of platelet products
    a) Pooled random donor platelets are equivalent to platelets pooled from 8 to 10 U of whole blood. These products are adequate and less expensive.
    b) Single-donor platelets have the advantage of reducing alloimmunization and transmission of infection. Cost considerations are a factor when deciding whether to use this type of product.
    c) HLA-matched products are single-donor apheresis products.
  3. Platelet refractoriness
    a) Platelet alloantibodies, particularly anti-HLA antibodies, are the most common cause of platelet refractoriness.
    b) Detection of alloantibodies: The median time from first transfusion to time of detection of alloantibody is four weeks. This can occur earlier if the recipient has been immunized previously by blood transfusions or pregnancy.

c) Anti-HLA antibodies can disappear after the discontinuation of transfusion or after switching to HLA-matched platelet transfusions.

d) Repeat HLA antibody testing is important in patients receiving prolonged platelet support.

e) Prevention of platelet refractoriness consists of leukocyte depletion and administration of single-donor platelet products. This reduces the number of HLAs the patient is exposed to.

4. Nonimmune platelet consumption can occur in disseminated intravascular coagulation, amphotericin B administration, splenomegaly, bleeding, fever, hemolysis, and antibiotic administration.

5. Administration

a) Patients should not receive routine premedications prior to the transfusion of platelets.

b) If there is no history of a nonhemolytic febrile reaction, routine premedication is not required.

c) If there is a history of a hemolytic febrile reaction, routine premedication is required.

d) Platelet products should be agitated gently at room temperature until they have been administered.

C. Granulocyte transfusions

1. Indications: Granulocyte transfusion use in the transplant patient remains controversial. Granulocyte transfusions may benefit the severely neutropenic patient with a documented life-threatening infection unresponsive to antibiotics.

2. Administration

a) Concurrent administration with any medications or IV fluids except 0.9% normal saline solution is contraindicated, since hemolysis can occur.

b) Amphotericin B should not be administered within four hours of a granulocyte transfusion.

c) The primary precaution of granulocyte transfusions is noncardiogenic pulmonary edema due to sequestration of granulocytes in the lung and transmission of infection, particularly CMV.

III. Transfusion reactions (Table 8.2)

Table 8.2 Transfusion Reactions

Type of reaction	Cause	Manifestations	Management
Acute immune hemolysis	Red cell incompatibility	Back pain, dyspnea, fever, hemoglobinemia, renal failure, anxiety, nausea, vomiting, hypertension	Isotonic fluids, forced diuresis, other measures for renal failure and dyspnea
Delayed immune hemolysis	Red cell incompatibility	Usually only hyperbilirubinemia but may progress to renal failure, etc., as above	Supportive care
Nonhemolytic febrile reaction	Leukocyte or platelet antibodies	Fever, chills	IV meperidine for rigors, PO acetaminophen if febrile
Leukoagglutinin reaction	Leukocyte antibodies	Noncardiac pulmonary edema, fever, chills	IV meperidine for chills, O_2 etc., as for adult respiratory disease syndrome
Port-transfusion purpura	Antibodies to platelet antigen	Thrombocytopenia, bruises, hemorrhage	P1-negative platelets
Urticaria	Antibodies to proteins in plasma	Hives	IV diphenhydramine
Anaphylaxis	Antibodies to IgA	Anaphylaxis	Epinephrine, O_2, etc., as usual for anaphylaxis
Septic shock	Bacterial contamination	Fever, chills, hypotension	Isotonic fluids, IV meperidine for chills, antibiotics, pressors, if needed
Volume overload	Rapid infusion or infusion of large volumes of cells	Cardiac pulmonary edema	IV furosemide

A. A rise in temperature of $1°$ to $2°F$ is considered a transfusion reaction.

B. Not all transfusion reactions are accompanied by a fever, and not all fevers during a transfusion are considered transfusion reactions.

C. In the neutropenic transplant patient, sepsis must always be considered in addition to a transfusion reaction.

D. If any transfusion reaction occurs, stop the transfusion. If the patient is febrile and neutropenic, initiate a fever work-up and management.

IV. Nutrition support

A. Systematic nutritional assessment identifies nutrition-related problems in the transplant patient.

B. Usual weight
   1. Prediagnosis weight: In patients who have been ill for several years, prediagnosis weight is not the best indicator.
   2. Obese patients: Usual weight may be determined by what weight the person equilibrates when not dieting or by the ideal body weight.

C. Weight change
   1. Evaluate rate and cause of weight loss or gain since the onset of the disease presentation, and consider factors that could influence weight change (e.g., exercise, change in activity, complications of treatment).
   2. Interpretation of weight loss from usual body weight
      a) > 5% in 6 months represents a moderate weight loss.
      b) > 10% in 6 months represents a significant loss.

D. Diet
1. Eating problems: Assess any active problems interfering with food intake.
2. Food allergies or therapeutic diets
3. Food preferences: Elicit general meal preferences, including likes and dislikes and any faith-based dietary practices.
4. Lactose intolerance: Identify any preexisting symptoms with ingestion of lactose-containing foods and beverages and whether lactose therapy has been beneficial in the past.
5. Children: Identify the stage of eating development (pureed food versus table food, cup versus bottle, and infant formulas including concentrations).

E. Review past medical history, such as gastrointestinal diseases, hepatitis, surgeries, and family history of chronic diseases (i.e., diabetes, heart disease, hyperlipidemia, hypertension).

F. Height
1. Bone marrow transplant has been associated with poor growth.
2. In children who are prepubertal at the time of transplantation, decreased growth velocity is first detected at age 8 to 9 years. If a decrease in serial growth of more than two channels or growth velocity below the 10th percentile is observed post-transplant, any contributory effects of inadequate nutrition deserve evaluation.

G. Ideal weight
   1. Ideal body weight (IBW) is estimated and its
      determination is more of an art than an exact science.
   2. Appropriate age- and sex-based guidelines have
      been developed and are shown in Table 8.3. These
      guidelines are interpreted as follows:
      a) Less than 90% IBW is mild depletion.
      b) Less than 80% IBW is moderate depletion.
      c) Less than 70% IBW is severe depletion.
   3. Multiple myeloma patients may lose stature due to
      vertebral compression; however, their body mass may
      not have been significantly altered. Their previous
      height should be used to estimate IBW. If current
      weight falls between the ideal ranges of past and
      present heights, this weight may be used as IBW.
   4. In patients who are currently taking steroid therapy,
      weight may be elevated due to fluid retention or fat
      deposition without any lean tissue weight gain. It is
      recommended that IBW not be adjusted, but instead,
      weight should be based on usual weight prior to
      steroid therapy.

   5. Interpretation of obesity
      a) Adjusted IBW reflects the increased lean tissue
         associated with obesity and is used to determine
         dosages for the drugs and the calculation of a
         patient's energy and protein requirements.

IBW = adjusted IBW + (actual IBW - IBW) (0.25)

      b) Weight above 125% IBW: Consideration of
         exercise, weight history, upper arm anthropometry,
         and physical appearance may help to determine
         whether IBW should be adjusted.

Table 8.3 Ideal Body Weight Charts*

Height (cm)	Weight (kg)	Height (cm)	Weight (kg)	Height (cm)	Weight (kg)
Males					
145	51.9	159	59.9	173	68.7
146	52.4	160	60.5	174	69.4
147	52.9	161	61.1	175	70.1
148	53.6	162	61.7	176	70.8
149	54.0	163	62.3	177	71.6
150	54.5	164	62.9	178	72.4
151	55.0	165	63.5	179	73.3
152	55.8	166	64.0	180	74.2
153	56.1	167	64.6	181	75.0
154	56.6	168	65.2	182	75.6
155	57.2	169	65.9	183	76.5
156	57.9	170	66.6	184	77.3
157	58.6	171	67.3	185	78.1
158	59.3	172	68.0	186	78.9
Females					
140	44.9	150	50.4	160	56.2
141	45.4	151	51.0	161	56.9
142	45.9	152	51.5	162	57.6
143	46.4	153	52.0	163	58.3
144	47.0	154	52.5	164	58.9
145	47.5	155	53.1	165	59.5
146	48.0	156	53.7	166	60.1
147	48.6	157	54.3	167	60.7
148	49.2	158	54.9	168	61.4
149	49.8	159	55.5	169	62.1

*Ideal body weight for height. This table corrects the 1960 Metropolitan Standards to nude weight without shoe heel. (Adapted from Jelliffe DB: The Assessment of the Nutritional Status of the Community. Geneva, WHO 1986). Reprinted with permission from Fisher DS, Knobf TS, Durivage HJ (1993). *The Cancer Chemotherapy Handbook.* 4ᵗʰ ed.

6. Adolescents (females > 12 years or > 137 cm; males > 14 years)
    a) The postpubertal period is defined in males as in or past growth spurt and in females as after the onset of menarche.
    b) The postpubertal IBW is estimated between the 25th and 75th percentiles of weight for height by age and sex for 12- to 17-year olds as published by U.S. Vital Health Statistics.
7. Children and infants
    a) Prepubertal IBW is determined at the 50th percentile weight for height. In children less than 2 years old, IBW is determined by the weight for length on the age- and sex-appropriate National Center for Health Statistics growth grids (see Figures 8.1 and 8.3).
    b) Children with weight for height between the 35th and 75th percentiles may be considered at IBW if there is no known weight loss or inappropriate gain (e.g., due to steroids) and they are described by family as always being lean or husky.
    c) Interpretation of weight for height or weight for length
        (1) Below 5th percentile is severe depletion.
        (2) 5th to 10th percentile is moderate depletion.

H. Body surface area
    1. Body surface area is used in the calculation of drug dosages and fluid needs for patients whose weight exceeds 40 kg and is calculated from the following equation:

Body surface area (m²) = actual weight (Kg) X height (cm)/60

    2. This data will determine an adjusted IBW that is more appropriate in the calculation of body surface area for obese patients.

I. Nutrient requirements
   1. Energy requirements
      a) Indirect calorimetry provides the most accurate estimate of energy needs, but is often unavailable. Futhermore, obtaining reliable measurements in marrow graft recipients may be difficult. Equation-derived estimations are used in lieu of direct measurements. In adults and children greater than 45 kg, Harris Benedict energy expenditure equation is used to estimate basal energy needs:

Male: 66 + (13.7 X ABW) + (5 X Ht) - (6.8 X age)
Female: 665 + (9.6 X ABW) + (1.7 X Ht) - (4.7 X age)

      Where ABW is actual body weight in kilograms, Ht is height calculated in centimeters, and age is calculated in years.

      b) Energy requirements need to be adjusted downward for afebrile patients with hematologic evidence of engraftment, without metabolic complications such as GVHD or disseminated infection, and on bed rest.
      c) Energy requirements can be caluated at 1.3 X basal needs for adults and 1.4 X basal needs for children. These energy estimations provide approximately 1.1 X basal needs as nonprotein calories for weight gain until the patient is medically stable.
      d) Factors that require an increase in energy requirements: weight loss despite adequate nutritional support; disease process suggestive of increased metabolic needs like acute or chronic GVHD, disseminated infection, or pulmonary insufficiency; or patients in whom nutritional repletion is a realistic goal

2. Protein requirements
   a) Protein requirements for transplant patients are estimated to be twice the normal recommended dietary allowance.
   b) This requirement provides substrate for tissue repair after conditioning therapy and minimizes the breakdown of lean body mass.
   c) Protein requirements are based on IBW in obese individuals, on adjusted IBW.
3. Energy needs with stress
   a) Factors that influence energy needs: In the early postgrafting period, energy needs reflect increased requirements due to the conditioning regimen, fever, infections, acute GVHD, and other metabolic complications.
   b) Factors that will lower calorie needs include reduced muscle mass, obesity, low activity level, absence of fever, and normal organ function.
   c) Factors that may increase calorie needs include large muscle mass, low adipose reserves, high activity level, severe acute GVHD, persistent high fevers, and infections.
   d) In debilitated patients, it is difficult to achieve nutritional repletion during periods of metabolic stress; therefore, it is recommended not to provide additional calories for weight gain until the patient is medically stable.
   e) Measurements of energy needs: Stress requirements are estimated to be generally no more than a maximum of 1.7 X basal needs for adults and 1.8 X basal needs for children (providing 1.5 X basal needs as nonprotein calorie or a nonprotein calorie to nitrogen ratio of 150 : 1 or less).

4. Total parenteral requirements
   a) Energy and protein are usually given as glucose and a mixture of amino acids.
   b) Energy is generally estimated as 25 to 35 kcal/kg.
   c) Protein intake should be 1.2 to 2.0 g/kg.
   d) Fat provides 25% to 30% of kilocalories, with a maximum glucose oxidation rate in the septic patient of 5 mg/kg/min.
   e) Caloric needs: It has been recognized that hypermetabolic and septic patients do not need the massive caloric loads that were once recommended. The complications of excess calories can lead to hyperglycemia, excess carbon dioxide production, and liver failure.

J. Fluids and electrolytes
   1. Intravenous (IV) fluid hydration maintenance fluid recommendations:

Patient weight	Fluid requirements
> 40 kg	1500 mL/m2/24 h
21–40 kg	1500 mL plus 20 mL/kg for each kg > 20 kg/24 h
11–20 kg	1000 mL plus 50 mL/kg for each kg > 10 kg/24 h
< 10 kg	100 mL/kg/24 h

   2. Fluid needs will be dictated by clinical circumstances.
   3. Factors requiring increased fluid volume (hyperhydration)
      a) Forced fluid administration is required to prevent or lessen renal insufficiency or hemorrhagic cystitis with cyclophosphamide containing conditioning regimens.
      b) IV fluids are administered at a rate of 3000 mL/m2/24 h, twice the maintenance requirements.

4. Weight measurement as frequently as every eight to 24 hours is needed. Intake and output should be ordered and monitored.
5. Urine output
   a) Adults: If urine output declines less than 600 mL over four hours, normal saline boluses or furosemide is recommended.
   b) Children: If urine output declines to less than 2 to 3 mL/kg/h a 10 mL/kg bolus of normal saline is recommended over 20 minutes. If no response is observed in two hours, furosemide, 0.5 mg/kg is given.

V. Growth charts and pediatric calculations and values[1,2] (Figures 8.1–8.8)

A. Growth charts

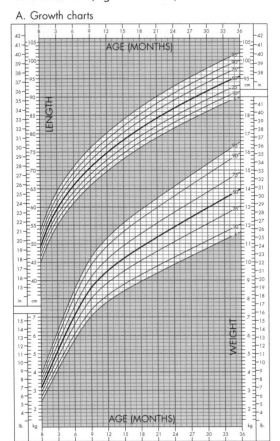

Figure 8.1 Girls, birth to 36 months: Length and weight.

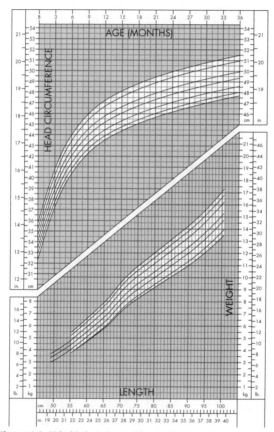

Figure 8.2 Girls, birth to 36 months: Head circumference and length-weight ratio.

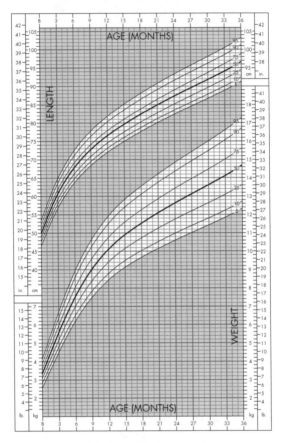

Figure 8.3 Boys, birth to 36 months: Length and weight.

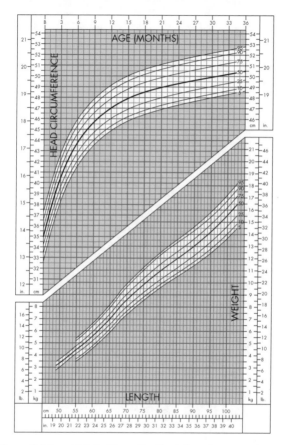

Figure 8.4 Boys, birth to 36 months: Head circumference and length-weight ratio.

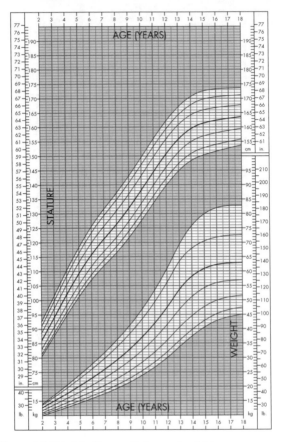

Figure 8.5 Girls, 2 to 18 years: Stature and weight.

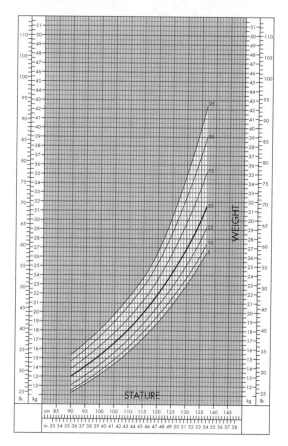

Figure 8.6 Girls, 2 to 18 years: Stature-weight ratio.

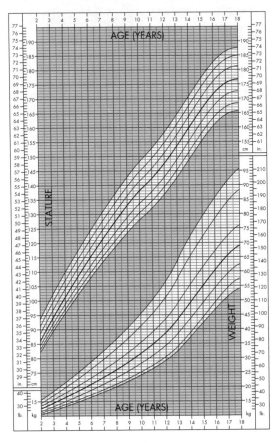

Figure 8.7 Boys, 2 to 18 years: Stature and weight.

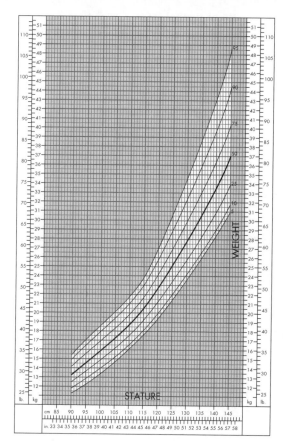

Figure 8.8 Boys, 2 to 18 years: Stature-weight ratio.

B. Body surface area in children

    1. Calculating body surface area in children (Figure 8.9): In a child of average size, find weight and corresponding surface are on the boxed scale to the left, or use the monogram to the right. Lay a straight edge on the correct height and weight points for the child, and then read the intersecting point on the surface area scale.

    2. Body surface areas (BSA) formulas:

BSA (m2) = height (in) X weight (lb)/3131
BSA (m2) = height (cm) X weight (Kg)/3600

C. Average weight and surface areas: See Table 8.4.

Table 8.4 Average Weight and Surface Area of Infants and Children

Age	Average weight (kg)	Approximate surface area (m²)
Months		
3	5	0.29
6	7	0.38
9	8	0.42
Years		
1	10	0.49
2	12	0.55
3	15	0.64
4	17	0.74
5	18	0.76
6	20	0.82
7	23	0.90
8	25	0.95
9	28	1.06
10	33	1.18
11	35	1.23
12	40	1.34
Adult	70	1.73

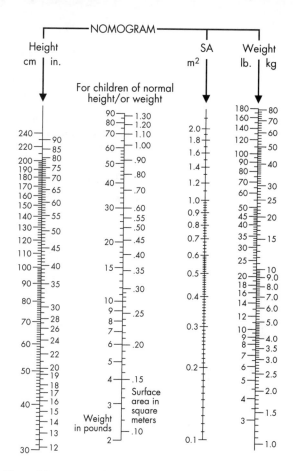

Figure 8.9 Nomogram for calculating body surface area in children.

D. Physical development
   1. Growth in first 6 weeks: 20 g/d
   2. Birth weight is regained by day 14, doubles by age 4 months, triples by age 12 months, and quadruples by age 2 years.
   3. Length increases 50% by age 1 year, doubles by age 4 years, and triples by age 13 years.
   4. Head circumference is 35 cm at birth, 44 cm by 6 months, and 47 cm by 1 year. Growth is 1cm/mo for first year and 0.3 cm/mo for second year.
   5. Teeth: first tooth at 6 to 18 months

 # teeth = age (in months) - 6 until 30 months

   6. Sexual development: See Table 8.5.

Table 8.5. Tanner Stages of Sexual Development

Stage	Characteristics	Age of onset (mean + SD)
Genital stages: male		
1	Prepubertal	
2	Scrotum and testes enlarge; skin reddens, and rugation appears	11.4 ± 1.1 years
3	Penis lengthens, testes enlarge further	12.9 ± 1 year
4	Penis growth continues in length and width; glans develops adult form	13.8 ± 1 year
5	Development completed; adult appearance	14.9 ± 1.1 years
Breast development: females		
1	Prepubertal	
2	Breast buds appear; areolae enlarge	11.2 ± 1.1 years
3	Elevation of breast contour; areolae enlarge	12.2 ± 1.1 years
4	Areolae and papilla form a secondary mound on breast	13.1 ± 1.2 years
5	Adult form	15.3 ± 1.7 years
Menarche Pubic hair: both sexes		
1	Prepubertal; no coarse hair	
2	Longer, silky hair appears at base of penis or along labia	F 11.7 ± 1.2 years M 12 ± 1 year
3	Hair coarse, kinky, spreads over pubic bone	F 12.4 ± 1.1 years M 13.9 ± 1 year
4	Hair of adult quality but not spread to junction of medial thigh perineum	F 13 ± 1 year M 14.4 ± 1.1 years
5	Spread to media thigh	F 14.4 ± 1.1 years M 15.2 ± 1.1 years
6	"Male escutcheon"	Variable if occurs
Maximal growth rate		
		Males at 14.1 ± 0.9 year Females at 12.1 ± 0.9 year

E. Normal blood values in children
   1. Red blood cells: See Table 8.6.
   2. White blood cells: See Table 8.7.

Table 8.6 Normal Red Blood Cell Values in Children

Age	Hgb (g/dL) Mean	Low/nL	Hct (%) Mean	Low/nL	MCV (fL) Mean	Low/nL	High/nL
Cord	16.5	13.5	51	42	108	98	118
1-3 d	18.5	14.5	56	45	108	95	121
1 wk	17.5	13.5	54	42	107	88	116
2 wk	16.5	12.5	51	39	105	86	114
1 mo	14	10	43	31	104	85	113
2 mo	11.5	9	35	28	96	77	106
3-6 mo	11.5	9.5	35	29	91	74	108
6 mo-2y	12	10.5	36	33	78	70	86
2-6 y	12.5	11.5	37	34	81	75	87
6-12 y	13.5	11.5	40	35	86	77	95
12-18 y F	14	12	41	36	90	78	102
12-18 y M	14.5	13	43	37	88	78	98
18+ F	14	12	41	36	90	80	100
18+ M	15.5	13.5	47	41	90	80	100

Hgb = hemoglobin; Het = hematocrit; MCV = mean corpuscular volume.

Table 8.7 Normal White Blood Values in Children (Caucasian)

Age	Total WBC Mean	Low/nL	Abs polys Mean	Low/nL	Abs lymph Mean	Low/nL	High/nL
Cord	18	9	11	6	5.5	2	11
12 h	23	13	15.5	6	5.5	2	11
24 h	19	9.5	11.5	5	5.8	2	11.5
2 wk	11.4	5	4.5	1	5.5	2	17
1 mo	10.8	5	3.8	1	6	2.5	16.5
6 mo	11.9	6	3.8	1	7.3	4	13.5
1 y	11.4	6	3.5	1.5	7	4	10.5
2 y	10.6	6	3.5	1.5	6.3	3	9.5
4 y	9.1	5.5	3.8	1.5	4.5	2	8
6 y	8.5	5	4.3	1.5	3.5	1.5	7
8 y	8.3	4.5	4.4	1.5	3.3	1.5	6.8
10 y	8.1	4.5	4.4	1.8	3.1	1.5	6.5
16 y	7.8	4.5	4.4	1.8	2.8	1.2	5.2
20 y	7.4	4.5	4.4	1.8	2.5	1	4.8

WBC = white blood cells; Abs polys = absolute polymononuclear count;
Abs lymph = absolute lymphocyte count.

References

1. Children's Hospital of Boston. Hospital Formulary; Hudson, OH: Lexi-Comp, Inc; 1996.

2. Johnson K, ed. The Harriet Lane Handbook. 13th ed. St. Louis: Mosby; 1993.

Bibliography

Aker SN. Bone marrow transplantation: nutrition support and monitoring. In: Bloch A, ed. *Nutrition Management of the Cancer Patient*. Rockville, MD; Aspen Publishers; 1990:199–222.

Barton RG. Nutrition support in critical illness. *Nutr Clin Pract*. 1994;9:127.

Bersinger WI, Buckner CD, Clift RA, et al. Comparison of techniques for dealing with major ABO incompatible marrow transplant. *Transplant Proc*. 1987;19:4605–4608.

Bishop JF, Mc Grath K, Wolf MM, et al. Clinical features influencing the efficacy of pooled platelet transfusions. *Blood* 1988;71:383–387.

BMT/PBSCT *Nutrition Care Criteria:* From Fred Hutchison Cancer Research Center. Seattle, WA: 1995.

Cheney CL, Weiss NS, Fisher LD, et al. Oral protein intake and the risk of acute graft–versus–host disease after allogeneic marrow transplantation. *Bone Marrow Transplant*. 1991;8:203–210.

Fisher DS, Knoff TS, Durivage HJ, eds. *The Cancer Chemotherapy Handbook*. 4th ed. St. Louis: Mosby; 1993: 498.

Herrmann VM, Petruska PJ. Nutrition support in bone marrow transplant recipients. *J Parent Enter Nutr*. 1993;8:19.

Klumpp TR. Immunohematologic complications of bone marrow transplantation. *Bone Marrow Transplant*. 1991;8:159–170.

Moe GL. Enteral feeding and infection in the immunocompromised patient. *Nutr Clin Pract*. 1991;6:55–64.

Morgan M, Dodds A. ABO incompatibility and blood product support. In: Atkinson K, ed. *Clinical Bone Marrow Transplantation.* Cambridge, England: Cambridge University Press. 1994:291–296.

Stern JM, Lenssen P. Food and nutrition services for the BMT patient. In: Buchsel PC, Whedon MB, eds. *Bone Marrow Transplantation: Administrative and Clinical Strategies.* Boston: Jones and Bartlett; 1995:113–136.

CHAPTER 9

Long-Term Follow-Up

The appropriate time for discharge from the inpatient setting is determined by each transplant center and should be individualized to each patient situation. There is a trend, however, toward earlier discharge and even to transplantation in the outpatient setting for certain types of transplant. These trends have been made possible because of increased knowledge and skill in transplantation technology as well as major advances in supportive modalities.

I. Ambulatory management following bone marrow transplant (BMT)

A. The schedule of post-transplant outpatient visits will differ from center and by type of transplant. Generally, allogeneic transplant patients will be seen at least twice weekly for the first 100 days post-transplant, and autologous transplant patients will be seen at least once weekly for the first several weeks post-transplant. Patients undergoing outpatient transplant may require daily visits to the outpatient clinic until they reach a level of stability that would be consistent with discharge for a traditional transplant patient.

B. Each outpatient visit involves a thorough assessment of laboratory parameters, subjective data, physical status, and psychosocial status as well as review of medication list with appropriate adjustments.

    1. Routine laboratory studies

        a) Complete blood count (CBC) with differential

        b) Platelet count

        c) Reticulocyte count

  2. Interim history

    a) Subjective data

    b) Review of medication list

  3. Physical examination

    a) Weight

    b) Vital signs

    c) Affect/behavior

    d) Skin

    e) Oropharynx/oral mucosa

    f) Lymph nodes

    g) Heart

    h) Lungs

    i) Abdomen (bowel sounds, hepatosplenomegaly)

    j) Peripheral or central edema

  4. Nutritional assessment

  5. Psychosocial evaluation

C. Repeat bone marrow aspirate and biopsy may be performed as part of routine follow-up. The scheduling and frequency of this procedure will be determined by each transplant center and is dependent upon disease process, type of transplant, treatment protocol, and individual patient situation (e.g., delayed engraftment, clinical indication of disease relapse).

D. Many patients require hospital readmission at least once during the post-transplant period. Symptomatic criteria for readmission are as follows:

  1. Fever greater than 100.5°F

  2. Shaking chills with or without fever

  3. Active bleeding

  4. Respiratory distress

  5. Unstable blood pressure

  6. Cardiac arrhythmia

7. Failure to thrive (>10% weight loss in adult; > 5% weight loss in child)
8. Severe fluid loss/dehydration
9. Intractable vomiting or diarrhea
10. Alteration in mental status
11. New, acute, or flair of GVHD

E. Patients with a diagnosis of acute myelogenous leukemia, chronic myelogenous leukemia in blast crisis, certain types of lymphoma, or any disease with risk of central nervous system (CNS) involvement require a series of lumbar punctures with instillation of a chemotherapeutic agent (usually methotrexate) to prevent CNS relapse of disease. This series consists of at least five lumbar punctures scheduled weekly when platelet recovery is sufficient (> 70,000/µL).

II. Psychosexual adjustment following BMT

A. There is generally no restriction of sexual activity with a monogamous partner after transplant. Condoms should be used.

B. Some level of sexual dysfunction after transplant is not uncommon among both male and female patients. This dysfunction may be related to low sexual desire, difficulty with arousal, or dyspareunia. Often, dysfunction begins with one factor but eventually involves other factors.

C. Low sexual desire in the post-transplant patient may be related to fatigue, depression, alteration in hormonal levels, medication effect, or concern about body image.

D. Difficulty with arousal may occur in both male and female patients. In the male patient, this may be characterized by the inability to achieve or maintain erection, which is apparently psychogenic in origin. In the female patient, physiologic changes related to ovarian failure and decreased estradiol appear to affect arousal.[1]

E. Dyspareunia, or painful intercourse, is a common complaint in female patients post-transplant. This is most likely due to atrophy of the vaginal mucosa and decreased vaginal lubrication, which results from ovarian failure.

F. To facilitate discussion of specific problems, a general discussion of potential for sexual dysfunction should take place in the context of the pretransplant work-up. Additionally, general questions regarding sexual function should be a routine part of post-transplant follow-up visits.

G. When specific problems with sexual dysfunction have been identified, appropriate treatment strategies can be implemented. In cases of complex dysfunction, a sex therapist should be consulted.

H. Both male and female patients undergoing BMT are at significant risk for infertility, due both to prior standard chemotherapy and radiotherapy and to the dose-intense conditioning therapy administered for transplant. The risk to a female patient increases with increasing age, as the patient approaches natural menopause.

I. Total body irradiation and total lymphoid irradiation will cause sterility in most patients, both male and female. Although testosterone levels remain within normal limits, follicle-stimulating hormone (FSH) and luteinizing hormone (LH) levels will be elevated, and semen analysis will reveal azoospermia.

J. In female patients, ovarian function can be evaluated post-transplant by measuring serum FSH and LH. Most often, these hormonal levels will be elevated, consistent with a menopausal state. Many women will complain of associated menopausal symptoms such as hot flashes, vaginal dryness, and urethral irritation. Regardless of age, they are also at risk for cardiovascular disease and osteoporosis, as any woman who has experienced menopause. Hormone replacement therapy is effective treatment in these patients, but may be contraindicated in some patients (e.g., history of hormone-sensitive carcinoma). In these patients, a long-acting water-soluble vaginal lubricant may provide symptomatic relief of vaginal-urethral atrophy.

K. In prepubertal children, gonadal function may recover allowing exposure to a single high-dose chemotherapeutic agent. Use of high-dose chemotherapy and total body irradiation, however, appears to delay puberty and may affect gonadal function permanently.

III. Long-term post-transplant testing and evaluation

A. Most centers will require follow-up visits at 6 and 12 months post-transplant. The following elements of follow-up may be performed at these visits:
1. Comprehensive history and physical examination
2. Assessment of growth and development in children
3. Review of medication list with alteration or tapering of dosages
4. Laboratory studies
   a) CBC with differential
   b) Platelet count
   c) Reticulocyte count
   d) Biochemical profile
   e) FSH, LH
   f) Human immunodeficiency virus (HIV)
   g) Thyroid function tests
5. Bone marrow aspiration and biopsy with appropriate testing, based on disease
6. Consider
   a) Pulmonary function testing with diffusing capacity of carbon dioxide in the lung (DLCO)
   b) Ophthalmologic examination
   c) Gynecologic examination

B. Autologous transplant patients are considered to be "disabled" (no work or school) for 6 months post-transplant. In patients undergoing allogeneic transplant, this period of disability is extended to 12 months. Additionally, patients must avoid any exposure to chemicals, radiation, solvents, and pesticides.

C. The use of interferon-α in patients with multiple myeloma and chronic myelogenous leukemia is currently accepted post-transplant practice at most transplant centers. Doses and dosage schedules will vary by center and by patient ability to tolerate the drug. The optimal length of post-transplant treatment is currently under study.

IV. Immunizations

A. At the one-year follow-up visit, the patient should receive diphtheria/tetanus vaccine, Pneumovax, *Haemophilus influenzae* B vaccine (HIB titer), Salk polio vaccine, and influenza vaccine (if the visit is conducted during "flu season").

B. Patients should be advised that they must avoid any live virus vaccine for the rest of their lives (e.g., MMR, Sabin polio).

Reference

1. Ostroff JS, Lesko LM. Psychosexual adjustment and fertility issues. In: Whedon MB, ed. *Bone Marrow Transplantation: Principles, Practice, and Nursing Insights.* Boston: Jones and Bartlett; 1991.

Bibliography

Flowers MED, Sullivan KM. Preadmission procedures, transplant hospitalization, and posttransplant outpatient monitoring. In: Atkinson K, ed. *Clinical Bone Marrow Transplantation: A Reference Textbook.* Cambridge, England: Cambridge University Press; 1994.

Lonergan JN, McBride LH, Kelley CH, Randolph SR. *Homecare Management of the Bone Marrow Transplant Patient.* 2nd ed. Boston: Jones and Bartlett; 1996.

Randolph S, Leum E, Buchsel P. Long-term complications of BMT. In: Buchsel PC, Whedon MB, eds. *Bone Marrow Transplantation: Administrative and Clinical Strategies.* Boston: Jones and Bartlett; 1995.

Psychosocial Issues

Daniel Shapiro, Cynthia Monheim

For patients, families, and staff, the bone marrow transplant experience is psychologically challenging. This chapter presents guidelines for recognizing and addressing mental health issues common to these complex patients.

I. Evidence of major depression

A. Intervene early. At the first signs of depression a referral to mental health professionals is indicated.

B. Features of depression in bone marrow transplant (BMT) populations

1. The following symptoms are indicative of depression in BMT patients:
   a) Pervasive sadness (every day, nearly all day)
   b) Excessive guilt
   c) Suicidal ideation in the absence of hopeless medical circumstances
   d) In children, depression often manifests as withdrawal, irritability, or prolonged periods of quietness or inactivity.[1]

2. The following symptoms of depression occur in most BMT patients,[2,3] and may be better accounted for as side effects of treatment:
   a) Anorexia
   b) Insomnia
   c) Poor concentration
   d) Anhedonia
   e) Low energy

C. All patients should be monitored for depression during long periods of isolation or pain.[1]

II. Mania

A. Intervene quickly, as manic patients may engage in risky behaviors.

B. Mania is unusual in BMT populations.

C. In bipolar populations, mania is typically followed by severe depression. Symptoms include
   1. Inflated self-esteem
   2. Decreased need for sleep
   3. Pressured or rapid speech
   4. Flight of ideas
   5. Psychomotor agitation
   6. Excessive involvement in pleasurable activities that have a high potential for painful or dangerous consequences

III. Substance abuse

A. Occasionally, a patient will be admitted who has a long history of substance abuse and who is detoxing while also starting transplant.

B. Referral to mental health professionals who specialize in substance abuse is indicated.

IV. Psychosis or delusions

A. Actively psychotic or delusional patients are generally unable to participate in their own care and may have difficulty adhering to treatment recommendations (e.g., could remove central line, leave isolation rooms).

B. Definition of psychosis: Evidence that the patient is not oriented to reality. Constructions of reality that violate the natural laws as they are known (e.g., thoughts are broadcast into the patient's head from the radio).

C. Definition of delusions: Implausible constructions of reality that do not violate the natural laws as they are known (e.g., patient claims the President is going to marry her).

V. Overwhelming anxiety

A. In addition to descriptions of anxious feelings, symptoms include:
1. Restlessness
2. Difficulty concentrating
3. Muscle tension
4. Difficulty sleeping (both insomnia and early morning awakening), irritability

B. Most common reason for referral to mental health professionals in the BMT population

C. Anxiety typically increases when patients are in transition stages of transplant:
1. Immediately before transplant
2. At onset of graft-versus-host disease (GVHD)
3. Prior to discharge

VI. Suicidal ideation in the absence of hopeless medical circumstances

A. Mental health professionals should conduct suicide assessment.

B. Suicide assessment includes following:
1. Intensity and frequency of suicidal thoughts
2. Presence of plan
3. If plan, lethality of plan
4. Degree of intent
5. Degree of desperation
6. Degree of anger

VII. Staff-patient conflicts

A. Splits

    1. Splits occur when one or more members of the treatment team disagree or are angry with other members of the treatment team.

    2. Splits are to be expected. There are few other medical procedures that parallel the intense emotional bonds that develop between staff and transplant patients.

    3. As a result of these bonds, staff members are likely to feel very invested in the progress of patients.[2] This investment magnifies the intensity of disagreements between staff members.

B. Why splits must be addressed: Team splits often result in poorer care being offered the patient. The decisions made during the care of the transplant patient are complicated enough without added pressures of personal conflicts.

C. Team splits between junior physicians and experienced nurses

    1. Residents, fellows, and junior attending physicians are often in the unenviable position of making decisions with which other team members (i.e., nurses) may disagree. These nurses are often very experienced.

    2. A common but unfortunate response to this situation is for the physician to exert authority without carefully considering the legitimacy of the medical opinion of the experienced nurse.

    3. The savvy junior physician or nurse practitioner walks a fine line between empowering the more experienced nursing staff and still taking responsibility for decisions.

    4. Great physicians sacrifice enduring humiliation for the betterment of patient care.

    5. Preventing splits between junior physicians and experienced nurses:

     a) Transplant requires considerable nursing interventions.

     b) Strong transplant physicians understand enough of the details of these interventions to be able to balance the nursing effort required in a given situation against the needs of the patient.

     c) Strong transplant physicians do not require nurses to needlessly perform procedures or, at the other end of the spectrum, sacrifice patient care.

D. Team splits between nurses

1. Because transplant requires considerable technical nursing skill and time, and this skill can be the difference between positive and negative outcomes in patients, and because not all nurses are equally committed, resentment sometimes results.

2. Interventions are indicated that
   a) Encourage open dialogue
   b) Minimize competition
   c) Rapidly punish indirect communication (e.g., assigning difficult patients to nurses with whom one is angry)

3. The savvy physician or nurse practitioner speaks for patient care always.

E. Splits between the team and the patient

1. It is common for patients to argue with staff over a myriad of issues such as visiting hours, mouth care, or unexpected side effects. The following interventions will limit these arguments in many cases:

   a) Maximize the patient's control. The more patients perceive they have control over their environment, the better they feel. When opportunities for patient collaboration exist, they should be utilized.

   b) Make experiences as predictable as possible. The majority of patients will seek information. For these patients (roughly 85%), the more they understand what is likely to happen to them in the near future, the better they are likely to feel.

   c) Maintain a stance of respectful collaboration. Talking about patients in the "third person" in their presence, making decisions without telling patients, or violating trust will often escalate anger.

2. In some cases, patients will express their fears and anger at having to go through the experience on the people nearest them: family and staff. Because most health professionals enter the field to be helpful this can be painful and unpleasant. The following interventions are indicated:

   a) Set appropriate limits. Abuse of staff should never be tolerated. While most health professionals prefer to avoid confrontation, abuse by patients plants the seeds for burnout, which both hurts patient care and is expensive.

   b) Unit staff in leadership positions should intervene on behalf of involved staff to set appropriate limits with abusive patients.

F. Splits between the team and the family

1. The family is the primary source of support for severely ill patients and are often vital in maintaining the patient's will to survive.[4]

2. Parents and family staying at the hospital for extended periods of time during treatment can present the BMT staff with unique challenges. Family members face the overwhelming stress of witnessing a loved one struggle with difficult treatment. Often, they show common stress responses, including

   a) Insomnia or early morning awakening

   b) Fatigue

   c) Chronic worry[5,6]

   d) Forgetfulness

   e) Poor concentration

3. Staff must sometimes label these symptoms of stress and assist family members in taking care of themselves. The understandable urge to simply remove family members from the unit should be restrained in all but the most detrimental of circumstances.

4. Often, the frustrations, guilt, and fears that family avoid sharing with the patient will be released on the staff. In many cases, staff will find it necessary to accept this burden and find ways to help family vent in more appropriate forums.[4] These include the following:

   a) Family support groups
   b) Mental health staff
   c) Other social supports outside of family

5. In some situations, family members will blame the staff for poor patient progress. Staff should

   a) Avoid defensiveness.
   b) Acknowledge disappointments.
   c) Spend some time with the family.

VIII. Pain medication abuse

A. Philosophies regarding pain medication and abuse vary among health-care providers.

B. Some ascribe to a "survival philosophy," that is, anything that helps the patient get through the experience is indicated. Others view use of excessive pain medication as an abuse of the team-patient relationship and as potentially hazardous to the patient.

C. Because each case differs, and patient pain complaints must be balanced against the risks of potentiating abuse, consultation with mental health professionals specializing in substance abuse is indicated.

IX. Interventions helpful for all patients

A. Relaxation and distraction are powerful psychological interventions and have been found to reduce pain reports, improve immune function, and give a sense of "well-being."[1,3] These techniques are particularly useful during painful procedures (e.g., bone marrow aspirations, lumbar punctures, central line removal).

1. Relaxation during procedures

a) Teach patients to concentrate on taking slow deep breaths, in through the nose and out through the mouth, and to imagine a peaceful scene.

b) With children, instruct them to imagine blowing bubbles or blowing out candles.

c) Children may also be asked to imagine the difference between a rag doll and a tree. Then ask the child to act like a rag doll during the procedure. This is an effective way to demonstrate the difference between a tense body (which will experience more pain) and a relaxed body (which will experience less pain).

2. Relaxation for anxiety

a) Progressive muscle relaxation: Tell patient to make a fist and then to relax the hand completely. Slowly go through muscle groups, starting with the feet and working through the entire body, first tensing and then relaxing.

b) Help patient develop the ability to observe the difference between how it feels to have muscle tensed and muscle relaxed.

3. Distraction for both procedures and anxiety

a) Invite patients to use whatever distractions are available and work for them (e.g., television, magazines, knitting).

b) For children, video games are often effective.

4. Optimize touch.
   a) Patients and families often avoid touching during transplant for fear of transferring germs.
   b) Clear messages regarding allowable and unallowable touch, including sex, will assist patients in negotiating these confusions.
5. Maintain as normal a sleep/wake cycle as possible.
   a) Night nursing staff should be coached to be as unobtrusive as possible.
   b) Encourage activity during daylight hours.
   c) Encourage patient to use bed only for sleeping.

B. Help patients to communicate with team more effectively. BMT transplant patients have demonstrated a greater need for information and involvement in their treatment than the typical medical patient.[7]
   1. Patients should be acculturated to the specific medical system they will be living in.
      a) Roles of the varied professionals with whom they will interact
      b) Whom to ask which questions
      c) What aspects of treatment are negotiable and which are not (e.g., Can patients avoid 4 A.M. wakings for vitals? Are visiting hours flexible?)
   2. While patients are more sophisticated today than ever, a sizable proportion are still intimidated by physicians and their brethren. Encouraging questions in one-on-one meetings and in rounds will optimize the chances that patients will interact effectively.[8-10]
   3. Vast majority of patients are information seeking. Because mild memory difficulties are common during transplant, encouraging patient to write down questions or inviting family members to ask questions is effective.

4. Techniques for improving communication include the following:
   a) There is evidence that oncologists speak on a level that is too sophisticated for the average patient.
   b) Words such as *remission, stem cell,* and *harvest* should be explained, and nonthreatening queries regarding comprehension should be used (e.g., suggesting that many people find much of the language confusing may be helpful).
   c) The use of short words and sentences improves recall regardless of how information is presented.
   d) Material presented first or last is remembered better.
   e) Specific, definite advice rather than suggestions is more likely to be adhered to.
   f) Summarize the most important information at the close of interaction.
   g) Patients often find rounds, when they include numerous professionals, intimidating. One-on-one interactions should be used to supplement rounds.

C. Prepare patients in advance. Despite having thorough informed consent meetings, most patients do not retain accurate information about their upcoming treatment.[1,10] While tempting, it is a mistake to minimize the realities of painful procedures. Doing so jeopardizes the legitimacy of all medical professionals. For example, prior to performing aspirations, line pulls, or lumbar punctures, tell patients what to expect for discomfort, duration, and procedure.

D. Optimizing control
   1. Research has found that perceived control is a powerful predictor of physical and psychological health status in BMT patients.[3,11]
   2. The isolation and waiting associated with BMT seem to increase control issues.

3. Often, patients attempt to regain control over their uncertain situation by fighting with family and staff over medications, procedures, or daily routines.[5,11,12]
4. Give patients as much control of their environment as is realistically possible.
5. Decisions about the timing of mouth care, meals, routine blood draws, privacy, and visits should be left to the patient.

X. Interventions helpful for family

A. Encouragement to rest, maintain contact with other supports, maintain adequate nutrition, and get time away from hospital

B. Parents may prefer to stay in the hospital with children. This is reasonable as long as sleep is not disrupted for either. Rooming-in policies vary by transplant center.

C. Power of attorney should be discussed early in treatment rather than later. This prevents the stress of attempting to second-guess patient's wishes.

XI. Interventions helpful for donors

A. Donors often worry that their marrow may be inadequate. Clarification regarding the role of the donor and the chances of recovery should be provided to the donor.

B. Excessive guilt by donors during GVHD or other complications is to be expected. Continued reassurance or referral to mental health professionals is indicated.

XII. Pretransplant screenings

A. Many BMT units incorporate a psychological screening into their routine pretransplant program. While screenings are generally not used as criteria for accepting or rejecting a BMT candidate, screening can be useful in a number of ways.

B. Screening prepares the patient for the psychological experiences common during transplant.

C. Learning how candidates have coped with prior stressors will shed light on coping style.

D. Information gleaned can be used to prepare team for patient needs.
   1. Patient's information preferences (wanting to be involved in all decisions and gathering all information versus low information seeking)
   2. Degree of family support
   3. Compliance issues (low cognitive ability, substance abuse history, poor social support)[13]

E. Major psychological illnesses that may affect treatment will be identified. Specific factors should include
   1. Any likely impediments to compliance, including low intellectual functioning, substance abuse history, history of psychosis or delusions, poor relationships with staff
   2. Having little or no social support from family or friends
   3. Unusual preferences (e.g., family's desire not to tell the patient that the patient has cancer)
   4. Cultural preferences
   5. Depressed mood pretransplant. Depressed mood pre-BMT is predictive of shorter post-BMT survival time.[14]

XIII. "Difficult patients"

A. Difficult patients are those who "would try a saint's patience."

B. Somatization
1. Patients who are hypervigilant about their condition may misinterpret bodily sensations to mean that they have new serious conditions
2. Patients who appear to have low pain threshold or complain about mild irritants
3. Treating somatic patients:
   a) Consistent reassurance is the only intervention that minimizes complaints in this population. First, acknowledge the discomfort the patient is experiencing and address it.
   b) Within the bounds of what is true and reasonable, remind patients that they are doing well.

C. Noncompliance
1. Noncompliance that jeopardizes the patient's life must be addressed immediately.
2. Behavioral plans that tie reinforcers to compliance should be implemented (e.g., the patient must do mouth care before television or visitation is permitted, the patient must spend 30 minutes out of bed to get 30 minutes in bed).
3. For behavioral plans to be effective, all team members must agree to follow them to avoid placing inconsistent expectations on the patient.
4. Communication across shifts should be systematically conducted so that team splits are avoided.
5. The benefits of interventions when noncompliance is not dangerous must be carefully weighed.
   a) Some patients "act out" in a misguided effort to exert control.
   b) Some patients adopt educated nonadherence (do not comply for rational reasons).

D. Anger
1. Expressions of anger directed at team members is common during BMT.[5]
2. Fear of death, discomfort, dependence, changes in appearance, loss of freedom of movement, disappointments in the rapidity of progress, unexpected complications, symptoms of GVHD, steroid therapy, isolation, and loss of privacy are powerful psychological experiences that challenge the most hearty of personalities.
3. Most expressions of anger may be unprovoked, unexpected, and misdirected. Taking most such expressions personally is a mistake for staff and family members alike.[4]
4. Other expressions of anger are targeted at specific staff behaviors (e.g., not responding to call buttons in a timely fashion, waking patients up in the early hours of the morning, inability to get a central line to draw blood).
5. Acknowledging real mistakes and apologizing minimize distrust and hostility. Professionals should guard against the urge to "brush over" patient complaints.

E. Illness parenting
1. Fear that their child may not survive can influence parents' reponse to their child's behavior.[15,16]
2. Many parents respond to their child's illness by reducing discipline, not encouraging autonomy, and not preparing the child for procedures.
3. Unfortunately, this understandable response to the child's illness may enhance children's tendency to "act out." Rather than expressing themselves to get what they need, and comforting themselves when immediate satisfaction is unavailable, children may indirectly express themselves by whining, having tantrums, or throwing things.

4. At the first signs of such behavior, rapid intervention is indicated. A three-step approach is indicated:
   a) Acknowledge the parents' desire to make things as easy for the child as possible.
   b) Inform the parents that children need limits and boundaries to feel safe and cared for. If parents feel unable to set such limits (optimal), then the staff will set the limits for them.
   c) Limits should be established and instituted for misbehavior. Time-out is effective. Time-out refers to the removal of reinforcers from the environment. Reinforcers are usually parent or staff attention. Time-out (1 minute per year of age) should be explained to the child as "quiet time" that will be used whenever the child does the identified misbehavior. All staff members must be alerted to the institution of time-out procedures and use them consistently.

F. Dangerous behaviors
   1. Dangerous behaviors (hitting, biting, throwing things at people, pulling at the central line) should be punished immediately.
   2. Blowing air into the face of a child or squirting water is an effective punishment but must be used immediately after the misbehavior and should only be used in dangerous situations.
   3. In very rare circumstances, and only after all other options are exhausted, chemical (tranquilizers) or physical restraints must be used to settle an uncontrollable patient.
   4. Staff should carefully examine if such methods are warranted and may choose to convene an in-house ethics committee.

G. Drug seeking
1. Many patients experience the transplant as overwhelming and attempt to use pharmacologic agents to "blot out" or escape from their discomfort.
2. Balancing the need for patients to be coherent (so that they can complete mouth care, get some exercise, independently use the restroom or make decisions) against their desire to escape is often difficult.
3. Individual nurses and physicians given the same patient in the same circumstances will make different decisions.
4. Negotiate with the patient so that comfort is maximized without sacrificing too much of the patient's independent functioning.

XIV. Emotionally difficult circumstances

A. The dying patient
1. One of the most difficult decisions health-care professionals must make in this culture is when to move from curative to palliative measures.
2. Technology has provided an impressive arsenal of "long shot" and dramatic procedures that can prolong life.
3. This can often lead physicians and other health professionals to see death as a sign of failure rather than a natural life process.
4. While it is certainly the case that patients should be involved in as many decisions as possible, the reality is that how options are presented greatly impacts patient decisions.[10,17] In addition, in some circumstances, the patient is no longer cognitively capable of making decisions.
5. Health professionals should consider and acknowledge what their true preference is before attempting to present an unbiased menu of options to the patient or patient's family.

6. The health professional's own sense of failure, regret, loss, and unrealistic hopes must be contained in these circumstances so that the patient or family member can make unbiased and informed decisions.

7. Palliative measures
   a) After the decision has been made to move to a palliative frame the health professional has a new obligation to prepare the patient for death.
   b) Despite the frequency of death in medical settings, many health professionals skirt the issue of death, assuming that patients will figure out their situation on their own. This is erroneous.

8. Our society lacks social rules for the last goodbye. While it is taboo to miss birthdays, anniversaries, and greetings, it is not to avoid saying goodbye, finally, to loved ones. Social taboo and general discomfort on the part of the staff and family often limit the dying patient's opportunities to explore or express their own feelings in the face of death.

9. Most patients and their families want to know what to expect in simple biologic terms. When talking with dying patients:
   a) Be very clear regarding impending death.
   b) Ask the patient and familiy to ask you questions.
   c) Generally, most patients and families want to know if death will be painful or slow and how they will know when it is happening.
   d) From a psychological standpoint, patients should be urged to talk about death with their loved ones. Many patients are unwilling to discuss issues of death with family members, hoping to avoid increasing the tremendous emotional burden already placed on them.

e) The same honesty and directness should also be directed to children. Unlike adults, children are more likely to indirectly express their fears of dying. An openness to discuss the topic is often helpful.

10. Transfer to the intensive care unit (ICU)

a) On some units, critically ill patients are not treated on the unit but are transported to the ICU. Staff who have been emotionally attached to patients and their families may have to abruptly end relationships during the most intense phase of treatment.

b) Families may experience these changes as particularly noxious.

c) Ongoing contact with families who feel displaced is indicated.

B. Coping with death

1. Most BMT units have acute mortality rates of approximately 10% to 20%.

2. Professionals who hope to remain in BMT must find a way to express and let go of these losses.

3. An organized venue for the staff to regularly express their feelings regarding the loss is indicated. Informally expressing one's sense of loss to other caregivers is an effective way to avoid "burnout." Staff may also choose to attend funeral services.

4. It is not uncommon for inexperienced staff to feel shock at the process of death or the appearance of the deceased. Preparing inexperienced professionals for the experience in advance or allowing them a venue to discuss their reactions is psychologically helpful.

C. Discharge

1. Patients are ambivalent at discharge because the constant vigilance offered by the team is abruptly ended.

2. Patients near the end of treatment may suddenly increase physical complaints, display more anxiety, or have other overt manifestations of distress.

3. Reassurance and follow-up visits scheduled close to discharge from the transplant center will help to wean the patient from the team.

4. Caregivers who anticipate bearing the majority of the patient's care after discharge may express anger or concern regarding their ability to successfully care for the patient.

5. Family members should have the opportunity to practice all necessary skills prior to discharge.

6. Clinicians should be vigilant for sudden crises immediately prior to discharge and carefully consider the possibility that psychological distress in response to leaving can sometimes be a factor.

References

1. Brown H, Kelly M. Stages of bone marrow transplantation: a psychiatric perspective *Psychosom Med.* 1976;38:439–446.

2. Brack G, LaClave L, Blix S. The psychological aspects of bone marrow transplant: a staff's perspective. *Cancer Nurs.* 1988;11:221–229.

3. Gaston-Johansson F, Franco T, Zimmerman, L. Pain and psychological distress in patients undergoing autologous bone marrow transplantation. *Oncol Nurs Forum.* 1992;19:41–48.

4. Artinian B. Fostering hope in the bone marrow transplant child. *Matern Child Nurs J.* 1984;13:57–71.

5. Pot-Mees C, Zeitlin H. Psychosocial consequences of bone marrow transplantation in children: a preliminary communication. *J Psychosoc Oncol* 1987;5:73–81.

6. Andrykowski A. Psychiatric and psychosocial aspects of bone marrow transplantation. *Psychosomatics.* 1994;35:13–24.

7. Rodrigue J, Boggs SR, Weiner RS, et al. Mood, coping style, and personality functioning among adult bone marrow transplant candidates. *Psychosomatics.* 1993;34:159–165.

8. Kiss, A. Support of the transplant team. *Support Care Cancer.* 1994;2:56–60.

9. Haberman M. The meaning of cancer therapy: bone marrow transplantation as an exemplar therapy. *Semin Oncol Nurs.* 1995; 11:23–31.

10. Morrow G, Hoagland A, Carpenter P. Improving physician-patient communications in cancer treatment. *J Psychosoc Oncol.* 1983;1:93–101.

11. Wikle T, Coyle K, Shapiro D. Bone marrow transplant: today and tomorrow. *Am J Nurs.* May 1990:48–56.

12. Gardner G, August C, Githens J. Psychological issues in bone marrow transplantation. *Pediatrics.* 1977;60:625–631.

13. Farkas Patenaude A, Rappeport J. Collaboration between hematologists and mental health professionals on a bone marrow transplant team. *J Psychosoc Oncol.* 1984;2:81–92.

14. Andrykowski M, Brady M, Henslee-Downey P. Psychosocial factors predictive of survival after allogeneic bone marrow transplantation for leukemia. *Psychosom Med.* 1994;56:432–439.

15. Atkins D, Farkas Patenaude A. Psychosocial preparation and follow-up for pediatric bone marrow transplant patients. *Am J Orthopsychiatry.* 1987;57:246–252.

16. Heiny S, Neuberg RW, Myers D, et al. The aftermath of bone marrow transplant for parents of pediatric patients: a post-traumatic stress disorder. *Oncol Nurs Forum.* 1994;21:843–847.

17. Street R Jr. Physicians' communication and parents' evaluations of pediatric consultations. *Med Care.* 1991; 29:1146–1152.

Index

Page numbers followed by a *t* or *f* indicate tables or figures respectively.

A

Acetaminophen, 363*t*, 385
Acid-fast stain, 269
Acyclovir, 62*t*, 331–32*t*
  for CMV prophylaxis, 96
  for HSV prophylaxis, 95
  for HSV therapy, 95
  for mucositis, 219
Adenovirus infection, 182–83
Adrenal disorders, 279–80
Airborne bacterial contamination, marrow aspiration and, 114
Albumin (human), 365*t*
Alloantibodies, platelet, 386
Allogeneic bone marrow, 113–15
Allopurinol, 364*t*
Amikacin sulfate, 292*t*
Aminocaproic acid, 343*t*
Aminoglycoside antibiotics, 370
Amitriptyline hydrochloride, 334*t*
Amoxicillin, 292*t*
Amoxicillin-Clavulanate potassium, 292–93*t*
Amphotericin B, 56, 64*t*, 90–91, 323*t*
Ampicillin, 293*t*
Ampicillin/sulbactam, 293*t*
Analgesics, 334–42*t*
Anaphylaxis, 388*t*
Anemia(s), 47*t*, 48–49, 132–34, 255–56
Anesthesia, bone marrow harvesting, 113
Anger, of patient(s), 432
Anhedonia, 419
Anorexia, 58–61, 419

Anthracycline cardiac toxicity, 210–11
Antibacterial agents, 64*t*, 293–314*t*
Antibacterial prophylaxis, 87–90
Antibiotic(s), used in gut decontamination, 87*t*
Anti-CD34 monoclonal antibodies, cell purging with, 117
Anticytokine agents, for GVHD prophylaxis, 106
Antidiarrheal agents, 315–16*t*
Antiemetic agents, 316–21*t*
Antiemetic management, 371–73, 372*t*
Antifungal agents, 64*t*, 322–24*t*
Antifungal prophylaxis, 91–93
Antigen(s)
  HLA type, 31–33
  red blood cell, 384
Antihistamine, 61*t*
Antihypertensive agents/diuretics, 325–31*t*
Anti-interleukin-2 receptor antibody (aIL-2), 106
Antilymphocyte globulin, 105
Antimicrobial(s)
  for diarrhea, 216
  selection of, 375–77
Antimicrobial prophylaxis, 85–86*t*, 87–99, 88*t*
Antiprotozoal agents, 293–314*t*
Antiprotozoan prophylaxis, 93–95
Anti-T-cell monoclonal antibodies, for resistant GVHD, 105
Antithymocyte globulin, 359*t*
Anti-tumor necrosis factor (TNF) agents, 106
Antiviral agents, 64*t*, 333–35*t*
Antiviral prophylaxis, 94–98